DATE DUE

GAYLORD			PRINTED IN U.S.A.

VICTORY DEFERRED

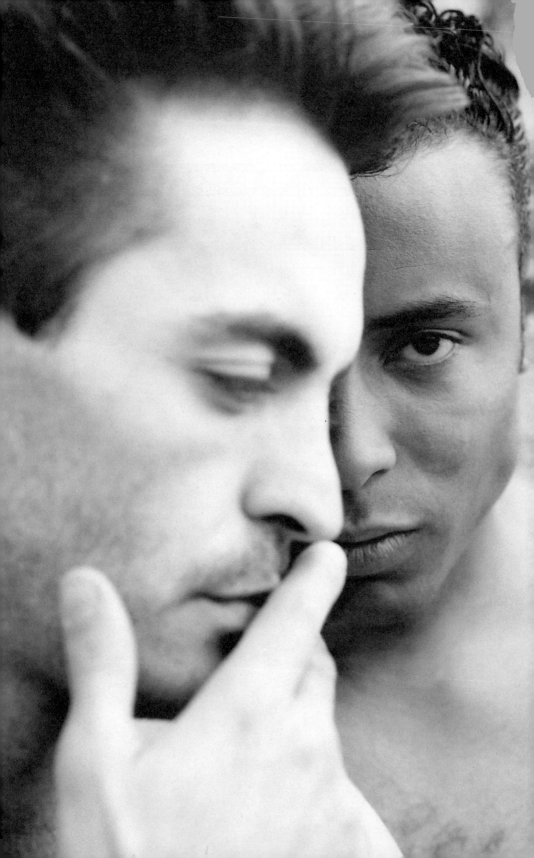

VICTORY DEFERRED

how AIDS changed gay life in AMERICA

JOHN-MANUEL ANDRIOTE

THE UNIVERSITY OF CHICAGO PRESS
CHICAGO AND LONDON

John-Manuel Andriote is a Washington-based journalist who has written about AIDS and gay-related issues since the early eighties for newspapers, magazines, AIDS advocacy organizations, and the U.S. Public Health Service. His articles have appeared in a variety of publications, ranging from the *Advocate* to the *Washington Post*.

The University of Chicago Press, Chicago 60637
The University of Chicago Press, Ltd., London
© 1999 by John-Manuel Andriote
All rights reserved. Published 1999
08 07 06 05 04 03 02 01 00 99   5 4 3 2 1

ISBN (cloth): 0-226-02049-5

Library of Congress Cataloging-in-Publication Data

Andriote, John-Manuel.
    Victory deferred : how AIDS changed gay life in America /
John-Manuel Andriote.
        p.   cm.
    Includes bibliographical references and index.
    ISBN 0-226-02049-5 (cloth : alk. paper)
    1. AIDS (Disease)—United States—History.   2. Gay men—United
States—Diseases.   3. AIDS (Disease)—Social aspects—United States.
4. Gay liberation movement—United States.   I. Title.
RA644.A25 A523   1999
362.1'969792'00973—ddc21   98-46236
                                                         CIP

This book is printed on acid-free paper.

In memory of
Dad, Allen, and Bill

As I ponder'd in silence,
Returning upon my poems, considering, lingering long,
A Phantom arose before me with distrustful aspect,
Terrible in beauty, age, and power,
The genius of poets of old lands,
As to me directing like flame its eyes,
With finger pointing to many immortal songs,
And menacing voice, *What singest thou?* it said,
Know'st thou not there is but one theme for ever-enduring bards?
And that is the theme of War, the fortune of battles,
The making of perfect soldiers.

Be it so, then I answer'd,
I too haughty Shade also sing war, and a longer and greater one than any,
Waged in my book with varying fortune, with flight, advance and retreat,
victory deferr'd and wavering,
(Yet methinks certain, or as good as certain, at the last,) the field the world,
For life and death, for the Body and for the eternal Soul,
Lo, I too am come, chanting the chant of battles,
I above all promote brave soldiers.

—WALT WHITMAN

Contents

Preface

I wrote *Victory Deferred* because, despite the abundance of books written about AIDS, no one until now has examined both the "big picture" and its finer details in considering the many ways AIDS affected the nation's hardest hit community, gay men. *Victory Deferred* looks at how AIDS changed gay life in America in almost every conceivable way: culturally, medically, politically, and socially. It traces the transformation of a disorganized collection of despised individuals into a self-affirming community and a full-fledged civil rights movement. It tells the story of a people who practiced the adage "Charity begins at home" by developing volunteer-run service organizations, designing novel and effective prevention campaigns, raising millions of dollars for research and care, creating memorials to the stricken, and wielding the tools of political pressure to wake up national leaders who wanted nothing to do with a disease perceived as afflicting "undesirables."

Although other books have explored particular aspects of AIDS among gay people, only *Victory Deferred* links with extensive first-hand accounts the personal impact of AIDS on gay people and their supporters and the emergence of the national gay political movement. In Randy Shilts's *And the Band Played On*, the effects of AIDS on gay America are only a subtheme of the author's overall look at the politics of American medicine and science. Elinor Burkett's more recent book, *The Gravest Show on Earth*, polemically (and mistakenly) equated the political efforts of gay people in defending their lives with the efforts of religious conservatives to exploit AIDS in promoting their antigay agenda. Gabriel Rotello's *Sexual Ecology* and Frank Browning's *Culture of Desire* examined the role and meanings of sexuality in gay male culture. In many ways, *Victory Deferred* elaborates upon Urvashi Vaid's point in *Virtual Equality* that "The AIDS epidemic so transformed the gay and lesbian political movement that, as with our personal lives, we can mark two distinct eras: life before AIDS and life after AIDS."

My aim is to provide an "inside" look at the effects of AIDS on gay people and the gay civil rights movement—and how gay people have pushed and pulled a reluctant nation into action in combating the epidemic. With few exceptions, I have intentionally "painted" from a palette of grays a picture of the people and events of the nearly two decades since the start of the epidemic. Like life itself, few things in the AIDS epidemic have been black or white in their moral or medical certitude, and few people have been exclusively heroic or cowardly. I expect readers will draw their own conclusions from this depiction of people, places, and moments in time. I believe, however, they will recognize that the story of gay people in the AIDS epidemic is not merely a story of the 1980s or 1990s but of human history as it is played out in all times and everywhere.

The book is a work of journalism, and represents one writer's attempt to organize and explain a complex and multifaceted cultural, medical, political, and social phenomenon. It is not a treatise on AIDS activism, fundraising, politics, prevention, psychiatry, sexuality, or any other specific topic; each of these is considered in the text because it is a facet of my overall subject. In telling the story, I draw mainly upon the more than two hundred interviews I conducted throughout the United States. People with AIDS, activists, caregivers, doctors, fund raisers, lawyers, scientists, and volunteers speak in these pages about their experiences, the lessons they learned, and the losses they sustained. I have woven their accounts together with material gleaned from extensive research in the existing literature on AIDS to tell the story, offer assessments of why things happened as they did, and suggest how they fit into a larger scheme. The book is organized thematically because of the vastness of my subject. Each chapter focuses on a particular aspect of AIDS and gay life and politics; together they make up the bigger story.

It is important to state that I have written a sympathetic account—but not an uncritical one. This will rankle those who insist on particular points of view, or "political correctness," even when they contravene the facts. I do not toe anyone's line, whether talking about bathhouses and sex clubs, ACT UP, or lobbying efforts in Washington. I will irritate those who feel that any challenge to what I call a "ghetto mentality" is a homophobic assault against all gay people. I will annoy those who believe that AIDS fund raisers should be "left alone" and not held accountable because they "are doing God's work." I will also touch a nerve in addressing the tensions between AIDS organizations run by people of color and the so-called "AIDS establishment" that includes the larger and wealthier groups started primarily by white gay men and women.

Despite my commitment to calling spades spades by challenging the "PC," or status quo, version of events, individual actions, or earlier interpretations, I believe that astute readers will take away an appreciation of what gay people have struggled against, how they have been affected by it, and why they gained in social and political stature because of the humanity and strength they demonstrated in responding to AIDS. If they keep an open mind, both gay and non-gay readers alike will be impressed by the ability of gay people to pull together to find solutions to the multitude of problems that AIDS brought upon them.

As a Washington journalist writing about AIDS and gay politics and culture since the early eighties, I have had an ideal vantage point from which to observe the unfolding of the national gay civil rights movement and the nation's response to AIDS. I have watched with a combination of horror and fascination as I have seen AIDS devastate so many lives and as I have watched so many people—including, most remarkably, those living with the disease itself—come forward and demonstrate repeatedly that charity and nobility are more than old-fashioned virtues. I have seen too much mortal illness and death, among too many of my friends and colleagues, at too young an age. I have also been privileged to witness truly extraordinary displays of heroism.

Against criticism that the current volume is incomplete because AIDS is still with us, I take shelter in Camus' point that any record of a plague "could not be one of final victory." As *The Plague*'s narrator, Dr. Rieux, explains, "It could be only the record of what had had to be done, and what assuredly would have to be done again in the never ending fight against terror and its relentless onslaughts, despite their personal afflictions, by all who, while unable to be saints but refusing to bow down to pestilences, strive their utmost to be healers."

In naming the names of those who made *Victory Deferred* possible, I must first thank all the people I interviewed for the book. I am grateful for their time and willingness to share with me the intimate, often painful, details of their personal stories that made my telling of this story possible. I am sorry to say that several have died since our interviews. I hope this book will help them to live on in our collective memory.

I think that Doug Mitchell, a jazz drummer moonlighting as my editor, must understand humanity so well because rhythm itself is central to all we know as humans, from the beating of our hearts to the music of the spheres. I thank him for passionately championing my portrayal of the human drama in the pages that follow. Thanks to others at the University of Chicago Press for their hard work on my and the book's behalf, including Doug's assistant Matt Howard, production editor Claudia Rex, copy editor John McCudden, designer Marianne Jankowski, publicist Erin Hogan, and marketing director Carol Kasper.

My thanks to Warren Frazier, my agent with the perfect name and wonderful voice, for sharing both my vision for this book as well as a love of books. Thanks also to Tom Murphy for not only reading and liking the manuscript, but for recommending it to Warren.

A picture may be worth a thousand words, but some of the photos provided for *Victory Deferred* leave me speechless. I am particularly thankful to Jane Rosett and Rink for their powerful images. Jane gave 150 percent as my informal photo editor, and I am grateful for her excellent counsel and judgment.

My deepest thanks to Dr. Delvin L. Covey, an ardent supporter of this book and reader of its drafts. "Doc" has not only set high standards for me since he was my adviser in college two decades ago, but he has consistently provided the loving encouragement I needed as I strived to measure up to them.

For reading the proposal for what became this book, as well as individual chapters, I thank my friends and colleagues Judy Auerbach, Curt Decker, Anne Lewis, (the late and greatly missed) Judy Pollatsek, Jane Silver, and Steve Taravella. I particularly thank Curt Decker for his heart of gold and sly humor, and for offering to throw the book launch party if I would write the book. Thanks to Doug Elliott for cajoling me and providing work projects to keep body and soul together during the writing; to John D'Emilio for reading drafts, introducing me to Doug Mitchell, and for his friendship; to Karl Goodkin for arranging all of my interviews in Miami; to Jim Holm for believing I was "just the right person" to write this particular book, and for his encouragement along the way; to Randy Miller for his friendship, and for sharing the risk of talking honestly together about his experience of being black and gay in a society that undervalues both; and to Gene Morris for listening to and encouraging me to follow a more effective course.

My gratitude to Arnie Kantrowitz, the "alpha and omega" of *Victory Deferred*. Arnie's candor, goodness, and love alone could change the world even without his passionate zeal for justice. I am blessed by his friendship and wisdom. I was profoundly moved as I stood with Larry Mass, Arnie's lover, at the Newseum, in Arlington, Virginia, to look at his 1981 article on display, "Cancer in the Gay Community"—the first news feature ever written about AIDS. Larry's boldness in writing about AIDS and cofounding GMHC make him a great hero of the story told in this book, and a personal hero of its author.

I couldn't have made it intact through the sorrow over my own losses in the plague years, or sustained the energy and passion it took to write *Victory Deferred*, if I wasn't blessed so extravagantly with wonderful people who encouraged and loved me throughout the years it took to bring the project to fruition. I am especially grateful for the love and support of my very dear friends Scott Foster and Kenny Hill, the life partner Scott for a decade has called the "exquisite center of his universe." They are both exquisite men and central to my own little world. Thank you to my friends Ron Caringi, Laura Goldstein, Jim Halloran, Charlie Harrison, Rod Mercer, Gregg Peterson and his partner Larry Teolis, Dennis Pfaff, Rich Rasi and his partner Jonathan "Jeb" Bates, my cousin Cindy Raedeke and her husband, Art Raedeke, and to Herb Schultz.

Mere words are inadequate to thank those whose lives continue to cast long shadows across my own life, but words are all I have to say what I feel. My mother, Anna Andriote, is simply the most generous and loving person I have ever known. Thank you, Mom, for loving me so generously. My sisters, Pamela Day and Susan Gladue, have always encouraged me—even when I think they haven't known what to make of me. My college professor and mentor, Thomas Howard, admonished me never to neglect my talent for writing and inspired me to know the Great Myth Come True. My eighth-grade English teacher, Dorothy Cramer, first showed me the power of literature and told me "Hitch your wagon to a star." I did, and the ride has been excellent (if a little bumpy at times).

Finally, I abide in honor, love, and loss "too deep for tears," as Wordsworth put it, for the three men to whose memory I have dedicated *Victory Deferred,* each of them a powerful force in shaping the man I am and the work I do today. My father, Manuel John Andriote, urged me to question what I don't understand and to ask for help when I need it. Allen Satterfield showed me by example what a life of integrity looks like, and wrote poetry for me. My former lover Bill Bailey urged me to write about AIDS, and fought so valiantly to prevent others from contracting it even as it stole his own life.

I am forever indebted to all of you. Thank you.

Introduction

Not long before his own death from AIDS, Randy Shilts, our best-known chronicler of the early years of the epidemic, said that the ability of gay people to forge solutions even as they coped with the horrors of AIDS remained "one of the great untold stories of the nineteen-eighties." In fact, to tell the story of gay people in the AIDS epidemic is to describe variations on the very theme that reverberates throughout human history: the brave few struggling against a powerful enemy as the silent majority chooses ignorance over involvement because they don't see themselves as personally at risk.

The solutions gay people forged have served as models for the nation and the world. Their common element, and most striking quality, has been the extraordinary level of volunteerism behind them, the time and commitment given because "someone has to do it." Gay people and their supporters demonstrated the "love in action" that, as Mother Teresa saw it, truly is God. When AIDS first struck gay men, in 1981, activists quickly rallied to share information, provide services, raise money, prevent new infections, and demand assistance from a skittish federal government. Within a month after the first cases of AIDS were reported, New York writer Larry Kramer wrote in the *New York Native,* "This is our disease and we must take care of each other and ourselves." In early 1982, Kramer and five other well-known gay men met in Kramer's living room to make plans for Gay Men's Health Crisis, a volunteer-run organization that would raise money for research and offer services to gay men afflicted with what was then called "Gay-Related Immune Deficiency," or GRID.

1

The same year, leaders in San Francisco's gay Castro area formed the Kaposi Sarcoma Education and Research Foundation. Within a few years, hundreds of organizations were formed throughout the country and around the world, modeled to one degree or another after these two early groups. Similarly, Pat Norman's AIDS Coordinating Committee, a group of mainly gay and lesbian community leaders in San Francisco in the early eighties, provided the earliest model for the now $1 billion-plus comprehensive AIDS services program funded by the federal Ryan White CARE Act.

My overarching conviction, which permeates this book, is that what the gay civil rights movement fundamentally seeks is a society in which individuals are able to love themselves as nature and nurture have combined to make them, and everyone can enjoy the freedom to love regardless of the sex of their beloved. If being gay is about love, an essentially private experience, it follows that life for gay people is an essentially private business—just as it is for heterosexuals. But because homosexual love is so feared and reviled in American society, gay life traditionally has been doubly private, the love and often the actual lives of gay men and lesbians hidden from the eyes of disapproving heterosexuals. Given the human need for connection with others, though, the "love that dare not speak its name" drew together people in similar circumstances as friends and lovers who could freely speak the name of their love.

Before AIDS forced open so many closet doors, gay life revolved mainly around circles of friends and lovers, and their interconnections with other similar circles across the country, even around the world. Despite the personal contacts, however, there was little sense of belonging to a "national" gay community. When hundreds of thousands of gay and lesbian marchers filled the streets of Washington in 1979, 1987, and again in 1993, Americans—including many gay people themselves—were astonished at the size and diversity of the gay community in this country. AIDS brought the gay community *as* a community out of the closet. The privately supportive circles linked publicly with other similar ones to form a nationwide "army of lovers," a term borrowed from Greek antiquity and used in the early seventies to describe the emerging gay community.

The story of gay America in the AIDS epidemic is ultimately that of a people who cared for their own and showed the world that neither disease nor human kindness has sexual preferences. Gay people and their nongay allies banded together in sorrow and rage, boldly demanding recognition of their loves and losses, even as activists and lobbyists fought for money to conduct research into AIDS, care for the sick, and prevent others from becoming infected with HIV. Gay people in the AIDS epidemic showed their heart: that it was capable of great love, that it quickened with anger and fear, and that it broke, too, from the weight of so many losses. As Virginia Apuzzo, former director of the National Gay and Lesbian Task Force, said when I interviewed her about political issues for the book, "Talk about our institutions, the legislation, and appropriations—it's important and I hope you do a good job on it. But if you do all of that, and don't talk about the grief and pain, and the fact that we still fight for the right to love—if you think of anything less—you miss the whole point."

An inescapable and discomfiting point in describing gay people in the AIDS epidemic is the fact that many gay men in the early years of the epidemic—some of them still today—ignored the dangers of AIDS because, among other things, it meant having to change their sexual behavior. Forced to be "sexual outlaws" by an oppressive American society, many homosexuals defined themselves as society defined them, by the very trait that distinguished them from heterosexuals: their sexuality. It was one thing they fully possessed, and they were damned if they'd let anyone take it away from them. But the question ultimately became, plainly and simply, whether sex was worth dying for. In the process of answering that question, the community devised ways to help men change their behavior—while reinterpreting sexuality and redefining what it means to be gay in affirmative, life-saving terms. Perhaps the greatest of gay people's many accomplishments in addressing AIDS has been the creation of a diverse community that nurtures its members to see themselves as distinctive for many reasons besides their sexuality alone.

Camus tells us in *The Plague* that the essence of heroism is caring for others as "a matter of common decency." Even as they were derided as "immoral" by religious conservatives merely for their sexual orientation, gay people were driven to the forefront of the war against AIDS by a strong sense of common decency, the will to survive, and love. The boldness that homosexuals gained after the 1969 Stonewall uprising meant that neither the shame of the closet nor the stigma of a fatal sexually transmitted disease would stop them from speaking out about the medical and political injustices they were experiencing. They deflected homophobic assaults as they pressed on toward the goal of surviving—and ultimately conquering—the scourge that afflicted them so cruelly and disproportionately.

As we hope, pray, and fight for ultimate victory over both the viral enemy and the oppression of antigay hatred, the struggle with AIDS itself has changed us and reshaped the way many of us think about ourselves, our health, our sexuality, our community, our nation, and our future. Gay people during the AIDS epidemic have experienced in a compressed fashion—and mostly at a young age—the physical and emotional suffering that priests and poets from time immemorial have described as part of the "human condition." The hatred and condemnation of self-appointed judges, on top of efforts to remain uninfected or to live with the physical and psychological challenges of the disease itself, have made life in the era of AIDS a moral crucible, an unwelcome and severe test of our individual and collective mettle.

I hope you will read *Victory Deferred* as the remarkable story of a people who were determined to survive the biological catastrophe of AIDS and the spiritual violation of oppression. The story is set at the juncture where culture, medicine, morality, and politics intersect—as volatile, even dangerous, a battlefield as ever existed. It's about learning to speak the language of politics and science in order to save lives. It's about the efforts of well-intentioned but inexperienced people who founded and ran AIDS organizations that, over time, became part of a vast, multimillion dollar industry. It's about our successes, mistakes, the battles we won, and the terrific losses we sustained. It's about individuals and a community's coming of age under the most extraordinarily difficult circumstances and against the greatest odds. It's ultimately about people whose battle against an epidemic was propelled by their love for one another and their desire to be able to love freely.

The book also is a witness to the gay men who have lived and died in the epoch of AIDS, and a legacy to future generations of both gay and nongay people. Above all, it is the story of how the members of one community—an "army of lovers"—were conscripted into service in a war that neither they nor any other human being ever chose to fight. They were, of supreme necessity, made extremely brave soldiers, engaged in a fight against both a faceless viral enemy and human enemies whose faces were too often contorted with hatred. Fierce as it has been, we can never forget that the struggle with AIDS is ultimately but one skirmish in the war in which every living thing is engaged, against what St. Paul called the last enemy that shall be destroyed: Death.

THE FIELD

Is this not a night of nights! It's the beginning of the summer of our lives!

LARRY KRAMER, *FAGGOTS*

Being gay in the seventies meant hot men, cool drugs, pounding discos, and lots of sex. Urban gay communities in such cities as New York and San Francisco were magnets that drew men from America's small towns everywhere. The promise of acceptance and belonging was as alluring and exciting as the testosterone that seemed to ooze from the very pavement of streets with names like Christopher and Castro. Amidst the drugging, dancing, and fucking, political activists struggled to remind gay people that they would remain second-class citizens until they pulled together to fight the government for their civil and human rights—just as they had fought the police at the Stonewall Inn for their constitutional right to assemble, and the medical establishment for the right to live without the stigma of being considered "sick." As the party wore on, the glitter wore off for some men who wanted "gay" to mean something more than second-class, sex-crazed, and STD-infected. But the viral seed had already been sown right along with all those wild oats.

In 1973, Arnie Kantrowitz was riding high on a wave of gay pride, sexual freedom, and political possibility. As a charter member and former vice president of New York City's Gay Activists Alliance, this self-described "nice Jewish boy" from Newark, N.J., had found within himself a previously unknown self-confidence bolstered by the community he helped to create with his fellow activists in GAA. That year he wrote an op-ed piece for the *New York Times* which served notice on the world that this young gay man and many others like him were prepared, at last, to stand up for themselves with dignity and without shame. Kantrowitz recalls thinking at the time, "Yes, we could hide if we wanted to, but that bothered us and we would no longer accept that. So we elected to be open and face the oppression that would come with it because that was more dignified than being frightened and hiding."[1]

Kantrowitz also moved to New York's Christopher Street in 1973, after living for two years with fellow GAA members in a commune in SoHo. Now he basked in the revolutionary spirit of freedom that suffused the air of Greenwich Village with possibilities for all sorts of conquests—sexual, political, and, most important, the chance for a coup de grâce in the lifelong internal battle fought by most American gay men against the guilt and shame of being "different." In a few short years, gay people had gone from being timorous and furtive to bold and "out." The change was exhilarating, the camaraderie palpable. Kantrowitz celebrated the new sense of community he found in New York in his 1977 autobiography, *Under the Rainbow: Growing Up Gay*. "Chin held high and hopes higher still," he wrote, "I declared my solidarity with my people. Solidarity is not just a unioneer's catchword. It is a sense of belonging I have felt to my marrow, a kinship as thick as blood relation."[2]

Like many gay people in the early seventies, Kantrowitz had been inspired by the audacity and dignity of the patrons of the Stonewall Inn, who, after years of gratuitous harassment by the police, finally stood up and said "enough." On the night of Friday, June 27, 1969, New York police raided the Stonewall. As usual, they expected to intimidate the Christopher Street gay bar's patrons, reminding them once again that they were powerless pariahs in American society. But the cops got more than they expected when the pariahs stood up to them en masse and refused to play the old game in which they were always the losers. Gay people vented years of rage that night and in the nights of demonstrations that followed the raid. "Ain't gonna take it no more!" became a gay rallying cry after Stonewall, as much a statement about refusing second-class status in American society as about resisting police harassment whose only purposes seemed to be to mollify politicians and let straight cops feel macho—or possibly even avoid dealing with their own homosexuality.

Within days, gay New Yorkers organized the Gay Liberation Front, replacing years of polite "homophile" gay organizing with an in-your-face militancy never seen before among gay activists. GLF's rejection of "society's attempt to impose sexual roles and definitions on our nature" sparked the imaginations of homosexuals in Los Angeles and San Francisco, where GLF chapters also formed. Within a few months, a group in New York broke off from GLF to form Gay Activists Alliance, focusing only on gay rights and political action, rather than the panoply of leftist issues championed by GLF's band of gay hippies.

The gay rights movement offered Kantrowitz, and many other gay men and women, not only a sense of belonging but a political cause in which to channel their youthfully idealistic energy. As Kantrowitz described it, "The gay world was a consuming infatuation, and liberation a vision we were reaching for, a vision of a world in which everyone could be honest, a world without pretending, where men could love men and women love women openly."[3] GAA was a militant, though nonviolent, organization—"an army of lovers," as members called themselves—working for the civil rights of gay people, often through direct confrontation. The group organized petition drives to repeal sodomy laws, demonstrated against newspapers and broadcast stations over media accounts deemed inaccurate or derogatory, and "zapped" elected officials and political candidates by disrupting public forums and even seizing the microphone. GAA also continued the Stonewall rebellion's choreographed style of "street theater" (a decade and a half before ACT UP would take it to new levels in its own protests) including open displays of affection by same-sex couples and "gay-ins," in which large numbers of people picnicked and danced together in public parks and open spaces.[4]

Besides GAA chapters that sprang up in cities throughout the country, gay political clubs, mostly Democratic, were also organized at the local level during the seventies. The first was the Alice B. Toklas Democratic Club, formed in San Francisco in 1971. Other early groups included Seattle's Dorian Group, organized in 1972, and the Washington, D.C., Gertrude Stein Democratic Club, formed in 1976 as an East Coast counterpart to the group in San Francisco.

The "army of lovers" fighting for gay liberation would have an endless supply of new troops because of the post-Stonewall emphasis on publicly revealing one's homosexuality, or "coming-out." As gay historian John D'Emilio has noted, "To come out of the 'closet' quintessentially expressed the fusion of the personal and the political that the radicalism of the late nineteen-sixties exalted."[5]

Despite the formation of political groups and community organizing at the local level, gay people in the seventies had no sense of a national movement or community. The only place a "national" gay community existed was in the pipe dreams of activists. After political ripples spread across the country from singer and former beauty queen Anita Bryant's successful effort in 1977 to overturn a gay rights ordinance in Dade County, Florida, gay activists throughout the country saw a need to step up their community organizing. Again, though, the organizing was at the local level; the goal was simply to stamp out the antigay brush fires that Bryant's "Save Our Children" campaign had ignited in other states. The campaign represented one of the earliest organized antigay drives by right-wing religionists—it would hardly be the last, and certainly not the most hate-filled.

Until Anita Bryant's anti-gay campaign, the gay rights movement was little more than a loosely connected ragtag band of committed individuals scattered throughout the country. Paul Boneberg, at the time vice president of the gay student union at the University of California in San Jose, later a prominent AIDS activist in San Francisco, said, "When I began doing gay politics in the mid-seventies, I would suspect there were a hundred people [engaged in gay political organizing] in the country, and if you knew those hundred people then you knew everyone who was doing lesbian and gay politics in America. Of those people, maybe two were employed—and not very well employed—in struggling organizations."[6] Bryant's campaign served notice that gay people had best wake up to the growing threat from the emerging "Christian" right.

Gay organizing in California was further catalyzed when Bryant protégé State Senator John Briggs in 1978 launched a statewide referendum, Proposition 6, known as the Briggs Initiative, that would have prevented gay people from working in public schools. The state field coordinator for Briggs was Lou Sheldon, today head of the rabidly homophobic Traditional Values Coalition. As is still the case, it was only when gay people realized that politics truly has personal ramifications—in this case, the risk of being barred from a job—that they joined the budding community's political efforts.

In November 1978, the Briggs initiative was defeated at the polls. That same month, San Francisco was rocked by the assassinations of Mayor George Moscone and openly gay city supervisor Harvey Milk. On November 27, 1978, Milk's fellow supervisor Dan White shot and killed Moscone and Milk in their offices at City Hall. Forty thousand people gathered that night for a candlelight vigil to honor the slain leaders. When an all-heterosexual jury found White guilty of voluntary manslaughter (his attorneys used the now-infamous "twinkie defense" to argue that White's mental capacity had been diminished by eating junk food) and the judge sentenced him to just seven years and eight months in prison with a chance for parole after only five years, the gay community exploded in rage.

On the evening of May 21, 1979, about three thousand gay demonstrators marched on City Hall, chanting, "We want justice!" and "He got away with murder!" A dozen police cars were burned, one hundred sixty people, including fifty policemen, were injured, and about $1 million in damage was inflicted. "Society is going to have to deal with us not as nice little fairies who have hairdressing salons," said one protester, "but as people capable of violence." Meanwhile, the police celebrated the verdict. Shouting "Fucking faggots!" they trashed the gay bars in the Castro area.[7]

While the mainstream media condemned the gay rioters, the gay press throughout the country was far more sympathetic. An editorial in the *San Francisco Sentinel* concluded, "If our justice system allows for a Dan White, it must also allow for rioters." As Rodger Streitmatter notes in his history of the gay press, an article in *Seattle Gay News* following the assassinations "left no room for doubt that lesbian and gay America was a single community unified in its grief at the loss of a magnificent leader."[8]

The unity among the gay press on the assassinations in San Francisco and the ensuing riot, as well as the press's support for successful local efforts to resist antigay spinoff organizations associated with Anita Bryant's "Save Our Children" campaign, went far toward creating a sense of belonging to a cause that extended across the country among the many otherwise unaffiliated local gay and lesbian communities. A spokesman for Boston's *Gay Community News* said in 1979,

"The greatest success of the gay press has been to foster community."[9] The role of the gay press as a conduit of information to and among gay men in the AIDS epidemic would prove to be one of the community's most important resources in mobilizing a nationwide network of AIDS programs in the 1980s and 1990s.

The first gay political group to take a national focus was the National Gay Task Force, which was formed in New York City in 1973. Now called the National Gay and Lesbian Task Force, or NGLTF, the group since 1986 has been based in Washington, D.C. According to the task force's founding codirector, Bruce Voeller, its mission was "to reeducate society, including its homosexual members, to esteem gay men and women at their full human worth and to accord them places in society which will allow them to attain and contribute according to their full human and social potential." In response to Anita Bryant's "Save Our Children" campaign, the task force launched its own national education program, underfunded but right on the money, which it called "We Are Your Children."[10]

The task force succeeded in having a gay rights measure introduced into Congress when New York Representative Bella Abzug introduced a bill on March 23, 1975, that would prohibit discrimination based on sexual or affectional preference. The bill languished in Congress in the coming years, trotted out annually to collect a few more sponsors but never actually voted on. Other than its involvement with this bill, NGLTF didn't have an ongoing presence in Washington in the 1970s. In fact, it wasn't until 1978 that there was even one full-time lobbyist in the nation's capital representing the collective interests of gay people nationwide.

Steve Endean, a young man from Minneapolis, formed the Gay Rights National Lobby in Washington in the fall of 1978. Endean was a forerunner of the kind of coat-and-tie gay and lesbian activists who operate in today's relatively large, well-off national gay rights groups in Washington. In an interview with Edmund White, Endean was quoted as saying, "The movement needs patterned, mature, planned programs—not just rage and marches. That energy is good—but it needs to be harnessed. Otherwise, when the anger subsides, it turns out nothing has been accomplished."[11]

After feeling like walking targets of the radical right, and after seeing Harvey Milk literally become an assassin's target, gay people were certainly enraged—and they were ready for a march of historic proportions. On October 14, 1979, more than one hundred thousand gay men and lesbians and their supporters converged on Washington for the first-ever National March on Washington for Lesbian and Gay Rights. A historic National Third World Lesbian and Gay Conference, sponsored by the one-year-old National Coalition of Black Gays, held at the time of the march, brought together gay blacks, Hispanics, Asians, and Native Americans. Five hundred people attended the conference, at which poet and author Audre Lorde delivered the keynote address.[12]

Brian McNaught, who at the time wrote a regular column for the gay newspaper in Boston, and would become the mayor's first liaison to the gay community and play a pivotal role in Boston's early response to AIDS in the eighties, described his impressions of the march shortly afterward. McNaught's words spoke for many of the gay men and lesbians at the march who, for the first time in their lives, felt a part of a real community, national in scope. "It was like nothing I had ever been a part of before," he wrote. "It was magic. It was spiritual. It was energizing. . . . 'We are everywhere,' we chanted as we marched to the beat of kazoos and tambourines. 'We are everywhere,' we screamed as we danced and skated and skipped like children. We embraced each other with shiny-faced grins of excitement. We renewed each other with winks and squeezes and outstretched arms. 'We are everywhere,' we insisted, 'and we will be free.'"[13]

Eric Rofes, who in the eighties would lead the world's largest gay organization and then one of the most renowned AIDS service organizations, in the late seventies was a member of a Boston activist group known as the GCN collective (from *Gay Community News*, a leftist gay newspaper)—a group that would produce a number of nationally prominent gay leaders. As one of the key organizers of the 1979 march, Rofes recalls that in 1979, "your typical gay person wasn't involved in gay politics." What's more, he added, "the typical gay political person was involved locally. It was a tough argument to make to get people to understand the need for a national movement." A lack of state-level gay organizations meant that even within individual states, local groups typically didn't work with others in neighboring communities. The energy and commitment that organizing the national march required of Rofes and the others who pulled it together can't be overstated. The outcome, though, was an increasingly national sense of gay solidarity. As Rofes told me, "The challenge of that march, and I think the accomplishment of that march, was to create a foundation for awareness on the part of your ordinary movement gay person that there were national issues of importance."[14]

Of course there is a substantial gap between awareness of national issues and preparedness for a major catastrophe like AIDS, as Rofes hastened to point out about the epidemic then on the verge of erupting among gay men. "This wasn't a disease visited upon a highly organized, powerful national movement," he emphasized. "The march was both a key trigger for what little national networks were being established at the start of the epidemic, and also a good bellwether of how unorganized we were and how little interest there was in a national movement."[15]

Urvashi Vaid, another member of the *GCN* collective, called the 1979 march "perhaps our biggest cultural success to date." But she noted that the end of the 1970s marked the beginning of a period of political losses spurred by the rise of an organized antigay opposition. Nevertheless, said Vaid, "the same decade saw gay and lesbian culture, community, and life breaking new ground."[16]

*

For many gay men, the seventies were a time of great possibility as they joined others like themselves in major cities to carve out a place where they could be open about who they were and feel safe from the hatred that threatened to oppress them as American society continued to force them to the margins of its awareness. Some were fortunate to find acceptance even among heterosexuals, and bonds were formed that would become stronger in the tribulations of the years ahead. Nowhere was there a greater willingness by both gay and heterosexual people to reach out and care for one another than in San Francisco, where a visitor might leave his heart and residents could find their heart's desire in the city's scenic beauty and air of openness and acceptance.

After arriving in San Francisco in 1971, Armistead Maupin says he was "shocked to discover that there were straight men and women who were utterly blasé about the fact of homosexuality." Both hetero- and homosexual people had long been attracted to the gentle city by the bay. Maupin, who portrayed life in 1970s San Francisco in his colorful and well-loved *Tales of the City* series of novels, added that because of the acceptance of differences among people in San Francisco, coming-out for him meant living as an openly gay man in the world at large. "It had nothing to do with burying myself in a ghetto and surrounding myself only with my own kind. There were enough people here not like me who accepted me [so] that I was able to feel good about myself."[17]

For people like Maupin and his friends, the freedom they en- joyed in San Francisco in the seventies meant they could build alter- native "families" and a true community. He points out that when AIDS struck the city, "it would have been even worse than it was if we didn't have those families in place." Unfortunately, albeit pre- dictably, it wasn't the domestic and community-building aspects of gay life that the news media focused on in the years before AIDS. Given the media's penchant for the anomalous and outré, Americans whose impressions of gay people came only from what they read in magazines or saw on television could easily believe that all gay people dressed in drag or leather, took drugs, copulated in public parks, and, for all they knew, probably kept Dorian Gray-like portraits hidden in the attic to deflect from their youthful faces the ravages of a de- bauched lifestyle.

In an April 26, 1980, *CBS Reports* news special about gay people in San Francisco called "Gay Power, Gay Politics," CBS reporter George Crile asked gay activist Cleve Jones, "Isn't it a sign of deca- dence when you have so many gays emerging, breaking apart all of the values of a society?" Although a media standards board later ac- knowledged that the show was biased against homosexuals, the im- pressions it conveyed were damaging. Armistead Maupin had played host to the CBS news team, showing them around the city and ex- plaining the many facets of gay life. But he said, "I had no idea they were doing a hit piece."

It certainly hit its mark. As Urvashi Vaid puts it in *Virtual Equal- ity,* "The tone of the CBS show was alarmist and seemed to suggest that gays would soon head out of the Castro, out of the gay bars and bushes that had been their 'traditional' domain, and into government offices, boardrooms, and, eventually, the playgrounds of America."[18]

Looking back at the pre-AIDS image of gay people painted by the media, Maupin says, "The thing that annoys me most is the revisionist attitude that gay people didn't discover the bonds of family until AIDS and impending death forced it upon them. Nothing could be further from the truth. There were, as early as the mid-seventies in San Francisco, gay lawyer groups, gay doctor groups, gay needlepoint groups, gay sports teams, and people forming viable, loving families."[19] Throughout the country, notes John D'Emilio, there were already more than one thousand gay and lesbian organizations by the mid-seventies. "Activists," he writes in *Sexual Politics, Sexual Communities,* "created newspapers, magazines, health clinics, churches, multipurpose social centers, and specialized businesses—in short, a range of institutions that implied the existence of a separate, cohesive gay community."[20]

Pat Norman, a veteran black, lesbian, and human rights activist in San Francisco, recalled her experience of working with the city's Gay Counseling Service in the early seventies. The transition from in-the-closet-and-ashamed to out-and-proud was not an easy one for many (if not most) gay people to make, and psychotherapy often became an important tool in adjusting to their newfound freedom. "It was a group of young gay men and me," said Norman, "who set up services outside the [mainstream] institutions in order to help people come out, deal with relationship issues, depression, anxiety, their problems within that particular era in coming out." She added, "It seemed to us then that everybody was coming out. It was a revolutionary time."[21]

The revolution wasn't only in the healing of psychological wounds, but in the increasing boldness of gay people to assert their rights as American citizens. One of the most important battles in the revolution was against unprovoked harassment and entrapment by police, an alarming feature of urban gay life in the years before Stonewall. John D'Emilio says the combination of a decline in police harassment and an increase in gay people coming out of the closet made for "a pretty vibrant urban sexual subculture of gay men that actually was a continuation of things that were going on in the sixties." Earlier gay subcultures could be found in places like San Francisco and New York, but they were hidden behind shaded windows. "Now," said D'Emilio, "the doors were open and people were half in and half out of the bar; it was part of public life, rather than just closeted life."[22]

The revolutionary spirit of freedom drew many gay men westward to San Francisco. A sense of expectation, adventure, and the chance finally to fit in somewhere gave the city the allure of a "gay mecca," as the city had become known by the seventies. As *Chronicle* reporter Randy Shilts observed, "The promise of freedom had fueled the greatest exodus of immigrants to San Francisco since the Gold Rush." He noted that between 1969 and 1973, at least nine thousand gay men moved to San Francisco, followed by twenty thousand more between 1974 and 1978. "By 1980," said Shilts, "about five thousand homosexual men were moving to the Golden Gate every year. The immigration now made for a city in which two in five adult males were openly gay."[23]

For thousands of gay men, San Francisco represented safety, literally a refuge from the insults, beatings, and moral condemnation they had suffered throughout their lives merely for being homosexual. Vast numbers of them made the Castro district the center of their world. Even in the 1990s, one can still hear the intersection of Castro and Eighteenth streets, the heart of the area, referred to as "the crossroads of the gay world." A pamphlet, called *Refugees from Amerika: A Gay Manifesto,* written by gay liberationist Carl Wittman in 1970, described San Francisco as "a refugee camp for homosexuals." After fleeing small towns, blackmailing cops, families who disowned or "tolerated" them, after being thrown out of schools and the armed services, fired from jobs, beaten by punks and policemen alike, Wittman wrote, gay people "have formed a ghetto, out of self-protection."[24]

The ghetto, however, was not universally regarded by gay men as a positive development. In an interview with Edmund White in the late seventies, then *Advocate* publisher David Goodstein described two large groups of gay men in San Francisco. One consisted of men over thirty who had lived in the city at least a decade, served on opera committees, worked in the professions, showed an interest and concern for the community. "They're not so different from gays everywhere," he said, "though more of them here are out of the closet and they're better organized than in most places." The second group was the "Castro clones," gay men who, as Goodstein put it, "are convalescing in the ghetto from all those damaging years in Podunk." He said they were a rough crowd, hanging out like teenagers, drinking too much, taking too many drugs, fucking day and night, infecting each other with venereal diseases, "and of course radical politically." Worst of all, said Goodstein, "They have a *shtetl* consciousness—you know, like the Jewish ghetto. They patronize Castro Street businesses; in fact, they seldom leave the area."[25]

Even if Goodstein's observations were accurate, they smacked of economic elitism. And criticism of the rampant promiscuity in the gay ghetto was ironic coming from the publisher of a newspaper supported largely by advertising paid for by bathhouses and other sexual services that fostered the very activities he deplored. The ghetto certainly was teeming with refugees, but merely condemning or mocking them, as Goodstein did, failed to address the oppression that these men felt had forced them there in the first place—and did nothing to aid their "convalescence." Shut away from a disapproving world, the ghetto flipped an angry middle finger at the society that had forced its creation, adopting its own value system and asserting a sense of pride that was far preferable to the shame that gay men had been told was their lot in life.

White observed in *States of Desire* that in San Francisco "gays constitute such a numerous and well-organized minority [an estimated 20 percent of the city's 335,000 registered voters were gay] that the life of the city is to a remarkable degree within their power to shape." In the gay ghetto, however, the reverse was true: the lives of gay men there were shaped by the life and values of the ghetto. As Randy Shilts put it in *The Mayor of Castro Street: The Life and Times of Harvey Milk*, "Gays no longer came to the Castro to create a new lifestyle, they came to fit into the existing Castro Street mold."[26] White's final take on San Francisco was that it was "where gay fantasies come true." But, he said, "the problem the city presents is whether, after all, we wanted these particular dreams to be fulfilled— or would we have preferred others? Did we know what price these dreams would exact?"[27]

The visibility of gay people in the ghettos made them easy targets for homophobes, capitalists, and social diseases that thrived on the vulnerability of people trying to find their place in the world. Describing the men who filled the ghettos, and whose minds were in turn filled by the ghetto way of thinking, Canadian writer Ian Young notes that few of these "refugees" had the skills they needed for emotional equilibrium—or even survival—in the big city. "Isolated gay boys from small towns," he said, "they arrived in the Village or the Castro lacking the discernment and abilities necessary to maintain real friendships or meaningful ties."[28]

Being smart capitalists, the owners of bars and bathhouses—frequently heterosexual and affiliated with the Mafia—gained control over the attitudes, behaviors, and spending habits of their gay patrons. They created a "need" for their services and then met that need in the dark and drug-addled anonymity of their establishments. The proliferation of these outlets in the seventies, and the pressures from peers and advertising in the gay press alike to avail oneself of them as socially acceptable alternatives to, say, relationships, led many gay men to define their lives in the very terms with which heterosexuals often stereotyped them. In this truncated view of homosexuality, one's attitude toward promiscuity became a kind of litmus test for how "out" he was; if one was uncomfortable with promiscuity, went the reasoning of the day, it was because he hated being gay.

How far gay men, at least the segment of them in the urban ghettos, had strayed from the visionary ideals of gay pioneers like Harry Hay, founder in 1950 of the nation's first "homophile" organization, the Mattachine Society! Though perhaps more cerebral than most, Hay had laid a fairly solid foundation for gay men to stand on in knowing who they were: homosexuals are unique, he asserted, and they have something important to offer to humanity in general. Hay believed that the gender of their sex partners was not the only thing that distinguished gay men from heterosexuals. Sex was certainly an important part of being gay for Hay, but it was years from becoming the part and parcel of gay ghetto life it became in the seventies.

"Who are gay people?" asked Hay. "Where have we been in history? What might we be for?" Hay spoke of homosexuals as "spirit people," who, throughout the ages, had served society through their roles as "messengers and interceders, shamans of both genders, priestesses and priests, imagemakers and prophets, mimes and rhapsodes, poets and playwrights, healers and nurturers, teachers and preachers, tinkers and tinkerers, searchers and researchers."[29] Hay believed that gay people had something special to teach nongay people about human life, and for that reason should be nurtured, rather than reviled, by society. He postulated that "gay people represent a genetic mutation of consciousness whose active fostering is now required for human survival."[30] It hardly seems likely that the "*shtetl* consciousness" of the gay ghetto was the "mutation" that Harry Hay had in mind.

Gay writer John Rechy, author of the extraordinary 1963 novel *City of Night,* called homosexuals "sexual outlaws," forced into a life at the social fringe whose main feature was promiscuity. "In this context, the sexual outlaw flourishes," wrote Rechy in his 1977 book *The Sexual Outlaw.* "The pressures produce him, create his defiance. Knowing that each second his freedom may be ripped away arbitrarily, he lives fully at the brink. Promiscuity is his righteous form of revolution."[31] The problem with this assessment, though, is that true revolutionaries don't just rebel, they push to bring about a society molded according to their own vision of how things ought to be. The "sexual outlaw" simply acted out of the pain of his pariah status without having anything other than a very myopic vision that couldn't see beyond the walls of the ghetto.

The lifestyle offered in the urban ghettos was, as Ian Young puts it, "the ultimate consumer product—a permanent sex holiday."[32] And it wasn't only the "clones" who enjoyed this holiday. Even politically active men who were working for gay liberation frequently equated freedom with the right to have prodigious amounts of sex with anyone, anytime, anywhere. Arnie Kantrowitz, who had found personal liberation in his work in the gay rights movement, said, "I came to define myself by my sexuality. And I valued myself by my sexuality. Sex came first." When he developed syphilis, he recalls, he wept because he had to stop having sex for a while. "Who would I be if I wasn't going to be the hot sex partner, the great pursuer or pursued?" he wondered.[33]

After moving from Michigan "to be gay" in San Francisco in the seventies, Chuck Frutchey said, "the sex, the political organizing, they were really jumbled up, there wasn't a lot of separation between them." Frutchey and many others believed that "gay lib" would benefit everyone by liberating sexuality from American puritanism and integrating it into ordinary life. "In the seventies," said Frutchey, "people didn't see any sort of philosophical clash between holding down their job during the day, volunteering for some political activity in the evening, and going to a bathhouse with people they met at the volunteer activity at night."[34]

Michael Callen, a musician who would become one of the best-known and longest-surviving people with AIDS in the country, recalled, "At first, I had been promiscuous because the only information I had about gay men was that we were all promiscuous *by nature.*" After discovering gay liberation, he "proudly and defiantly" celebrated the promiscuity that mainstream society so disapproved of. "During the seventies," said Callen, "I considered myself a lowly private doing battle on the front lines of the sexual revolution. I joked that I was a fast-food sex junkie. For me, being gay *meant* having lots of sex."[35]

For many urban gay men, the venues that facilitated sex—from the decaying piers at the end of Christopher Street, to the dark backrooms in gay bars, to the bathhouses and sex clubs—served as community centers of sorts: the more you frequented them, the more "social" you were (and, not coincidentally, the more "social diseases" you likely contracted). The Canadian gay magazine *The Body Politic* observed, "Promiscuity knits together the social fabric of the gay male community." The catch to this way of thinking was that "community," as it is usually defined, presumes at the barest minimum that people know one another's names. Anonymous sexual encounters in the dark, while they may have inspired a feeling of priapic brotherhood with other men in the same situation, were hardly the stuff of which a real community is made.

What Arnie Kantrowitz called "the freedom of facelessness" flourished in the darkened backroom bars and the baths. As gay sexuality was commercialized in the seventies, a range of sexual establishments arose to cater to increasingly specialized tastes. For many, the baths were places where a man could be held, if that's what he needed, or where he could test the limits of bodily endurance if that was his inclination. For men who were not open about their homosexuality, the baths might be the only place they felt free to act on their desire for other men. Because of this anything-goes atmosphere, various envelopes were pushed regularly—and far.

There was also an air of unreality about the baths, at least partly intentional. The early seventies image of gay men in towels sitting around listening to Bette Midler, with Barry Manilow on the piano, all of them surrounded by straight people in evening dress who came for the show at the Continental Baths in New York (one of the reasons Midler was embraced early and strongly by the gay community) seems unreal, yet it happened. But the establishments themselves, with their dimly lit hallways, rows of small cubicles, orgy rooms, nap rooms, steam rooms, and whirlpools, were also refuges for many gay men from the struggle that was their lives. As Kantrowitz recalled, "It was always night at the baths, protected from the reality outside the door by a thick layer of gay imagination that sealed us in a secure environment as if we were in a huge magic theater where we could forget for a few hours what society thought of us."[36]

Armistead Maupin recalls the baths in the early seventies with wistfulness. He called them "places of extraordinary communion and coziness." He explained, "There was still enough of the old generous hippie spirit afoot to keep things from being too cold-blooded and mechanical." Maupin never saw the promiscuity he enjoyed back then as a bad thing, even after AIDS came along. "I was never ashamed of my promiscuity," he said, "because I saw it as a fundamentally innocent and wonderful and human thing. And because I had spent way too many years suppressing my sexuality, I had no intention of forbidding myself that pleasure any longer."[37] But by the end of the seventies, Maupin noted that there had been a change in the urban gay sex culture as the seventies progressed and the baths drew thousands of men a week in some cities. "As the bathhouses and bars became more institutionalized," he said, "they became lonelier places, and much less fulfilling."[38]

In New York, the Mine Shaft in the late seventies and early eighties was the bar-cum-sex-club that, as Douglas Sadownick notes, "almost every survivor from the seventies points to as a symbol of the fearlessness with which some gay men broke sexual taboos."[39] Every possible sexual fantasy—except, of course, the fantasy of sex with love—was enacted within the walls of the Mine Shaft, from being pissed on in a bathtub to being whipped by a "master" while chained to a wooden cross. The club's denizens included far more than just ghetto "clones." In my own earliest experience of gay life in New York, circa 1980, I recall affluent gay men excusing themselves from fancy Upper West Side dinner parties, and, bedecked in the requisite black leather jackets, heading downtown for "dessert" at the Mine Shaft.

One of the esoteric activities that became popular among some of the men who frequented the Mine Shaft went by names such as "hand-balling," "fisting," and "fist-fucking." After an elaborate ritual involving douching and imbibing enough drugs to deaden both the pain of the act and the better judgment that might remind them of its potential deadliness, men would submit to the invasion of their rectum by another man's fingers, hand, and even forearm. Ian Young notes that "fisting was *the* 'new' sexual act of the nineteen-seventies" and "a characteristic activity of ghetto gays from the mid-nineteen-seventies on."[40] Fisting invariably involved multiple snorts of "poppers," the amyl and other nitrite inhalants that became ubiquitous aphrodisiacs in the sex life of the ghetto.

In a bit of perverse irony, the patent on amyl nitrite, the medicinal form of the inhalant originally used by angina patients—packaged in capsules that were "popped" to release their vapors—was owned by none other than the British pharmaceutical giant Burroughs Wellcome.[41] Few would recall this fact in the early eighties when poppers became one of the first suspected causes of AIDS, or later in the decade when Burroughs was licensed to distribute AZT, the first approved treatment for AIDS. As Larry Kramer put it, "The company that made money by 'enabling' promiscuity, as it were, is now making a fortune by trying to stem its aftermath."[42]

As the seventies wore on, the gluttonous sex scene began to wear thin for some men. For Arnie Kantrowitz, the realization that he derived as much pleasure from his writing as from sex provided something of a second liberation. "I found it more gratifying to finish a piece of writing than to have gotten laid," he said. "I found myself going to the baths, or the Mine Shaft in the old days, and I used to keep a pad in my pocket and take notes by the light of the cigarette machine because writing was exciting. After a while, I realized that the writing was just as much of a satisfying high as the sex was."[43]

Other men who had participated enthusiastically in the life of the ghetto had grown tired of its anonymity and inverted values. They questioned why membership in the gay community had come to require that one be alienated from his family, take multiple drugs and have multiple sex partners, dance all night at the "right" clubs, and spend summer weekends at the "right" part of Fire Island. Rather than providing genuine liberation, gay life in the ghettos had created another sort of oppression with its pressure to conform to social expectations of what a gay man was "supposed" to be, believe, wear, and do. The "safety" offered by the ghetto began to seem too artificial, with the price of "belonging" one's renunciation of the belief that there could be fulfilling gay life outside the ghetto. As Kantrowitz put it, "We had come in search of protective anonymity, and we had all wound up in the same gigantic closet."[44]

Twin bombshells exploded over the New York ghetto in 1978, when two gifted writers focused their sights on a world of romantics whose minds had been anesthetized by too many drugs, and whose hearts' desire for love had been deadened by settling time after innumerable time for mere sex. In his first novel, *Dancer from the Dance*, Andrew Holleran told the story of the handsome and enigmatic Malone, described by Holleran as a "prisoner of love." Fixing his literary "gun" on the gay disco scene, with its fixation on youth and drugs, Holleran described the dancers in one of Malone's favorite hangouts: "Many of them were very attractive, these young men whose cryptic disappearance in New York City their families (unaware they were homosexual) understood less than if they had been killed in a car wreck. They were tall and broad-shouldered, with handsome, open faces and strong white teeth, *and they were all dead* [my emphasis]."[45]

In the summer these men headed out of the city to Fire Island, a spit of land off the Atlantic side of Long Island, and one of the loveliest beach resorts imaginable. The island and the beautiful men it drew, the drugs they took, and the sex they had were mythic among homosexuals. As Holleran described it, "Fire Island was for madness, for hot nights, kisses, and herds of stunning men."[46] But Malone was growing tired of the madness and dreamed of more. The constriction of the ghetto ultimately killed individuality as the men who melded their identities with ghetto life "disappeared in New York City" and its gay demimonde. In the end, at the age of thirty-eight, his golden beauty ripening into middle-aged handsomeness, Malone's dream of lasting love—the source of his charm and even his identity—is lost in the carnal immediacy of the ghetto. Like his friends, Malone wound up "living on faces, music, the hope of love, and getting farther and farther away from any chance of it."[47]

Like Malone, many gay men surrendered their dreams of love for the chance to belong in the ghetto world, no matter how exorbitant the price of membership. In his own 1978 novel *Faggots*, Larry Kramer asked whether the price of membership hadn't become too high—or whether membership was even desirable. On the eve of his fortieth birthday, Kramer's protagonist, Fred Lemish, makes the argument his creator would continue to make for years: "Why do faggots have to fuck so fucking much?! . . . it's as if we don't have anything else to do . . . all we do is live in our Ghetto and dance and drug and fuck." Lemish warns his philandering boyfriend, Dinky, to slow down "before you fuck yourself to death."[48]

The book was savaged by gay reviewers who felt Kramer had betrayed them by daring to challenge the "shtetl consciousness" of the ghetto. Gay novelist George Whitmore, writing in *The Body Politic,* urged a boycott of the book. New York's Oscar Wilde Memorial Bookshop refused to sell it. With the appearance of AIDS three years after its publication, *Faggots* would continue to ignite passionate arguments among some in the gay community who believed that Kramer was gloating that AIDS seemed to deliver into his hands a kind of medical "I told you so." But Kramer insisted that his main concern had been gay men and their quality of life.

If Kramer had touched a nerve with *Faggots*, an op-ed article he wrote for the *New York Times* shortly after the novel's publication practically caused a nervous breakdown among gay activists. Having just returned from a trip to San Francisco to promote his book—coincidentally the week that Mayor George Moscone and gay supervisor Harvey Milk were murdered and the gay community mounted a spontaneous and massive candlelight vigil to mourn them—Kramer was impressed by the solidarity and political activism of the city's gay community. "I am back in New York, missing, very much, the sense of community I felt in San Francisco," wrote Kramer. "I call several of my friends, but no one is home. I know that most of my friends are at the bars or the baths or the discos, tripping out on trivia." This much was familiar from his just-published novel, but Kramer went one step further. "The City Council was right," he continued, referring to a recently defeated gay rights ordinance. "We are not ready for our rights in New York. We have not earned them. We have not fought for them."[49]

But where had Kramer been all those years when other gay people were putting themselves on the line to stand up for their rights? Although he had never joined a gay political organization, Kramer had certainly participated in the scene he now condemned. His most vocal critics dismissed Kramer's criticism as nothing more than bitterness from his disappointment that the ghetto life hadn't provided him with the lover he longed for. "People felt betrayed," says Arnie Kantrowitz. "He was asking us to alter our behavior so we could demand a legitimacy that not all of us were sure we wanted. Some of us just wanted the government and the police and our employers off our backs so we could be free from prying eyes and hypocritical judgments. We were like children playing a new game, and we weren't ready to assume the responsibility of adulthood."[50]

Therein lay the problem, as Kramer saw it. But saying so, and in public at that, earned Kramer a pariah status within a community of pariahs. He was undeterred, however, and his message would remain the same for the next two decades. After recalling the uproar over *Faggots,* Kramer said, "Why are we so perennially focused on our dicks? It's a very peculiar 'community' that uses sexuality as the sole yardstick of action and thought and everything. It just seems to me so limiting and blind."[51] Driven to be an outsider—a role he seemed to relish, despite protestations to the contrary—Kramer's years of self-imposed "exile" after *Faggots* came out would, with the appearance of AIDS, provide the outsider with a second walk-on role, the one he lived for and the name by which he came to refer to himself in the plague years: Cassandra. Like the mythic daughter of King Priam warning of the downfall of Troy, Kramer seemed gifted with prophecy but was fated never to be believed.

Kramer wasn't alone in resisting the view that gay men are nothing more than constellations of sexual impulses. Even among some who were active participants in the sex- and drug-filled ghetto scene, the time seemed right to move on to another phase of their gay lives that didn't include some of the old ways that had become precisely that, old. Arnie Kantrowitz, a veteran of both the political and sexual revolutions of the seventies, said at the end of the decade, "I had explored my sexual fantasies enough, and I was ready to return to the life I had once led, but as a new person." Even on the street that symbolized gay liberation, he said, "More and more tourists are coming to Christopher Street to look, and it isn't as totally gay as it once was, or as glittering. Times change. America is growing up through the resignation of a president and the shaking of its dreams. And I am growing with it."[52]

In a few short years, many shaken dreams, and too many foreshortened lives, would force similar growth in considerably greater numbers of gay men. In the meantime, the party continued. The Saint, the most expensive wholly gay-owned enterprise in the country and perhaps the most famous gay disco ever in New York, opened in September 1980. The most successful export of gay ghetto culture, the Village People, titillated America with their costumed variations on the macho clone—and sold millions of records. "I'm ready for the eighties," they sang on their 1980 *Live and Sleazy* album, "ready for the time of my life." How very different the eighties and the "time of their life" would look. They could not possibly have imagined it.

*

To understand the uneasy relationship between gay people and the American medical establishment, one must look at the medical specialty of psychiatry and its shifting views of homosexuality over the years. From the time psychiatry emerged as a discipline, in the nineteenth century, it offered medical explanations of human behavior that, in earlier times, was explained and evaluated in religious terms. An increasingly secular society looked to psychiatry for guidelines on right and wrong. The religious language of sanctity and sinfulness was translated into the terminology of science. But the moralism of earlier times carried over into the translation, as psychiatrists spoke of behavior in terms of "normal" and "abnormal." Behavior that was different from that of the majority was deemed abnormal. Homosexuality, however natural it was for some people, was not merely labeled abnormal, but its difference from the heterosexual "norm" led psychiatrists to condemn it—in terms that may have seemed scientific but that would prove to have less in common with the rationality of science than with the irrationality of prejudice.

"Psychiatry is the enemy incarnate!" shouted Frank Kameny, seizing the microphone as he and other gay rights activists "zapped" a major session of the American Psychiatric Association's 1971 annual meeting in Washington, D.C. "Psychiatry has waged a relentless war of extermination against us," he continued. "You may take this as a declaration of war against you."[53] Kameny, a firebrand of the homophile movement—as the pre-Stonewall gay rights movement was known—decried the injury and voiced the anger of gay men and lesbians who, for decades, had been subjected to electroshock, lobotomy, "conversion" therapy, and commitment to mental hospitals by psychiatrists who believed they were "sick" and in need of cure. Kameny believed that psychiatry's designation of homosexuality as a mental illness was the prop holding up society's disdain of homosexuals. Remove it, kick it out, he reasoned, and the walls of discrimination would come tumbling down.

Two years later, in 1973, the American Psychiatric Association did remove homosexuality from its official list of mental illnesses. Describing how a combination of science and politics led the APA to change its mind, ethicist Ronald Bayer notes that the APA's diagnostic change "deprived secular society . . . of the ideological justification of its discriminatory practices." In 1990, the World Health Organization abandoned its definition of homosexuality as an illness. And England, the country that gave "the abominable crime of buggery" its name and drove its most famous practitioner, Oscar Wilde, to an untimely death, in 1994 finally stopped treating homosexuality as a mental illness. Today there are gay-affirmative theories and therapies and hundreds of openly gay and lesbian psychiatrists who enjoy voting representation within the APA's governing bodies. But it hasn't been this way for long.

Many homosexuals wore the pathology label with as much dignity as they could muster, preferring to be labeled sick rather than be considered sinful or criminal, as they had been for hundreds of years. Scientific speculation shuttled between theories of causality and remedies for cure, the beginnings of a preoccupation that continues to this day: What *causes* homosexuality? Nature? Nurture? Genes? Family relationships? The most influential early theory of causality came from Sigmund Freud, who believed that everyone passes through a homoerotic phase, but that for some reason homosexuals' development is "arrested" during this phase, leaving them stuck with a less than "normal" (i.e., heterosexual) sexual orientation. Still, Freud conceded in a famous letter to an American mother, concerned about her son, homosexuality "is nothing to be ashamed of, no vice, degradation, it cannot be classified as an illness."

Unfortunately, Freud's radical humanism was soon lost on the profession he pioneered—psychoanalysis, the psychiatric specialty devoted to theories of unconscious development—and the view of homosexuality as pathology dominated the psychoanalytic field. In fact, this view remained largely unchanged until recent years in the thinking and practice of U.S. psychoanalysts. Richard A. Isay, the first openly gay member of the American Psychoanalytic Association, notes that the orthodox psychoanalytic view was that, "homosexuality is abnormal because it is not heterosexuality."[54] This bit of circular logic was also the official position of American psychiatry. In 1952, the first panel ever to deal with homosexuality at a meeting of the American Psychoanalytic Association was titled "Perversion: Theoretical and Therapeutic Aspects." That same year, the American Psychiatric Association published the first edition of the *Diagnostic and Statistical Manual,* its guide to mental disorders, describing homosexuality as a "sociopathic personality disturbance."

Conveniently ignored by antigay psychiatrists was an expanding body of scientific literature that homosexuals would eventually use to challenge psychiatry on its own terms. Most prominent was the 1948 survey of male sexual behavior by sex researcher Alfred Kinsey and his colleagues. The study shocked the nation with its finding that some 37 percent of (white) men in the United States had engaged in sex with another male to the point of orgasm at some point in their lives. Kinsey noted that attempts to categorize sexual behavior as *either* heterosexual *or* homosexual were pointless because of the complexity of the human animal. Sexuality, he argued, was a continuum, with lifelong, exclusive hetero- and homosexuality at its poles and most people falling somewhere in between, capable of behaving sexually with either males or females under particular circumstances. Kinsey likewise rejected notions of "normal" and "abnormal" sexual behavior.[55]

Kinsey's points were underscored in 1951, when Cleland Ford and Frank Beach analyzed more than seventy cultures outside the United States. The researchers found that among cultures for which such information was available, forty-nine overtly sanctioned homosexual behavior as natural for some members of the community. And in 1957, psychologist Evelyn Hooker finally did justice to the notion of scientific objectivity, long missing from research on homosexuality. Earlier psychiatric studies of homosexuality had focused on psychiatric patients, prisoners, patients from mental hospitals, and the military. But Hooker used standard psychological tests to disprove the claims of so-called experts who said they could distinguish the results of nonpatient homosexual from heterosexual subjects. Summarizing her findings, Hooker wrote, "What is difficult to accept (for most clinicians) is that some homosexuals may be very ordinary individuals, indistinguishable from ordinary individuals who are heterosexual."[56]

Gay people slowly began to challenge psychiatry's "scientific" views of homosexuality—and psychiatrists reacted strongly. Edmund Bergler's 1956 book, *Homosexuality: Disease or Way of Life*, infuriated the loosely organized gay community. Bergler blamed Kinsey, whom he derided as a "medical layman," for stirring up homosexuals to the point that "they are now virtually asking for minority status." The psychiatric profession, and the American public who listened deferentially to what these men had to say, turned to people like Irving Bieber and Charles Socarides for a purportedly intelligent opinion on homosexuality.

In 1963, Bieber, a psychoanalyst known for his unsubstantiated claims of "curing" homosexuals, said that he "does not approve the attempt by organized homosexuals to promote the idea that they represent just another minority, since their minority status is based on illness." Socarides, another leading psychoanalyst outspoken in his view that homosexuality constituted "profound psychopathology," couched his hostility toward gay people in the guise of doctorly concern. He said, "The homosexual is ill, and anything that tends to hide that fact reduces his chances of seeking treatment. . . . If they were to achieve social acceptance, it would increase this difficulty."[57] Ironically, in view of his traditional psychoanalytic belief that a distant father is a "cause" of homosexuality, Socarides' own son, Richard, is a longtime gay activist—and President Clinton's liaison to the gay community.

The deference of gay men and lesbians to psychiatric authority began to dissipate in the sixties. The black civil rights movement, the women's movement, the antiwar movement, and finally the gay rights movement—all challenged America's preconceptions and shook up its categories of right, wrong, normal, and abnormal. The Mattachine Society of Washington, D.C., an early gay rights group led by Frank Kameny, decided in 1965 to let the psychiatrists know that there would no longer be a market in the homosexual community for their "pseudo-scientific" views. The group adopted a resolution asserting that, "in the absence of evidence to the contrary, homosexuality is not a sickness, disturbance, or other pathology in any sense, but is merely a preference, orientation, or propensity, on par with and not different in kind from heterosexuality."[58] Said Kameny, "We are the experts on ourselves."[59] Gay people were getting fed up with being labeled and dismissed as sick and second-class.

In 1970, the executive committee of the National Association for Mental Health declared that homosexual relations between consenting adults should be decriminalized. Within a year, the group's San Francisco affiliate adopted a resolution asserting that "Homosexuality can no longer be equated only with sickness, but may properly be considered a preference, orientation, or propensity for certain kinds of life styles." Braced by such affirmation, gay activists began to strike with vehement regularity at the American Psychiatric Association. Barbara Gittings, a veteran lesbian activist from Philadelphia, relishes memories of the zaps of the APA's conventions, beginning in 1970. "A year after Stonewall," said Gittings, "a lot of gay people were raring to go." Off they went to San Francisco, for the APA's annual meeting, where they disrupted a session on behavioral therapy. "We said, 'We want you to talk *with* us, not *about* us,'" recalls Gittings.[60] Disconcerted by such confrontational tactics, many psychiatrists fled the room.

Some, however, stayed to listen. As a result, Gittings and Kameny the following year staffed the first gay-positive booth ever to appear at an APA meeting. The exhibit, "Gay, Proud and Healthy: The Homosexual Community Speaks," included photos of happy lesbians and gay men—a novelty for most of the psychiatrists who stopped by the booth. "In the spirit of the times," as he put it, Kameny and others also zapped an exhibition on "aversion therapy," a meeting of Irving Bieber's, and the APA's prestigious Convocation of Fellows, where Kameny lambasted the assembled doctors as the incarnated enemy of gay people. The APA responded by inviting Kameny and Gittings to participate in the first APA panel ever to deal positively with homosexuality, during its 1972 annual meeting in Dallas.

Two decades later, John E. Fryer, M.D., is an openly gay professor of psychiatry at Temple University in Philadelphia. But in 1972, Fryer was so unnerved by Gittings's invitation to appear on the panel in Dallas that he agreed only on condition that he be disguised and his amplified voice distorted beyond recognition. "H. Anonymous, M.D.," bedecked in a rubber mask, wig, and oversized tuxedo, debuted to an audience of about five hundred psychiatrists, recalls Fryer, laughing now. At the time, however, he sadly lamented to his colleagues, "My greatest loss is my honest humanity. How incredible that we homosexual psychiatrists cannot be honest in a profession that calls itself compassionate and 'helping.'"[61] The *Advocate* noted that the Dallas meeting might well have marked a "turning point" in the relationship between psychiatry and the gay community.

After reviewing the scientific literature and working closely with gay rights advocates, including Bruce Voeller, from the newly formed National Gay Task Force, Robert Spitzer, a member of APA's nomenclature committee, prepared a background paper on homosexuality for the APA's board of trustees. In it he defined the simple standard by which psychiatrists to this day gauge mental illness: For a psychiatric condition to be considered a mental illness, it must either cause distress or impair an individual's social functioning. "Clearly," wrote Spitzer, "homosexuality, per se, does not meet the requirements for a psychiatric disorder since . . . many homosexuals are quite satisfied with their sexual orientation and demonstrate no generalized impairment in social effectiveness or functioning." For the record, he noted, "the terms 'normal' and 'abnormal' are not really psychiatric terms."[62]

The APA's board of trustees agreed with Spitzer's assessment, and voted unanimously in December 1973 to remove homosexuality from the *Diagnostic and Statistical Manual.* It acknowledged that "the unscientific inclusion of homosexuality per se in the list of mental disorders has been the ideological mainstay for denying civil rights" to homosexuals. As if to atone for the profession's many years of mistreating homosexuals, the board also called for the repeal of sodomy laws and for the passage of antidiscrimination measures to protect the rights of gay people.[63]

Not all psychiatrists welcomed the change in diagnosis, chief among them Bieber and Socarides. Hoping to overturn the APA board's decision, the two demanded a referendum for the entire membership. Bieber regurgitated the traditional pathology argument in a statement in *Psychiatric News,* the APA's official newspaper. "Homosexuality," he wrote, "is always a consequence of a disordered sexual development, usually the outcome of a singular kind of disturbed network of relationships within a family."[64] Fifty-eight percent of the ten thousand psychiatrists who voted in the referendum upheld the board's decision.

To placate traditionalists like Bieber and Socarides, the board created a new category of illness, "sexual orientation disturbance." In this obviously politically motivated classification, having a homosexual orientation was no longer a problem, but being unhappy to the point of wishing to be heterosexual was. Content to leave well enough alone, at least for the time being, even gay activists mostly ignored so-called "ego-dystonic homosexuality." As Kameny was wont to say at the time, "Anyone who is unhappy being gay *must* be crazy!" In 1986, the APA finally deleted even "ego-dystonic homosexuality" from the diagnostic manual, removing the last official medical impediment to homosexuality's being considered a normal and healthy variant of human sexuality. The fear and loathing of gay people—dubbed "homophobia" by George Weinburg in his 1972 book, *Society and the Healthy Homosexual*—was finally seen as the root cause of the psychic stress from which so many gay people suffered.

When he started writing for the gay press in the late seventies, New York physician Lawrence D. Mass says he was "fascinated with this business of what is homosexuality, how it's defined, where we stand scientifically."[65] Mass was particularly interested in psychiatry. In fact, after already practicing medicine, Mass at one point wanted to retrain as a psychiatrist but was rejected from several psychiatric residency programs because he was honest about his sexual orientation when asked. His own therapist while in medical school had been none other than Richard Pillard, the first psychiatrist in America to reveal himself publicly as a gay man. Mass saw himself as a kind of "watchdog of psychiatry," keeping up with developments in the field and duly reporting them in the gay press. Given his awareness of the tepid acceptance by many psychiatrists of the APA's decision to declassify homosexuality, Mass continually worried that psychiatry would find a way to return it to the list of mental illnesses.

In particular, Mass feared that the promiscuity and STDs so rampant among urban gay men in the seventies could be just the thing the APA needed to declare that homosexuals really are pathological after all. When AIDS appeared, Mass, by then an established medical writer in the gay press, had sharpened his critique of the medical establishment's history as the enforcer of society's wish to "control" homosexuality. Mass's well-informed views of both medicine and gay culture and politics, and a skepticism toward the medical establishment based on his own experience with psychiatry, would prove invaluable in the early years of the epidemic as thousands of gay people throughout the country depended upon his medical articles for the earliest news about the AIDS epidemic.

Like all medical doctors, psychiatrists had enjoyed a level of power and authority in American society accorded them because, at least to nonscientists, they seemed to hold the keys to the mysteries of human life. They were frequently likened to priests, and certainly their views were considered sacrosanct to the many who depended upon authorities to define for them what is right and wrong. It took enormous audacity and bravery for gay men and lesbians to stand up for themselves against the psychiatric profession. Howard Brown, M.D., formerly director of public health for New York City before he came out publicly as a gay man in 1973, noted in *Familiar Faces, Hidden Lives*, "The gay activists who converged on Washington on December 15, 1973, were the first group of patients in history to insist that they were not sick and to demand that the label be removed." When the APA agreed and voted to depathologize homosexuality, wrote Brown, "never in history had so many people been cured in so little time."[66]

The willingness of gay people to stand up for themselves against the medical establishment in the 1970s would reverberate into the eighties and beyond, as they once again stood up to demand attention for a deadly new disease that made people squirm in discomfort because of its connections to sex and drug use. But discomfort was nothing compared to the devastation of AIDS, and it would be homosexuals once again who pushed the medical establishment and American society itself to overcome their prejudices, this time to save lives.

*

Despite the shift in the American Psychiatric Association's position on homosexuality, "modern medicine," as it was often called with a note of awe, seemed unassailable in the seventies. The medical establishment was at the apex of a self-confidence tilting toward cockiness when it came to infectious diseases that had long plagued humanity. In the 1950s and 1960s, a number of deadly diseases were successfully treated and controlled, including polio, influenza, and tuberculosis. By the end of the seventies, modern medicine could claim an astounding success in the complete eradication from the world of smallpox, an ancient scourge that had killed and disfigured millions. It was a time of great optimism that medicine would eventually solve every biological affliction of humankind. As Pulitzer Prize-winning health reporter Laurie Garrett puts it, "Few scientists or physicians of the day doubted that humanity would continue on its linear course of triumphs over the microbes."[67]

Nearly drowned in the din of self-congratulation were the importunate voices of medical experts warning that it was far too soon for a victory celebration. In 1981, Richard Krause, director of the National Institute of Allergy and Infectious Diseases, published a book called *The Restless Tide: The Persistent Challenge of the Microbial World.* Krause warned that diseases believed to have been defeated could return to endanger the American people. The following year, Krause was asked in a congressional hearing why the country suffered from so many infectious diseases. He answered, "Nothing new has happened. Plagues are as certain as death and taxes."[68] Of course the appearance of a deadly new viral disease—sexually transmitted, no less—would shake up the medical establishment beginning in the very year Krause's book was published. As Mirko D. Grmek, former president of the International Academy of the History of Sciences, puts it, "The AIDS epidemic caught us unaware and aroused the return of irrational fears because it exposed the impotence of modern medicine just when we had begun to believe that the infectious diseases had been vanquished for good."[69]

Centuries before a minute retrovirus finally revealed the mortal limitations of the "all-powerful" Oz—like the wizard, "modern medicine" was seen as magical and all-powerful because of the wonderful things it did—the puritanism of some of the nation's earliest colonists was passed down through history to shape the peculiarly American attitude of shame and embarrassment about sex and sexually transmitted disease. With a light touch, H. L. Mencken defined "puritanism" as "the fear that someone somewhere is having a good time." Far more often the deep-seated distrust of pleasure and bodily life underlying America's collective sexual shame—even as its popular culture uses sexy bodies and the promise of "peak performance" to sell everything from toothpaste to automobiles—plays out in the darkness of denial. With such a schizoid attitude toward sex, can anyone be surprised that the U.S. has more sexual diseases and teenage pregnancies than any other country in the developed world?[70]

We insist on seeing STDs as one of the worst possible things that can happen to someone, or that an individual could give to another. STDs are regarded as a well-deserved "punishment" for daring to flout the norms to which most Americans adhere, even if their adherence is stronger in word than in deed. For men reveling in the sexual "freedom" of the urban gay ghettos, flouting social norms merely by being alive, the norm which condemned STDs as one of the worst things imaginable was brushed aside along with the "middle-class values" that were so often derided as antiquated. As Frank Browning puts it in *The Culture of Desire*, "Born into a society whose medical establishment told them that because they were homosexual they were diseased, then let loose into the orgy of the bathhouse era, when gonorrhea was a minor inconvenience dispatched with a shot of penicillin, gay men who came of age in the days before

AIDS have had good reason to see themselves as outsiders to the medical codes that most people live by."[71]

But gonorrhea was the least of the STDs that gay men were passing around amongst themselves in the seventies. By 1980, studies were showing that 93 percent of sexually active urban gay men were infected with cytomegalovirus, a herpes virus that had been linked to cancer. Epstein-Barr virus, a microbe best known for its connection to mononucleosis (the "kissing disease") but also linked to cancers, had become pandemic among gay men.[72] Because of the increased popularity of anal sex in the seventies, hepatitis B evolved from being a blood-borne pathogen into a sexually transmitted disease.[73] Amebiasis, the most serious STD among gay men after hepatitis B and before AIDS, was casually referred to as "gay bowel syndrome."

Like hepatitis B, amebiasis had not been a sexually transmitted disease prior to its getting into the "mix" of pathogens being transmitted regularly by and among gay men; it mainly afflicted poor people living in abject squalor in third world countries. Now it was challenging even modern medicine. Dr. Donna Mildvan, an authority on the disease, told Larry Mass in an interview, "The reason [amebiasis] has been so difficult to treat is that, often, it is not the only organism causing symptoms in gay males who have amebiasis. These patients may also have giardia, shigella, or other enteric pathogens."[74]

Gay historian Dennis Altman notes that in the "liberated" seventies, when promiscuity was seen as a virtue in some segments of the gay community, "being responsible about one's health was equated with having frequent checks for syphilis and gonorrhea, and such doubtful practices as taking a couple of tetracycline capsules before going to the baths."[75] To gay men for whom sex was the center and circumference of their lives, their only real health concern was that illness would prevent them from having sex—which, to their way of thinking, meant they would no longer be "proudly" gay. Michael Callen recalled a lecture he attended on the eve of the AIDS epidemic in which Edmund White, who coauthored *The Joy of Gay Sex*, said that "gay men should wear their sexually transmitted diseases like red badges of courage in a war against a sex-negative society." Said Callen, "I remember nodding my head in vigorous agreement and saying to myself, 'Gee! Every time I get the clap I'm striking a blow for the sexual revolution!' "[76]

For Larry Mass, supporting the sexual revolution came naturally, though it required that he reconcile some unpleasant realities. While he believed that sexual and gender issues—including homosexuality, women's rights, sex education, sexual freedom, birth control access, improvement of research and treatment of STDs—were "part of an interrelated package," he also tried to understand the STD epidemics of the seventies in a larger context. "This meant pointing out that while gay people were having high rates of STDs, heterosexuals also were having epidemics of herpes and gonorrhea," he said.[77]

True as it was, the fact is that gay men accounted for vast majorities of the patients at many urban STD clinics. Pat Norman recalls that in San Francisco 85 percent of the people going to STD clinics in the seventies were gay men.[78] And the number and types of STDs gay men regularly contracted surprised even medical professionals. When David Ostrow recruited Northwestern medical student Gary Remafedi in 1977 to help him provide STD screening in Chicago's bathhouses, the future pediatrician had no idea what awaited him. Ostrow took Remafedi, now an assistant professor of pediatrics and nationally recognized expert on gay adolescents at the University of Minnesota in Minneapolis, to Man's Country, a Chicago bathhouse, and taught him how to draw blood. "I was astounded by what I was seeing," says Remafedi. "It looked like everyone had warts or herpes. It was dreadful."[79]

In 1978, *The Gay Health Guide* warned that "the mere fact that you are homosexually active exposes you to greater risk of VD than the person whose activity is exclusively heterosexual because your partner, if not also you yourself, is likely to have had more opportunities to contract a venereal disease." Written by New York urologist Robert L. Rowan and psychologist Paul Gillette, the guide delineated the sexual risks for gay men—and indeed they were manifold. The authors noted, "They range from the merely inconvenient, such as infestation by parasitic insects, to the severely limiting, such as fecal incontinence resulting from irreversible stretching of the anal sphincter muscle. They include, chiefly among males, rupture of the walls of the rectum and possibly fatal infection of the abdominal cavity."[80]

The guide certainly didn't paint a picture of a sexually healthy community, to put it mildly. As Michael Callen described it, "Unwittingly, and with the best of revolutionary intentions, a small subset of gay men managed to create disease settings equivalent to those of poor third world nations in one of the richest nations on earth."[81] In the late seventies, Selma Dritz, an infectious disease specialist for the San Francisco Department of Public Health, used to warn that "too much is being transmitted here."[82] Urban gay American men were infected with diseases that were previously considered problems only in poor, undeveloped areas of the world. After repeated bouts of these diseases, treatment with increasingly powerful antibiotics, and use of the recreational drugs that for many were just another "normal" part of ghetto life, the immune systems of many gay men were suppressed to dangerously low levels. As Ian Young puts it, "Years before AIDS, the health crisis of gay men could be seen daily in the lengthening lines at the VD clinics, the same men returning again and again."[83]

Where were gay doctors at the time? Why didn't they take a leadership role in telling gay men to mind their health, possibly even to use condoms to protect themselves against the range of microbes waiting to invade another warm body during sex? Dennis Altman says that most gay doctors were reluctant to warn their gay male patients about the negative consequences of repeated STDs lest they be dismissed as just another mouthpiece of the oppressive medical establishment.[84] Michael Callen recalled another reason for the doctors' silence. "Many of these physicians," he said, "could themselves be observed in the bathhouses and backrooms leading the same fast-lane lifestyle as their patients. Even if they had warned us, who would have listened?"[85]

In some cities, gay physicians moonlighting as "clap doctors," as they were known in the community, were the first to provide "gay-sensitive" STD screening and treatment for gay men, often through an arrangement with a local bathhouse. In 1972, David Ostrow was approached by Horizons, a community social services organization in Chicago, where Ostrow was then a medical student, to offer testing and treatment one night a week. At the time, Ostrow recalls, "there weren't any gay doctors or others willing to hang out a shingle saying that they specialized in gay medicine. I know many gay doctors who were afraid that if they got known for seeing gay patients they were going to lose their straight patients." Ostrow described how gay men typically were razzed by health authorities. "The biggest problem at the time with the Department of Health VD clinics," he said, "was that if you went in for anything other than penile discharge, and you asked for an oral or anal swab, they would go berserk—ask for names and numbers of every one of your sexual partners for the last ten years."

So Ostrow helped to start the Howard Brown Memorial Clinic (Howard Brown, the former New York City public health chief, died of heart disease in 1975), which—like the Fenway Community Health Center in Boston, the Seattle Gay Clinic, and the Whitman-Walker Clinic in Washington, D.C.—started out as an alternative to public VD clinics, offering gay men something that, for many of them, was as important in their health care as in their sex lives: anonymity. In a move that would echo into the era of HIV antibody testing, Ostrow noted that it was in the early gay clinics that confidential STD testing was born. "We invented the system of using confidential codes of their initials or their mother's maiden name and their birth date," he said. Something else the gay clinics had in common was their shoestring budgets. In Chicago, Ostrow recalls, "We met once a week above a grocery store across from the Biograph Theatre. Horizons had the coffee shop on one end of the room, and we had this set of curtains. I used to bring my kitchen table in and that's what we would examine people on. And the medicines were whatever we could rip off of the clinics we worked or studied in."[86]

Individually, the clinics were sometimes hard-pressed to keep pace with the demand for their services. But when they joined other gay clinics across the country, the fledgling organizations discovered the advantages of networking and sharing information. In the mid-seventies, community-based gay STD clinics such as Howard Brown banded together with others throughout the country to form the National Coalition of Gay STD Services. Howard Brown was at the center of a nationwide network of agencies and individuals working with gay men in the area of STDs. Ken Mayer, who worked with Ostrow at Howard Brown, while he also was a medical student in Chicago in the seventies, now conducts infectious disease research at the Fenway Community Health Center in Boston. He recalled

the national STD coalition as "a bare-bones kind of organization—
a mimeographed newsletter a couple times a year to let people know
what others were doing."[87]

Within a few years, largely as a result of this networking and
keeping up with what others were doing around the country, a substantial national gay and lesbian health movement would emerge,
providing an important cornerstone of the gay community's response
to the AIDS epidemic. The gay clinics, together with gay men and
lesbians in the health professions, would serve as invaluable sources
of information, treatment, and community organizing. Said Mayer,
"Particularly for gay men, it was fortunate for an emergency like
AIDS that [the gay and lesbian health movement] was built around
STDs."[88]

It was also fortunate for gay men that lesbians, steeped in the
feminist politics of the late sixties and early seventies, understood
the connection between personal health, the power dynamics of
health care, and one's position in society. Lesbians also seemed to
understand that gay liberation and gay rights were about vastly more
than the "right" to be promiscuous. Many of these women had
learned their own lessons about illness and health care by dealing
not only with homophobic health care providers, but often with the
public health system that was created in this country to provide basic
services to those with lower incomes, a category that, unfortunately,
includes many lesbians. Their political critique of the health care
system arose from firsthand experience as both gay people and as
women dealing with a system dominated by heterosexual men.

Of course there were gay men working in the health care professions, and it was through their joint efforts with lesbian colleagues
that the gay and lesbian health movement was able both to tap the
existing network of community-based gay clinics and to create a momentum within the health care professions to consider the health of
gay men and lesbians an issue worthy of serious attention. Gay and
lesbian health care professionals from a number of national organizations met in Philadelphia on May 30, 1976, where they formed the
National Gay Health Coalition. According to Walter Lear, a key
organizer of gay and lesbian members of the American Public Health
Association (APHA), the coalition was created to provide gay health
professionals with a means for sharing data and experience, and to

facilitate relationships between the groups they formed within their national organizations and the community-level gay health services, community centers, political organizations, and periodicals.[89]

From the day he walked down Thirteenth Street as a college student in Lawrence, Kansas, and saw a poster in a side window of a house that said, "Gay is Good—Stonewall," Lawrence "Bopper" Deyton said he knew "there was something out there that would allow me to integrate my sexuality with something that was positive." With a father and brother who were physicians, and a sister who was a nurse, Deyton seemed destined for a health career. But he also knew he wanted somehow to integrate his interest in the health field with his emerging gay political awareness. Finally it came together while he was in graduate school in Boston, earning a master's degree in public health. "I met a boy in a bar and went home and had a wonderful time," Deyton recalls. "He was a physical therapist and we talked about these issues. He said, 'There's this new group that's forming in the APHA. I just got this flyer, and there's this guy named Walter Lear and here's his phone number.' I called Walter the next day, and that's how I got involved."

For Deyton, Lear, and many other gay people in the health fields, the APHA's willingness to embrace its gay members allowed the association's gay and lesbian group to create what served as a model for gay people in other health organizations. Deyton explained that once a caucus of gay people came together within an organization—including social workers, nurses, physicians, medical students, psychologists, psychiatrists, and substance-abuse workers—they emulated the APHA model, first organizing themselves, then insisting upon integration with the larger organization. When AIDS appeared, he said, "there was a foundation—of relationships, of respect, of working together, of the gay and lesbian professionals in their organizations."[90] Today Deyton is a medical doctor and formerly a high-ranking official at the National Institute of Allergy and Infectious Disease, the foremost of the National Institutes of Health conducting biomedical research on HIV.

In May 1978, two hundred men and women crowded into the basement of All Souls' Unitarian Church, in Washington, D.C., for the first National Gay Health Conference, sponsored by the two-year-old National Gay Health Coalition. Dr. Paul Wiesner, from the federal Centers for Disease Control, delivered a keynote address about the "positive aspects and potentialities of the gay health movement." The late Howard Brown's sister, Jule Sibley, addressed the group before Walter Lear presented the first Jane Addams–Howard Brown Award for outstanding contributions to the health and welfare of the gay community—to none other than Evelyn Hooker, the psychologist who in the fifties revolutionized psychological research on homosexuals. The conference program notably reflected the fact that, six years after the American Psychiatric Association's decision to declassify homosexuality, gay people working in the mental health fields had begun to address the societal homophobia now blamed for the high levels of psychic stress among many homosexuals.

The networks of gay health care professionals would prove to be vitally important in the gay community's ability to mobilize services for people with AIDS and to mount a political response in Washington. But they were only part of the foundation laid in the seventies that would be built upon in the eighties as gay people were forced to address the AIDS epidemic. Equally important ties were established in the seventies between gay physicians, pharmaceutical companies, and government scientists when they collaborated in testing and, in 1978, licensing a vaccine to prevent hepatitis B.

David Ostrow's medical specialty in gay health was strengthened when Ortho Pharmaceuticals approached Howard Brown about participating in a test of hepatitis B immune globulin. "They'd heard we had a clinic in Chicago seeing a lot of men with hepatitis," he recalls, "and they figured that gay men recovering from acute hepatitis would be ideal sources for the antibodies" they needed for their vaccine. Ortho thus became the first drug company willing to work with a gay clinic in the U.S. The gay men seen at the clinic certainly were well-suited for the research: Ostrow said that not only did 10 percent of his patients have chronic hepatitis B, but upwards of 60 percent of them had the disease at one time or another.[91]

In San Francisco, gay men were recruited at the bathhouses for the hepatitis B studies. Some sixty-eight hundred blood samples were taken in the city in 1978, and stored for possible use in the future. Of course no one knew at the time that a few years later, hepatitis B would seem like the common cold in comparison to the lethal STD about to appear. By the time it did so, scientists like Donald

Francis, with the Centers for Disease Control, would already have had years of experience working with gay men around hepatitis B and other STDs. As Francis told me, "We were already studying diseases of gay men, which made a huge difference in terms of the federal government's having at least some communication and inroad to the gay community. We had long-term close relationships following literally tens of thousands of gay men."[92]

The hepatitis B studies also would prove to have enormous importance in tracking the early spread of HIV. When an HIV antibody test finally became available several years into the AIDS epidemic, Don Francis went back to the San Francisco blood samples he'd taken for the hepatitis B trials in 1978 and 1980. Of the one hundred ten samples from 1978 that he tested, only one was positive. But 25 percent of the fifty samples from 1980 that he tested were infected with HIV. It seemed apparent that HIV had appeared among gay men in the city in the late seventies and spread rapidly.

Through the hepatitis B studies, gay physicians developed rapport and credibility with the government researchers—and vice versa. As Ken Mayer explained, "It was the first partnering of the government and gay community, and it created a cadre of health professionals who were considered responsible leaders in the gay community around health issues, and a certain amount of trust and bridge building."[93] The working relationships between gay doctors and government scientists would prove mutually beneficial in the coming years, providing researchers with at least a basic understanding of gay sexuality and access to community leaders, and would offer the gay community a link to emerging scientific information about AIDS. These relationships would contribute significantly to bringing gay people into the "mainstream" of medical research. Clearly there had been some progress since the medical establishment viewed gay people as abnormal and mentally ill merely for being homosexual. Too bad it would have to take a deadly epidemic to bring them together.

As the silent killer made its insidious way among unsuspecting gay men, the doctors and scientists focused their attention on the health crisis that was already building in the urban gay ghettos by the late seventies. At a 1979 meeting in Chicago to celebrate the success of the hepatitis B vaccine, David Ostrow recalls Dr. James

Curran, then head of the CDC's VD division and soon to become director of its AIDS program, telling the group, "If you people who represent the gay clinics in America think the vaccine is the answer to your problems, you're making a big mistake. If hepatitis B can go from *not* being an STD to *being* an STD because of behavior in the gay community, what *else* can do the same thing?" Then he warned the gay doctors of the possible social consequences. "If you as the gay community's health leaders don't clean up its act, sooner or later the health care problems will get such that they're such a threat to the larger society that they will force behavior change on the gay community."[94]

Before that happened, a rash of bizarre illnesses and brutal deaths among young homosexuals in the nation's large coastal cities would perplex physicians and frighten gay men into making changes of their own. In a few short years, the seventies would be rued as a decade of abundant opportunities for sex—and bungled opportunities for making changes that would have saved lives. They were a decade when liberation wavered in an uneasy balance with oppression, as gay people struggled to define themselves on their own terms. Gay thinkers like Larry Kramer, gay doctors like David Ostrow, and government scientists like Jim Curran—people with sufficient perspective to see causal relationships where others saw only individual STD cases and isolated events—warned of dire consequences, if gay people didn't finally liberate themselves from an oppression they had turned in upon themselves.

Like most prophets whose warnings disturb and alarm, the good counsel these people offered was mostly ignored. But the cost of ignoring a prophet has historically been high. Not even our latter-day prophets could have predicted just how high the cost would be this time.

A POX ON OUR HOUSE

Love casts out fear, but conversely fear casts out love.

ALDOUS HUXLEY, *APE AND ESSENCE*

When young men in the gay ghettos suddenly began to die of rare and bizarre diseases, theories about the cause abounded. Scientists tried to figure out why gay men seemed to be singled out by the apparently new and extremely deadly scourge. Gay men looked everywhere for an explanation—except at their own behavior. They were desperate. The first people to die of AIDS were no different than themselves. Would they meet a similar fate? Straight people also recognized that gay men were just like them—except for that part about loving other men. This not only challenged their stereotypes and bigotry but meant that they could "catch it" too.

As if fear alone wasn't challenging enough, those in the suddenly energized so-called Christian right—emboldened by their access to the highest levels of government—jumped on AIDS as if it was manna from heaven. They thrived on the fear and hatred of gay people that, for them, seemed a justifiable exception to Jesus' commands to love others and to care for the sick. Even mainstream Americans took part. News that the agent causing AIDS was transmitted in blood products provoked a level of irrationality and scapegoating in the general public that was indistinguishable from the rantings of the religious rightists.

Many gay men dug in their heels against the hysteria—and warnings within the gay community itself—refusing to yield one inch of what they viewed as their "freedom." Community leaders were verbally flayed for daring to suggest that perhaps gay liberation and sexual license had been conflated once too often. Newly formed AIDS organizations hesitated to tell gay men "how" to have sex in ways that might save their lives lest they, too, be dismissed as homophobic and puritanical. Many in the fast lane wouldn't or even couldn't slow down, addicted as they were to sex, drugs, and the rush of finally being accepted by others. Unlike Andrew Holleran's "prisoner of love" Mallone, though, the "sentence" for too many of these men was vastly more permanent than a broken heart.

In 1979, Donald Abrams was doing his medical residency in San Francisco, when gay men began coming into the clinic where he worked, complaining of swollen glands. A hematologist friend at the clinic suggested that Abrams biopsy the lymph nodes to see what was going on. They were "reactive," meaning that the men's immune systems were overcharged as though fighting off some kind of infection. Abrams recalls, "We advised people to slow down. This was at the end of the seventies in San Francisco, and gay men had many partners, did drugs, and had a lot of STDs. We told patients to shift out of the fast lane for a while to see if their lymph nodes went down." Looking back over the years and the more than half a million American AIDS cases that had been reported up to the time of our interview, Abrams added, "Retrospectively, that was one of our earliest indications that something was amiss."[1]

Everyone was puzzled by the deaths of the formerly healthy young gay men who were showing up with the unusually swollen lymph nodes, malaise, weight loss, fevers, thrush, rare tumors, and bizarre infections that would come to be associated with AIDS. The initial cases were thought to be isolated to New York and California, with no apparent link to one another. They were regarded as medical quirks signifying nothing. Some of the men had the purple lesions of Kaposi's sarcoma, a rare skin cancer that mainly afflicted older men of Jewish, Italian, or Ugandan extraction. The federal Centers for Disease Control (CDC), in Atlanta, became aware of the unusual cases of *pneumocystis carinii* pneumonia that were afflicting other young men when the centers received multiple requests in the spring of 1981 for pentamidine, the standard drug to treat the disease that was ordinarily found among the elderly, transplant patients, or others with weakened immune systems.

The CDC's first report on the AIDS epidemic was published on page two of the June 5, 1981, issue of its *Morbidity and Mortality Weekly Report (MMWR)*. The report, titled "*Pneumocystis* pneumonia—Los Angeles," described the cases in five gay men being treated by Drs. Michael Gottlieb and Joel Weisman, in Los Angeles. In the mainstream press, only the *Los Angeles Times* carried the Associated Press story on the *MMWR* report. But the gay press already was setting the pace for reporting on AIDS. Larry Mass was the first to note the AIDS epidemic. His reports in the *New York Native* were to become the gay community's first and best source of information in the epidemic's earliest years, as they were reprinted and circulated in gay newspapers throughout the country. In the May 18, 1981, issue of the *Native*—predating even the first CDC report—Mass wrote a news item about the "rumors that an exotic new disease had hit the gay community in New York."[2]

At first no one saw a relationship between the odd cases of KS and PCP, as the skin cancer and pneumonia respectively would become commonly known when they became all too familiar. But in a July 3, 1981, letter in the *MMWR*, Dr. Alvin Friedman-Kien, a professor of dermatology and microbiology at New York University Medical Center, drew the connection between the cases of KS and PCP in New York City and California. His report, "Kaposi's Sarcoma and *Pneumocystis* Pneumonia Among Homosexual Men in New York City and California," also announced the appearance of another ten cases of PCP among gay men, including six in the San Francisco Bay area.

Don Abrams heard a news report about the strange outbreak among gay men on the car radio as he drove to the airport for a flight to Seattle, where he was about to start a year-long fellowship in oncology. His experience with cancer would serve him well in the years ahead. Friedman-Kien's report in the *MMWR* also attracted the attention of Dr. Lawrence K. Altman, a former CDC staffer who was now a medical writer for the *New York Times*. Buried on page A20, Altman's fairly brief July 3 news article represented the first mention among "all the news that's fit to print" of a disease that, within two years, would be called the most serious health threat of the century.

The article, "Rare Cancer Seen in 41 Homosexuals," was a tragic postscript to the gay pride celebrations of the previous week. In one of the crueler ironies in the AIDS epidemic, the date of the article's publication was precisely twelve years to the day after the first mainstream news report about the importance of the Stonewall rebellion to the budding gay liberation movement.[3] For many gay men, this July 3, 1981, date would forever mark the line between innocence and experience—the exuberant innocence of gay life before AIDS, and the doleful experience of so many gay deaths because of AIDS.

Once the link was made between the PCP and KS cases that had appeared on both coasts, bigger questions presented themselves: What was causing these diseases? Why were gay men being singled out among the population? And, above all else, why now?

No one knew the answers, although everyone had their own theories. In an interview with Friedman-Kien for the *Native,* Larry Mass asked the question that would baffle scientists for some time to come: "Why should immunosuppression be such a prominent feature in these cases?" The cases of KS and PCP were being referred to variously as Gay Related Immune Deficiency (GRID), Kaposi's Sarcoma and Opportunistic Infections (KSOI), and Acquired Immunodeficiency (AID). Friedman-Kien suggested a few possible reasons, including multiple sexual partners, a history of numerous sexually transmitted diseases, and "poppers." One of the strongest candidates seemed to be cytomegalovirus, a member of the herpes virus family known to suppress immunity, which was far more prevalent in sexually active gay men than in heterosexuals.[4]

In "Cancer in the Gay Community," the first feature article ever written about AIDS, Mass described the consternation among medical observers of the early cases of KS and PCP among gay men. "Perhaps," he wrote, "certain homosexuals in certain urban areas have been breathing, eating, drinking, or wearing unusual things, behaving in unusual ways, or frequenting unusual locations." He went on to add, more presciently than he realized at the time, "The most immediately seductive environmental explanation of 'the gay cancer' is that it is being caused by an infectious or otherwise cancerous agent. Because of their community proximity and physical interaction, perhaps some homosexuals are transmitting a carcinogen, a virus, parasite, bacteria, or other microbe."[5]

There were other "candidate etiologies" as well. Certain sexual practices that injured the rectum, particularly "fisting"—even sperm itself—were implicated as possible causes. Because only homosexuals seemed to be affected, conspiracy theories abounded. Perhaps, went one theory, an agent of chemical warfare had been loosed upon "undesirables" in a diabolical government experiment. Among the more far-fetched notions was Dennis Altman's particular favorite: some sort of chemical agent "sprinkled like fairy dust on the floors of bathhouses where barefoot homosexuals would absorb it through their skin."[6] As Mass subsequently, and not entirely facetiously, noted, "On the superficial basis of numbers alone, of course, wearing handkerchiefed Levi's and having Judy Garland records in one's collection might also seem risky."[7]

Chief among the more serious theories was the view that some kind of overload, caused by too many drugs and too many STDs, had resulted in an immunological meltdown that left fast-lane homosexuals prey to the variety of bizarre infections associated with AIDS. Dr. Joseph Sonnabend, a physician with a large gay practice in Greenwich Village, became the leading proponent of this theory. Another respected theory to explain the apparent selectivity of the disease was that some individuals were unusually susceptible to whatever it was that caused it. STD expert Donna Mildvan, chief of the infectious diseases division at New York's Beth Israel Medical Center, said, "There could be a genetic predisposition or some other vulnerability among selected individuals."[8]

In an editorial that accompanied the first articles on AIDS ever published in an American medical journal, David T. Durack, writing in the *New England Journal of Medicine* on December 10, 1981, asked, "Why this group? Why now, and not before?" He noted that homosexuality was nothing new, and wondered, "Were the homosexual contemporaries of Plato, Michelangelo, and Oscar Wilde subject to the risk of dying from opportunistic infections?" Of course a few deaths caused by unusual microbes could have passed unnoticed among the billions of deaths predating modern microbiology. But what of recent times? *Pneumocystis* had been known for almost thirty years and was fairly easy to identify. "Present indications," concluded Durack, "are that we are seeing a truly new syndrome, not explainable by failure to diagnose earlier cases."[9]

Laurie Garrett notes that, "The emergence and spread of HIV

were ideal in the gay communities of the late nineteen-seventies in the U.S. and Europe, particularly because the population was highly mobile and extraordinarily sexually active." But something unusual must have happened that allowed a formerly obscure pathogen to suddenly find its way into America's gay communities. In fact, several things did happen. "Between 1970 and 1975," says Garrett, "the world offered HIV an awesome list of amplification opportunities." Among them were increased multiple partner sexual activity among gay men in North America and Europe and among urban heterosexuals in Africa; needles that were constantly reused in Africa because of shortages; soaring heroin, amphetamine, and cocaine use in the industrialized world; STD epidemics that lowered immunity and made the genitals and anus susceptible to HIV infection; and the burgeoning international blood market.[10]

The immune overload theory appealed to gay men who didn't run in the fast lane, take drugs, or have multiple partners, because they could comfort themselves with a belief that only selected homosexuals would get the disease. "It's only the 'clones,' " they'd say, reassuring themselves that they had nothing to worry about because they were "good" gays who only did one drug at a time, or were monogamous, or lived outside the early AIDS epicenters of New York, San Francisco, and Los Angeles. These men could hear the testimonials of early AIDS patients and not find any relevance to their own lives. But then, even some of those early patients were surprised to be diagnosed with AIDS because they didn't see themselves as fitting what already had become the stereotype of a "typical" person with AIDS.

In the first mainstream magazine article about AIDS anywhere, *New York* quoted the CDC's special Task Force on Kaposi's Sarcoma and Opportunistic Infections, headed by Jim Curran, in describing the "average AID victim." According to the task force, the individual—always a gay man, as those not fitting the "average" were simply not described—"is thirty-five years old, has a college degree, and makes between $20,000 and $25,000 a year. He is likely to be white, to have grown up outside New York City and migrated here somewhere between ten and fifteen years ago. He had been relatively healthy and always employed. He had led vigorous work and social lives—until about six months to a year before his diagnosis."[11]

Mark Wood, a gay man in San Francisco whose partner, Bobby Reynolds, was one of the city's earliest and best-known AIDS patients, was as surprised as anyone by his diagnosis. When asked what he had thought about his own risk for AIDS at the time of his lover's diagnosis the previous year, Wood said, "Almost nonexistent. I never, at that point, thought that it would be the remotest possibility." He didn't live a fast life and do lots of drugs and have multiple sex partners and kinky sex—the things he was led to believe would endanger him. "I didn't fit any of those criteria," said Wood. "I'd always been real healthy. I'd never had any lengthy illnesses other than the standard gay diseases of VD and some strep throat, but never anything that had debilitated my body for any period of time."[12]

Larry Kramer, who had kept a low profile since the uproar over *Faggots*, used his name recognition to call attention to the new disease. In a "personal appeal" that ran alongside Mass's "Cancer" article in the *Native*, Kramer wrote, "The men who have been stricken don't appear to have done anything that many New York gay men haven't done at one time or another. We're appalled that this is happening to them and terrified that it could happen to us. It's easy to become frightened that one of the many things we've done or taken over the past years may be all that it takes for a cancer to grow from a tiny something or other, that got in there who knows when from doing who knows what."[13]

At an April 8, 1982, dance benefit at the West Village's Paradise Garage for Gay Men's Health Crisis—the group that Kramer, Mass, and their friends formed to conduct research on AIDS, provide services to those with the disease, and educate others about it—GMHC's board president, Paul Popham, told the two thousand men and a few women who each had paid twenty dollars to attend the dance, "We are in the grip of a medical emergency. Something we have done to our bodies—and we still don't know what it is— has brought us closer to death. The finest minds in medicine are on our side, but the problem is still ours. The threat to our confidence is enormous. . . . We've got to show the outside world that we've got more than looks, brains, talent, and money. We've got guts too, and lots of heart."

New York magazine reported, "At the Paradise benefit, a saucy three-woman disco ensemble called the Ritchie Family closed its set with some motherly advice, counseling the men to stay out of the bathhouses, out of the back rooms, 'and, this is the cardinal rule, fellas: one lover per person.' The audience formed its own impromptu chorus, chanting back, 'NO WAY!' Everyone enjoyed a healthy laugh. It was, however, a laugh informed with fear."[14]

The fear would become palpable as the protective, often self-righteous, bubbles in which many gay men lived were burst within a year after the first reports of AIDS. By June 1982, CDC researchers had uncovered evidence to link GRID cases through a network of sexual relationships among forty gay men in ten different cities, including New York, Atlanta, Houston, Miami, San Francisco, and Los Angeles. The so-called Los Angeles Cluster Study offered powerful evidence that AIDS not only was transmissible—probably sexually—but that it was also likely to be the result of a single infectious agent. The study also offered clues about the seemingly long, asymptomatic latency period of the new disease.[15] The Fire Island summer house of Paul Popham was the site of one of the first "clusters" of cases.

What gay New Yorkers had taken to calling the "Saint's disease," because it seemed to afflict the men who frequented the popular disco called The Saint, suddenly became a disease of saints, sinners, and every other kind of homosexual—as well as growing numbers of heterosexuals. If, as was now suspected, AIDS was the result of sexual contact, any man who had ever had sex with another man was potentially at risk.

As of July 15, 1982, the CDC had received reports of 471 cases, and two new cases were being reported each day. The disease's various names—which included a fourth, Acquired Community Immune Deficiency (ACID), CDC's own name for it—were compressed into one dreaded and dreadful name by which the disease and the epidemic it spawned would be known, Acquired Immune Deficiency Syndrome, or "AIDS."[16]

With the evidence linking AIDS to sexual contact, the many questions that had confounded everyone from the beginning now were distilled to a mere two. The answers to these two questions—and it is important to bear in mind that no one knew the answers—literally meant the difference between life and death: How can I avoid getting it? And the other, shattering in its implications, what if I already have it?

Hundreds of gay physicians met in San Francisco for the second annual Gay Pride Week symposium, called "Medical Aspects of Sexual Orientation," at the end of June 1982. The meeting was sponsored by Bay Area Physicians for Human Rights (BAPHR), the oldest and largest organization of gay physicians in the country, with 350 members at the time. The newly formed American Association of Physicians for Human Rights (AAPHR, today known as the Gay and Lesbian Medical Association) held its first major membership drive during the symposium. Issues related to STDs and AIDS accounted for less than a quarter of the program.

Foremost among the physicians' STD-related concerns was the prediction of "a disastrous new gay cancer in the nineteen-eighties and nineties as a result of the increased incidence of hepatitis B in the nineteen-sixties and seventies." Those who become chronic carriers of the hepatitis B virus—upwards of 10 percent of infected individuals—have a high risk of developing liver cancer or cirrhosis. Dr. Patrick McGraw, cofounder and president of the Resource Foundation, a community organization committed to ending the epidemic of hepatitis B, said, "Unless we can use the immunization techniques that are now available to curtail the epidemic of [hepatitis B] virus, [gay men] will probably always have an unfortunate prevalence of this highly fatal carcinoma."

Reporting on the symposium for the *Native,* Larry Mass noted, "Both BAPHR and AAPHR are anticipating the forthcoming hepatitis B vaccine crisis. At $150 a shot, many of the young, sexually active gay men who would most benefit themselves and others from immunization, will not be able to pay for it." As though he could see ahead to what would happen in the AIDS epidemic in the coming years, Mass added, "As has so often been the case for important gay health care services, the money will have to be raised by the gay community."

As the gay doctors marched in San Francisco's annual Gay and Lesbian Freedom Day Parade, they saw members of the roller-skating Sisters of Perpetual Indulgence—a group of campy gay men dressed as nuns—handing out a leaflet called "Play Fair!" The sisters, many of whom were themselves health care professionals in "real" life, used whimsical language in this first attempt to define "safe sex" for gay men. "Don't put other people at risk by engaging in sexual activity," warned the leaflet. "Wait until you KNOW you can cum clean." Echoing the advice of the Committee to Monitor Poppers, which was formed in 1981 by San Francisco gay activist Hank Wilson when the nitrites were first implicated as a possible cause of AIDS,[17] the sisters warned, "The Reverend Mother has determined that popper inhalation may be dangerous to your health."[18]

Gay leaders met in New York on July 12 with Jim Curran, who traveled from Atlanta to brief the group on the AID (it was not yet called AIDS) situation, particularly the recent discovery of cases among nongay hemophiliacs. According to National Gay Task Force executive director Lucia Valeska, "Curran emphasized his feeling that leading gay organizations and individuals must become directly involved in the government's public information efforts on AID as well as in the formation of public policy for combating it." Valeska noted that Curran's request that the gay community formulate an "appropriate" response had thrown the group of leaders into a quandary. How, they asked, can you determine what is an "appropriate" response to a disease for which neither the cause nor cure is known? And because the political context of the new disease was "extremely tricky and volatile," as Valeska put it, any recommendations the leaders might make were likely to be interpreted in some quarters as "serving some special interest."

As the task force prepared to host the first national forum on AIDS, to be held during the annual gay and lesbian health conference in Dallas that August, another meeting was called later that month by Assistant Secretary for Health Dr. Edward N. Brandt. The task force put the gay community's best foot forward, sending "scientifically credible" gay community representatives—Dr. Roger Enlow, a respected immunologist, and Bruce Voeller, who held a doctorate in biology and was a savvy politico. Valeska noted that this meeting marked the first formal relationship between the gay community and the federal government in the eighteen months of the new Reagan administration. Going into the meeting, community leaders were concerned about the political ramifications of the new disease so disproportionately affecting gay men. As Valeska put it, "What if the disease is infectious and traveling from the gay community outward? We have to make decisions in the dark, but how we respond may have grave implications for our political as well as medical welfare."[19]

Larry Mass, Roger Enlow, and Dan William were invited as openly gay physicians to give presentations at the first international workshop on AIDS, held at Mount Sinai Medical Center in New York, on July 13, 1982. After noting that only a virus "would seem able to provide a unitary hypothesis that could explain the sudden appearance of AID in a growing number of distinctive populations," Mass voiced what he believed was an obvious and sensible cornerstone for any kind of prevention strategy that might be devised to prevent AIDS. He reasoned that instead of forcing gay people into a Catch-22 by condemning them as incapable of forming stable relationships, and then condemning them for having gay relationships—making them "sexual outlaws," as John Rechy put it—society should provide homosexuals with the legal, theological, and social opportunities to establish committed love relationships. Hoping others would see the reasonableness of his view, Mass concluded his remarks at the workshop by saying, "The passage of civil rights legislation for gay people will begin to be seen as a critical cofactor in the preventive medicine of sexually transmitted diseases, which probably include AID."[20]

Seeking to quell the rising fears of gay men, and to quash the homophobic backlash that gay leaders expected would be stirred up by the growing epidemic, Mass's copresenter Dan William told Mass in a *Native* interview, "What needs to be emphasized is that homosexuality per se is not a risk factor." William, a gay New York City internist specializing in STDs among gay men, foreshadowed two volatile issues that would take on lives of their own in the coming years: bathhouses and blood donations.

Noting that a significant portion of gay men with AIDS had visited bathhouses prior to developing the disease, William observed, "Restaurants are now required to post signs describing the Heimlich Maneuver, a simple, easily learned technique for saving the life of someone who is choking on food. Perhaps baths should post signs that warn their customers of health risks and advise them about precautionary measures." As for blood donations, William said, "I think I would advise promiscuous gay men with a prior history of multiple sexually transmitted diseases not to give blood until more information is available."[21]

Lesbian activist Ginny Apuzzo, then the director of the Fund for Human Dignity, an affiliate of NGTF, had warned at the July 13 workshop that, like other minorities that had been scapegoated, gay men risked being further stigmatized for having "bad blood" if they were singled out for exclusion from blood donations. But gay men were already stigmatized because of the perception—this was three years before an antibody test afforded the ability to know who did or did not have the mysterious pathogen lurking in their bloodstream—that every one of them was tainted by whatever "it" was causing AIDS. Despite the appearance of the disease in nongay people (besides homosexuals, the other three of the so-called "Four H" group believed to carry special risk were hemophiliacs, Haitians, and heroin injectors), the view that AIDS was a "gay disease" meant these others were discounted at first as simply unfortunate anomalies. Astonishingly, even scientists thought they were dealing with a disease that somehow had a sexual orientation, extrapolating to a microbe the prejudiced belief of many heterosexuals that more than just sexual orientation distinguishes homosexuals from "normal" human beings, which is to say heterosexuals.

Researchers continued to look for something unique about gay men in their efforts to deduce the cause of AIDS. To be fair, we should note that one of the main reasons they focused on gay men, rather than the others with AIDS, is that gay men demanded attention from medical care providers—and because a number of prominent gay leaders were themselves medical professionals. In an early 1982 article he originally wrote for the *Village Voice* titled "The Most Important New Public Health Problem in the United States," Larry Mass quoted Dr. Yehudi Felman, New York City's foremost expert on STDs, as saying that other groups—he mentioned women (who suffered more frequently than most from gonorrhea and nongonococal urethritis), blacks, and Hispanics (both groups that had disproportionately high rates of some STDs)—hadn't been as active as homosexuals in asking for better care because they didn't want the stigma attached to having STDs. Gay men were different, though.

Said Felman, "Gays, who are used to stigma, are willing to fight for their needs."[22]

In 1982, the fight had just begun.

*

America's blood industry will be tainted forever by the way it shirked responsibility in the early years of the AIDS epidemic. Thousands of people were put at risk of contracting AIDS—and thousands more actually did—because for several crucial years after the appearance of AIDS among hemophiliacs and transfusion recipients industry officials refused to acknowledge the probability that the nation's blood supply had been infected by the unknown pathogen believed to be causing AIDS, and refused to use tests available at the time that would have eliminated at least some of the infected blood. As early as July 1982, the CDC warned the blood industry of the problem and asked blood banks not to accept blood donations from gay men and injection drug users. It would be several years, and many transfusion-related infections later, before the industry finally listened.

In August 1982, the CDC recommended to the Public Health Service that all blood be tested for evidence of hepatitis B, using a test that measured for the virus itself, because there seemed to be a high correlation between symptoms of AIDS and the bloodborne hepatitis B commonly found among gay men and needle users. In December 1982, the first fully documented case of AIDS from a blood transfusion was reported, providing the strongest evidence to that point that the "it" causing AIDS was transmissible by blood as well as sex. Even so, the president of the New York Blood Center a month later denied the evidence that AIDS was transmissible in a blood transfusion.[23]

While the CDC and blood industry officials wrangled over guidelines for blood donations, gay leaders were vehement that any policy which excluded all gay men would risk not only stigmatizing the would-be donors but might also have such serious consequences as getting them fired from their jobs. Ironically, these community leaders made their argument against a blanket exclusion by invoking the very same denial of widespread risk among gay men with which so many of them had deluded themselves into thinking they were safe. Bruce Voeller, representing the National Gay Task Force at a meeting of CDC and blood industry officials on January 4, 1983, said, "So-called 'fast-lane' gays are causing the problem and they are just a minority of male homosexuals. You'll stigmatize, at the time of a major civil rights movement, a whole group, only a tiny fraction of whom qualify as the problem we are here to address."[24]

CDC researcher Don Francis was generally sympathetic to the gay community's efforts to win civil rights. This time, though, he strongly disagreed with the gay leaders. While he understood their point about the risk of stigmatizing a whole group of people for the "sins" of the few, his commitment to ensuring the public health superseded politics of any kind. "I agreed with them that a monogamous or abstinent gay man who's never had sex is a perfectly fine blood donor," Francis recalls. "But short of that I wasn't willing to accept a gay man as a blood donor if he didn't know all his sexual partners—because I knew what the sexual activity of gay men was."[25] As Francis saw it, "there is no civil right to donate blood."[26]

For gay people who too often felt their very humanity questioned, the "right" to donate blood had everything to do with the desire to be seen as human beings whose blood possessed the same lifegiving properties as that of nongay people. Gay men routinely participated in blood drives for the same humanitarian reasons as their heterosexual counterparts. Also like many heterosexuals, gay men often donated blood because of the same pressure to give that everyone else feels when, for example, there is an office blood drive. Ginny Apuzzo, who argued against excluding gay men, recalls, "My concern was that gay men who were fearful of losing their jobs or suffering from other things could feel pressure to donate blood during some kind of community blood drive. If you asked them to abstain, you could be asking them to identify themselves as gay and then people would conclude that they had AIDS." This unwitting "outing" of gay men might have real and dire consequences, Apuzzo and other gay leaders feared. As she said, "Look at what this country did to children with AIDS, not letting them go to school. What the hell would they do to a gay man in an office?"[27]

As usually happened in the early years of the epidemic, the first inclination of public health officials was to stop the spread of AIDS—no matter what. Gay leaders counterbalanced these otherwise laudable efforts to protect the public health by pointing out that the "what" in the AIDS epidemic might well be an insufferably high political price to be paid by an already despised minority. Pat Norman, who at the time was coordinator of gay and lesbian health in San Francisco's public health department, recalls, "The first reaction was 'let's identify them, let's mark them and make sure everybody knows them'—without taking into consideration the political ramifications of actions such as people losing families, jobs, or homes if some confidential information was put out."[28]

But gay people who saw the potential threat to their homes, livelihoods, and their very lives, were not about to accept passively the pronouncements of a medical establishment they felt had long since abandoned them to fend medically for themselves. Fortunately, as often happened in the crucial political moments in the epidemic, individuals who had feet planted on both sides of the issue were able to intervene in a way that ultimately resulted in a fairly reasonable compromise. One such person was Dr. Peter Page.

In 1983, Page, a gay man, was medical director for the American Red Cross blood bank program for Massachusetts and Maine, headquartered in Boston. The city of Boston at the time had the nation's first full-time liaison to the gay community, Brian McNaught, appointed by the mayor to serve as a bridge between his office and the community. Unlike his counterparts in other cities, Page considered himself fortunate because he at least had an individual to call upon who had the confidence of both the political establishment and the gay community. Page's own gayness also was an asset. As he told me, "Feeling comfortable with gayness and gay people, I had zero reluctance in diving right in and talking with people to learn about [AIDS]." He noted that others in the blood-bank industry weren't quite so comfortable around gay people.

Although Page is gay and Don Francis is not, they agreed that the public health was the number-one priority. For the general American public, said Page, "When they're sick and need to be transfused, they don't need to worry about the safety of the blood supply. And wrong though it is, they just don't need to have to worry about getting blood from a gay man who donated blood."

Page met with McNaught, telling him that he was concerned that "promiscuous gay men probably shouldn't be blood donors."

McNaught resisted. "Gay men are being picked on again," Page recalls McNaught saying to him. "It's not fair to discriminate." McNaught invited Page to meet with the AIDS task force he had organized. Page told the group of community leaders and medical professionals that together they needed to figure out a way to get people who might be at risk of being infectious and asymptomatic not to donate blood. Page suggested that gay men should self-defer from donations. At first the group demurred. Said Page, "The committee was not happy to hear this. They didn't believe it, they didn't like it, and they accused me of all sorts of bad things—discrimination, unfairness, and blame."

By the end of the meeting, though, Page recalls, "Somebody said, 'Now wait a minute, we ought to listen to this character, Page. Maybe there's something there, and we don't want to walk away from it. We don't want to be blamed for causing more of the problem. Let's think about how we can act responsibly.'" Working with Page and the Red Cross, the task force agreed to design an insert to be included in a brochure called "What You Should Know About Donating Blood," which would be given to all prospective donors. To the request for self-deferral by anyone who had ever had hepatitis, injected drugs, or traveled to a malarial area, was added the line "If you're a man with anonymous or multiple sexual partners, please don't donate." This self-deferral seemed a reasonable way to eliminate a significant number of potentially infected donations.

"As it turns out," said Page, "we found ways not to discriminate, but to base donor deferral upon objective descriptions of behaviors, which we fine-tuned and made more strict over the years. We made some people mad—but as we say, donating blood is not a right, it's a privilege." The AIDS task force agreed to help educate Boston's gay community about blood donations, so that at least those with known risk would be discouraged from donating. The level-headed approach that had been worked out by a gay doctor in the blood industry and gay community leaders in Boston became a model for other regions as Page's counterparts in blood banks in other parts of the country, particularly those in nonurban areas, called him for advice about what to do.[29]

While leaders in Boston's gay community were recommending that gay men not donate blood—my own doctor in Boston told me in January 1982 that I, as a gay man, should no longer donate blood—a group of New York gay medical and political leaders formed the AIDS Network to formulate and disseminate guidelines to the community urging gay men who believed themselves at risk to refrain from donating blood. The AIDS Network—which included Ginny Apuzzo, Roger Enlow, Larry Kramer, Larry Mass, and Dan William—issued a statement on January 17, 1983, supporting the testing of blood and blood products for agents such as hepatitis B, and self-screening by individual blood donors. It also acknowledged that mere questioning of donors was inadequate for safeguarding the blood supply, just as a policy excluding any group from blood donation would be ineffective and inappropriate.[30]

In San Francisco, the Bay Area Physicians for Human Rights urged gay men to cooperate with blood banks in screening themselves out as blood donors. But the national group, AAPHR, opposed the elimination of gay men from blood donation—other than those "who think they may be at increased risk for AIDS." Of course relying upon gay men to determine whether they were at "increased risk" was, in 1983, ineffective, as no one knew then how AIDS was caused or exactly how to prevent getting or transmitting it. Gay activists in Washington, D.C., persuaded the American Red Cross not to ask about sexual orientation per se in donor questionnaires. In fact, Frank Kameny advised gay men to lie if their local blood bank asked about sexual orientation.[31] At a time when homosexual relations were considered criminal acts in more than half the states, it was no small consideration to expect someone to answer "yes" to a question about private behavior that was considered illegal.

In March 1983, the Public Health Service recommended that donors from high-risk groups—all gay men and injection drug users were indiscriminately lumped into this category—voluntarily refrain from donating blood and plasma. In fairness, it must be acknowledged that no one at the time could know for certain whether a particular gay man or drug user had AIDS. The antibody test was two years in the future and there was no telling, other than by overt symptoms, who did or did not have whatever was causing AIDS. But in an extremely negligent move, Red Cross and other blood industry officials continued for well over a year afterward to refuse the use of other tests that would have prevented at least some HIV infections. Even more egregiously, they continued to deny that there was any risk at all from blood or blood products despite the mounting number of AIDS cases among transfusion patients and hemophiliacs that were attributable to these very causes. Beginning in 1984, heat inactivation was used to kill the virus in plasma products such as Factor VIII, which was used by thousands of hemophiliacs.[32] But it wouldn't be until April 1985 that the just-approved antibody test was used to screen all blood and plasma for HIV antibodies.

Eventually the blood-bank industry would pursue a three-pronged strategy for eliminating infected blood. Rather than focus on sexual orientation per se, a predonation questionnaire focused on more specific behaviors so donors, at least those who acknowledged their potential risk or actually knew they were HIV-positive, presumably would self-defer. A second method was introduced in the form of a simple box to check off whether one wanted his blood used only for research purposes rather than for actual transfusion. This "confidential unit exclusion" permitted those who felt pressured to donate to save face with coworkers, for example, while helping to minimize the risk to the blood supply by excluding their blood from actual transfusion. Finally, of course, was actual antibody testing of the donated unit of blood itself after the test became available in early 1985.[33]

Since 1996, the American Red Cross has used an even more sensitive test that actually measures for the presence of the virus itself, rather than the ELISA's measurement of antibodies to the virus. This cuts the time, from about twenty-two to sixteen days, in which it is possible to know whether an individual has been infected with HIV. Although it boosted the cost of a pint of blood by as much as three dollars, the new test was expected to cut the risk of HIV infection from a blood transfusion to 1 in every 660,000 blood donations— a significant improvement over the 1 in 100,000 ratio in 1983, before HIV antibody testing was available.[34] In fact, a study reported in the *New England Journal of Medicine* noted that the risk of HIV infection from a blood transfusion has now dropped to two in one million.[35]

The early foot-dragging of the blood industry and the manufacturers of Factor VIII would eventually cost not only thousands of lives but hundreds of millions of dollars in lawsuits as well. In late

1996, a federal judge approved a $640 million settlement by four drug companies accused of knowingly selling HIV-tainted clotting products to about six thousand hemophiliacs in this country alone.[36] There were similar cases in other countries. In Canada, for example, health authorities in 1996 stripped the Red Cross of authority over that nation's blood supply because of the deterioration of public confidence after an estimated twelve hundred Canadian citizens were infected with HIV through transfusions in the 1980s.[37]

Clearly, the blood and blood-products industries were responsible for circulating "bad blood" throughout the nation and the world. It cost them only money. It cost too many who trusted them their lives.

*

Once the public became aware that AIDS could be transmitted through the blood supply, fear, panic, and a pent-up hatred for homosexuals was unleashed in a sudden and virulent storm of media coverage. A June 1983 *New York* magazine cover-story reported, "At the city Bureau of Preventable Disease, the telephone began ringing as many as fifty times a day with inquiries from fearful citizens. One caller was reassured that mosquitoes are not known to carry AIDS. Another was told that there is no reason to fire a maid simply because she is Haitian. One doctor who works at the office was stopped by a neighbor who wanted to know if it was still safe to visit Greenwich Village. Another neighbor asked if she should worry about working with a homosexual." In a telling description of the fear that had gripped the city, the article noted, "New York in 1983 has become a place where a woman telephones Montefiore Medical Center and asks if her children should wear gloves on the subway."[38]

Amidst this hysteria, Ginny Apuzzo's fear that gay men would be stigmatized because of a belief that they all were tainted by "bad blood" proved to be more than well-founded. Now those already inclined to hate gay people cloaked the daggers of their bigotry in the guise of concern for public health. But gay men weren't the first—and hardly the only—targets of this kind of scapegoating for a public health crisis. As Dennis Altman notes, "The idea that the nation's blood supply was contaminated became a twentieth-century version of poisoning the wells (for which Jews were put to death during the Black Death)."[39]

On May 25, 1983, Assistant Secretary for Health Edward Brandt announced that AIDS had become the government's "number one health priority." For the first time in the epidemic's nearly two-year history at that point, the *New York Times* ran a front page article about it, reporting Brandt's announcement. And as James Kinsella writes in *Covering the Plague,* "If it is in the *Times,* it is widely regarded as fact."[40] Because the newspaper is considered to take a conservative approach to the news, and is required reading by executives in both print and broadcast media, the placement of a story on the front page of the *Times* has a powerful influence on what other newspapers, television, and radio reporters consider newsworthy and important. It is not surprising, then, that in the spring of 1983 the American news media suddenly "discovered" that there was an epidemic underway. The result was what Dennis Altman called "the great media panic of 1983."[41]

Although *Newsweek* was the first major print outlet to report on AIDS among others besides gay men—hemophiliacs, injection drug users, and children—the *Times* and other media continued to focus almost exclusively on gay men. This was due at least in part to the fact that white middle-class gay men with AIDS were the most accessible to reporters—and because they "looked like" the mostly white middle-class reporters themselves. But the focus on gay men had the unintended effect of perpetuating the view that they were the *only* victims of the epidemic—and that AIDS was, by extension, a singularly gay problem.

Not only that, but the prevailing stereotype of an AIDS victim as a *white* gay man who lived in one or another of the nation's urban gay ghettos meant that gay men of color—as well as gay men who lived outside the major cities—would remain at great risk for years to come because of a lack of information about the disease. Neither the mainstream media nor the white gay community troubled themselves to understand that the gay community included more than just white gay men, and that only a small fraction of all gay people actually live in the urban gay ghettos. For their own part, black,

Latino, and other nonwhite gay men could continue to deny their own risk—they were not, after all, white.

Gil Gerald, a longtime black gay activist, first realized that AIDS was disproportionately affecting people of color after a staffer of the Gay Rights National Lobby in spring 1983 sent him copies of the *Morbidity and Mortality Weekly Report.* Gerald learned, for example, that while blacks comprised 12 percent of the population, they already were accounting for more than 20 percent of the nation's AIDS cases. When Gerald shared this information with a group of black gay men who were board members of the National Coalition of Black Lesbians and Gays, they scoffed at it. At a reception in Gerald's home in Washington, D.C., he recalls the men saying, "No, Gil, this is all bullshit. They just want to change our sexuality—and [the only ones at risk are] guys like you who sleep with white guys." Ironically, Gerald notes, "Most of the people in that room went on to become prominent AIDS activists in D.C." On a more somber note, he added, "Most of the people in that room are gone."[42]

With the sudden interest in AIDS by the mainstream media, hysteria and sensationalism became the order of the day. They jumped all over an ill-informed and soon-debunked report in the *Journal of the American Medical Association* in May 1983 that AIDS could be transmitted through "routine household contact." Arch-conservative columnist and inveterate presidential candidate Patrick Buchanan poured his own bit of poisonous rhetorical gas on the growing fire when he wrote that month in his syndicated newspaper column, "The poor homosexuals; they have declared war upon nature, and now nature is exacting an awful retribution."[43] Somehow Buchanan's so-called "pro-life" views didn't extend to the lives of adults of whom he disapproved. And, of course, to acknowledge that AIDS was affecting others besides homosexuals would have further undercut his irrational and hateful diatribe.

Buchanan's compatriots in the Moral Majority found in AIDS an issue well suited to their efforts to wage cultural war against what they viewed as America's slide into godless immorality. In a 1983 fundraising letter, the Moral Majority argued: "Why should the taxpayers have to spend money to cure diseases that don't have to start in the first place? Let's help the drug users who want to be helped and the Haitian people. But let's let the homosexual community do its own research. Why should the American taxpayer have to bail out these perverted people?"[44]

On July 17, 1983, gay San Francisco psychotherapist and AIDS activist Gary Walsh faced Moral Majority founder Reverend Jerry Falwell in a transcontinental television hookup for a show by San Francisco's ABC affiliate, called "AIDS: The Anatomy of a Crisis." Falwell opened his discussion with Dr. Mervyn Silverman, then director of San Francisco's Department of Public Health, *San Francisco Chronicle* AIDS reporter Randy Shilts, and Gary Walsh by quoting from St. Paul's Epistle to the Galatians: "When you violate moral, health, and hygiene laws, you reap the whirlwind," he said. "You cannot shake your fist in God's face and get away with it."

Walsh told Falwell, "One of the most perverted uses of religion is to use religion to justify hatred for your fellow man." Falwell responded that he had "nothing but my compassion, love, and prayers" for Walsh. Falwell craftily dodged Walsh's invitation to visit him in San Francisco to see firsthand the life Falwell had automatically condemned as "perverted." To prove his concern, however, Falwell noted that his church had seven psychiatrists and counselors standing by to help "cure" homosexuals. Walsh assured him it wasn't his homosexuality that needed to be cured.[45]

Others in the so-called Christian right exploited the public's fear of AIDS and hatred of gay people to raise money for organizations that purported to represent "family values." The American Family Association in winter 1983 sent a direct-mail fundraising letter that said: "Dear Family Member, Since AIDS is transmitted primarily by perverse homosexuals, your name on my national petition to quarantine all homosexual establishments is crucial to your family's health and security. . . . These disease carrying deviants wander the street unconcerned, possibly making *you* their next victim. What else can you expect from sex-crazed degenerates but selfishness?"[46]

Naturally these moralists refused to acknowledge the selflessness and self-sacrifice that many homosexuals were exhibiting at the time in caring for friends and lovers who were dying from AIDS. To do so would have meant being confronted by the fact that they were, as John Fortunato puts it in *AIDS, the Spiritual Dilemma*, promulgating "this grotesque perversion of Jesus' message of compassion that markets itself under the guise of born-again Christianity."[47]

In view of the access and influence that the born-again right had in the Reagan White House—one of Reagan's inner circle, outspokenly antigay domestic policy adviser Gary Bauer, today is the director of the arch-conservative Family Research Council—it was with good reason that gay leaders feared a backlash that would irretrievably set back the community's efforts to achieve equal rights. As Jim Holm, a prominent gay activist in Seattle, recalls, "Everything we had—a modicum of civil rights in certain well-educated larger cities, some freedom in some places such as the Castro to show such minor affectations as holding hands, the acceptance by the media of our spokespeople as legitimate news sources, the cooperation of friendly straight politicians such as mayors who restrained their homophobic police forces—was seen to be on the line."[48]

Writing in the *New Republic* in the summer of 1983, pundit Charles Krauthammer said, "How much of a national scientific effort we devote to fighting an illness is a reflection of the political value we attach to it and to its victims. But that is only the most superficial issue aroused by AIDS. The deeper issue is the moral value we attach to an illness, and on that may hinge the fate of the homosexual movement itself." Krauthammer alluded to the former designation of homosexuality as a mental illness, noting, "Just as society was ready to grant that homosexuality is not illness, it is seized with the idea that homosexuality breeds illness."[49]

A week after Krauthammer's article appeared, *Newsweek* ran a long article called "Gay America in Transition." The magazine noted that, besides politicians using AIDS to justify antisodomy laws in Texas and Georgia, gay people had been told to leave restaurants, refused ambulance service, and evicted from their apartments simply because they were perceived as having AIDS. In October 1983, New York physician Joseph Sonnabend was evicted from his office building because of fear that his largely gay practice would bring down the building's market value. Boston's *Gay Community News* also reported that fall that corporate personnel managers were paying $395 each to learn how legally to fire people with AIDS from their jobs.[50] They could have saved their money, because a 1986 decision by the

Department of Justice, under Attorney General Edwin Meese, permitted the firing of anyone who was even *perceived* to have AIDS if coworkers were afraid of "catching" it.

The *Newsweek* article cited data from a Gallup poll indicating that 58 percent of Americans rejected homosexuality as an acceptable "alternative lifestyle." Taking a page from Jerry Falwell himself, the article went on to say "it is difficult for many straights to avoid the conclusion that nature or God is punishing homosexuals for defying sexual shibboleths that are as old as the Bible itself."[51] Even Joan Collins, the bitchy star of "Dynasty," a television soap opera that was popular with many gay men in the early eighties, blamed AIDS on what she called the "moral laxity" of gay men.[52]

Gay people who had only begun slightly more than a decade earlier to, as *Newsweek* put it, "enjoy, at best, a precarious tolerance in the public mind," also wrestled with the taunts of internal demons that, even today, can nag at the mind and spirit of the most self-accepting homosexual. Richard Failla, described in the *Newsweek* article as "a professed homosexual who is a prominent New York City judge," told the magazine, "The psychological impact of AIDS on the gay community is tremendous. It has done more to undermine the feelings of self-esteem than anything Anita Bryant could have ever done. Some people are saying, 'Maybe we are wrong—maybe this is a punishment.'"

A mere decade after the American Psychiatric Association had removed homosexuality from its official list of mental illnesses, gay people feared that public hysteria over AIDS could lead to an attempt to "re-medicalize" homosexuality. Larry Mass says he felt "the necessity to publicize the fact that we were dealing with this extreme health emergency that was quickly becoming unprecedented," while at the same time "feeling a lot of pressure from a lot of people who wanted to jump on a bandwagon to say there was something deeply and seriously wrong with gay people."[53] Mass had long feared that the antigay forces within psychiatry would cite the promiscuity and exorbitant rates of STDs among gay men as "evidence" of pathology, and try to reclassify homosexuality as a mental illness. What would they do now with a fatal STD that seemed to be targeting gay men so disproportionately?

In Provincetown, Massachusetts, the spit of land at the very tip of Cape Cod that for decades has enticed artists, bohemians, and homosexuals with its brilliant sunlight, stunning beaches, and acceptance of diversity, fear gripped heterosexuals and homosexuals alike. Alice Foley, a lesbian and longtime resident of the resort town, recalled in an interview how gay employees in her former restaurant, Alice's Cafe, reacted when a man with AIDS came in for dinner one night early in the epidemic. "An entertainer here in town who was obviously sick came in the restaurant and ate," said Foley. "I remember the staff and myself in the kitchen talking. We didn't know what to do with his dishes, so we threw them out. That's when I said I've got to get more information on this shit—I can't keep throwing dishes away!"

Foley, who at the time was also Provincetown's director of public health (technically the town nurse) not only got more information but went on to become the local hero in P-town's efforts to address AIDS among its heavily gay population. She fought, sometimes against other gay people and often with the town's Rescue Squad, to procure or create services for people with AIDS—and, above all, to overcome fear with factual information. Foley recalls that in the early eighties she used to have to park her car at least a block and a half away when visiting the home of someone known to have AIDS because the gay community was shunning those who were sick. "They were so frightened," she said. "Everyone was terrified."[54]

Obviously gay people were not immune to the panic that swept the nation, and the loyalty to the community by some gay men proved as fickle as that of all too many of their heterosexual supporters when they were confronted by AIDS. In a word, gay men were scared—and not merely of the much-feared political backlash. A bizarre and fatal disease of unknown origin and etiology had attacked them, the mysterious pathogen believed to cause it almost certainly transmitted through their most intimate acts of love and pleasure. They were scared for their very lives. Could any sexually active person at the time not have been frightened and at least a bit irrational?

*

Armed with a medical degree and a doctorate in retrovirology, experience working on feline leukemia virus—which causes an AIDS-like

immunosuppression in cats—and in the CDC's smallpox eradication program, Don Francis was in the right place at the right time
when the AIDS epidemic began. His background of working on epidemics and with gay men on the hepatitis B vaccine made him a
valued member of CDC's AIDS Task Force. But the globe-trotting,
San Francisco-born scientist remained puzzled about one basic
thing, and he knew he had to understand it if he, as a heterosexual
doctor–researcher, was going to succeed in working with gay men
being afflicted by AIDS: Why were gay men sexually attracted to
other men?

"I was comfortable with gay men," Francis says. When he realized he was going to be dealing with AIDS, he wanted to try to
understand homosexual orientation. So he asked his friend Marcus
Conant, a gay physician in San Francisco, "Why do you go around
having sex with other men?" Francis recalls Conant saying, "Remember when you were a teenager and you started fucking around sexually, and you started being turned on with girls? Well, I had the
same experience, but I was turned on with other boys." Francis was
incredulous. As the two walked together on the streets of San Francisco, a couple came walking toward them. Conant asked, "Now see
that, does that turn you on?" Francis answered, "Yes, when I see a
good-looking woman coming down the street I get a little primitive
urge." Said Conant, "No, no, no—the guy walking with her!"

The proverbial lightbulb came on for Francis. Still, he couldn't
understand why gay men—at least the ones he had observed in his
work, the men with many anonymous sexual partners and frequent
STDs—were so promiscuous. Although he had begun to understand
homosexuality and certainly knew firsthand the randiness of healthy
men in general, Francis remained baffled at why so many gay men
seemed to be drawn so easily into the world of sex clubs, bathhouses,
and cruising in public parks—particularly when there was a deadly
epidemic that seemed to be emanating from these very bastions of
anonymous sex. For Francis, it was clear that, as he said to me, the
"post-Stonewall commercialization of gay sex allowed an incredible
amplification of an otherwise relatively difficult-to-transmit disease."

Francis recognized the awkward position he was in, wedged between a gay community that was frightened and defensive, and a
conservative Republican administration that would have preferred

to see both gay men and their new disease quietly—and of course privately—eliminated from the nation's consciousness. Speaking to a gay group in Los Angeles early in the epidemic, Francis recalled thinking, "I'm sitting here as a straight man who is employed by Ronald Reagan, my boss, and I'm telling gay men that I thought lots of sexual activity was a dangerous thing to do today."[55] He realized he wasn't in the best position to be the bearer of such a message.

It certainly was a message many gay men did not want to hear. Some refused even to listen. For many homosexuals, gay liberation—and what it means to be gay—was inextricably linked to sexual freedom. The right to have sex anytime, anywhere, and with anybody they chose was, for them, inalienable. So to suggest that they needed to limit their sexual behavior in *any* way represented for them an abridgement of their hard-won freedom and an untenable compromise of their very identity as gay men. What's more, the fact that physicians—even if many of them were gay themselves—were urging gay men to restrain their sexual behavior brought back painful and angry memories from the recent past. After all it had been physicians, psychiatrists in particular, who considered gay people to be sick merely because they were not heterosexual.

Writing in GMHC's second newsletter in January 1983, Larry Mass reported that physicians were advising their gay patients, especially those in urban centers with large gay communities, to limit their sexual activity by having fewer partners and by selecting partners known to be in good health and themselves limiting the number of different partners with whom they had sex. He added, "It is the increasing number of *different* sexual partners, not sex itself, that apparently increases the risk of developing AIDS."[56] Mass had been committed to being "sex-affirmative" since the seventies. But the advent of what was looking increasingly to be an epidemic caused by a fatal sexually transmitted disease challenged his commitment. He put out a twofold message, saying that while gay people shouldn't abandon their political struggle and commitment to fundamental civil liberties, they also had to recognize that in the midst of a public health emergency, precautions were necessary. "I would not allow myself to be put in a position of being sex-negative," said Mass.[57]

GMHC itself didn't want to seem prudish. It certainly didn't want to be perceived as telling gay men how to have sex. After all, another of the agency's founders, novelist Edmund White, who co-wrote *The Joy of Gay Sex,* had been quoted in the seventies as saying that gay men should view their sexually transmitted diseases as "red badges of courage" in the sexual revolution.[58] Others in the community who were willing to speak out in support of more decisive changes in gay sexual behavior faced vicious criticism from gay men who were convinced they had "sold out" their gay birthright of free and easy sex—and that they likewise were selling the gay community down the river by not supporting the status quo of the ghetto. At the time that Mass's article appeared in the GMHC *Newsletter,* some vocal members of the gay community in New York were still enraged over an article published two months earlier by Michael Callen and Richard Burkowitz, both diagnosed with AIDS and patients of Joseph Sonnabend. The *Native* article, "We Know Who We Are: Two Gay Men Declare War on Promiscuity," was, in Callen's words, "a blunt, provocative warning to gay men about the possible consequences of continuing to expose themselves to the diseases that were epidemic among promiscuous gay men."[59]

Callen used his income tax refund in May 1983 to publish and distribute a forty-eight-page booklet, called *How to Have Sex in an Epidemic: One Approach,* one of the first publications ever to speak of "safe sex"—and to offer what even today is considered some of the best thinking about the meaning of the epidemic for gay men.[60] The booklet, written by Callen and Berkowitz, recommended "avoiding the exchange of potentially infectious bodily fluids," which would eventually become the cornerstone of safe sex advice. Callen and Berkowitz believed GMHC's advice to limit the number and assess the health of one's sexual partners was "dangerously inadequate." For their forward thinking, the men were roundly condemned—by GMHC and other gay men.

Like others in the community, GMHC feared that publicizing the facts about gay promiscuity would hasten the impending backlash everyone feared. Callen noted, "GMHC and other critics retorted that by focusing attention on the incidence of the many sexually transmitted diseases common among promiscuous gay men, we were 'shouting guilt from the rooftops,' " as Peter A. Seitzman, a gay physician, had put it in the *Native.*[61] Callen believed passionately—some say fanatically—that promiscuity per se, in addition to a run-down immune system, was the cause of AIDS. He held to this belief long after HIV was discovered and implicated as the actual cause of AIDS. But others, who were receptive to whatever possibility science might eventually suggest was the cause, still felt it essential to keep the high level of promiscuity under wraps. Don't air our dirty laundry in public, they reasoned, and the public will leave us alone. Of course they would learn all too soon that the American public and the federal government were only too willing to let gay men suffer and struggle to address the AIDS epidemic on their own.

In his own front-page article in the *Native* in March of 1983, called "1,112 and Counting," Larry Kramer echoed Callen and Berkowitz's views—in the hyperbolic Kramer style that led soon thereafter to his ouster from GMHC's board. "I am sick of guys who moan that giving up careless sex until this blows over is worse than death," wrote Kramer. "How can they value life so little and cocks and asses so much? Come with me, guys, while I visit a few of our friends in Intensive Care at [New York University]. Notice the looks in their eyes, guys. They'd give up sex forever if you could promise them life."[62]

Besides galvanizing many gay people around the country to respond to AIDS on a political level, Kramer's article emboldened other gay men to speak out against a sexual lifestyle that now could end abruptly and hideously in an early grave. In San Francisco, Bill Kraus and his fellow Harvey Milk Democratic Club members Cleve Jones and Ron Huberman—highly visible and well-liked gay men—published an article in the gay newspaper *Bay Area Reporter* that, as Randy Shilts put it, "drew the battle lines on which [Kraus] would wage his fiercest political fight." In the article, the men said, "We believe it is time to speak the simple truth—and to care enough about one another to act on it. Unsafe sex is—quite literally—killing us." They went on, "Unsafe sex with a number of partners in San Francisco today carries a high risk of contracting AIDS and of death. So does having unsafe sex with others who have unsafe sex with a large number of partners. For this reason, unsafe sex at bathhouses and sex clubs is particularly dangerous." Given their political bent, they added, "If the gay movement means anything, it means learning self-respect and respect for one another. When a terrible disease means that we purchase our sexual freedom at the price of thousands of lives, self-respect dictates it is time to stop until it once again is safe."[63]

For their boldness, and despite years of service to the community, Kraus, Jones, and Huberman were reviled in San Francisco as traitors to the "cause" by gay men who refused to distinguish sexual license from gay liberation. They were treated like pariahs by the community whose political interests they had championed. Jones recalls, "I had people spit on me on Castro Street, and call me a Nazi. And I thought I *was* a gay liberationist!"[64]

Many gay men believed that people like Jones and Callen had been co-opted by the government or some other "enemy" of homosexuals into participating in a plot that would prevent them from having sex. Pat Norman told me, "People were not going to hear the doctors, or hear their friends or other people. They thought [safe sex] was some kind of homophobic strategy to keep people from having sex, to keep people from each other and paranoid about each other. People did not want to believe they were going to have to make such 'severe' changes in their lifestyle."[65]

San Francisco's gay newspapers supported the denial of gay men who refused to believe that a major health crisis was underway. In large part this was because virtually all gay publications at the time depended upon the advertising revenue from bathhouses, bars, and sexually explicit services. The public health—and the very lives of gay men—mattered little to them in comparison to the money they stood to lose if they angered bathhouse owners by reporting honestly what was happening. The *Sentinel* trivialized the medical research being done on AIDS. Offering its own theory of the cause of AIDS, the newspaper suggested that one thing unique about gay men was a stereotypical assumption that they all enjoy brunch—hence, a front-page April Fool's joke: "Brunch Causes 'Gay Cancer.'" Another lead story a month later purported to be an investigation into the safety of bathhouses and sex clubs, but turned out to be about their lack of fire safety precautions rather than the sexual activity that went on in them. Rodger Streitmatter notes that the newspaper then "began waging a bare-knuckled attack not against the disease, but against an organization the community had created to *fight* the disease," the K.S. Foundation (now the San Francisco AIDS Foundation).

After the appearance of Kramer's "1,112 and Counting" stirred up discussion among gay men about the epidemic, the *Bay Area Reporter* promised to "up the noise level on AIDS." But, says Streitmatter, "rather than attacking the unrestrained promiscuity of the bathhouses, [*BAR* editor Paul] Lorch set his sights on AIDS patients and activists. Two weeks after upping the volume on the disease, Lorch denounced patients as freeloaders and activists as fanatics." After a group of twenty-two AIDS patients wrote *BAR* publisher Bob Ross to criticize Lorch's coverage—the *Sentinel* actually got hold of their letter and published it on its own front page—Lorch kept their letter and, in one of the more reprehensible acts of the epidemic, checked off the signers' names as they one-by-one succumbed to AIDS.[66]

The nationally circulated *Advocate* had been singled out by Kramer in "1,112 and Counting." He wrote, "I am sick of the *Advocate,* one of the country's largest gay publications, which has yet to quite acknowledge that there's anything going on. That newspaper's recent AIDS issue was so innocuous you'd have thought all we were going through was little worse than a rage of the latest designer flu. And their own associate editor, Brent Harris, died from AIDS. Figure that one out." In 1982, the *Advocate* had declined to publish Larry Mass's "Basic Questions and Answers About AID"—despite the fact that it was one of the only information sources available about the epidemic "during a period when no other such information was being featured," as the magazine's own history reported it.[67] In fact, it wasn't until April 1983 that the *Advocate* tepidly suggested that the "use of condoms may be helpful" for gay men engaging in anal intercourse.

At the *San Francisco Chronicle,* Randy Shilts began in May 1983 to focus attention on the bathhouses—and to become himself a lightning rod for the wrath of those in the community who considered them sacrosanct. Shilts was demonized for daring to question the judgment of some gay people in the pages of a so-called "straight" newspaper, rather than simply bowing to the pressures of gay activists to keep it as it were "in the family."

As the city's annual Gay Freedom Day Parade approached, Shilts's May 27, 1983, article "Gay Freedom Day Raises AIDS Worries" quoted public health director Mervyn Silverman as saying, "There has been some pressure on me to close the bathhouses." But

Silverman left it to gay men to monitor their own behavior, and trusted that out-of-town visitors coming for Gay Freedom Day "will realize they can't do the kinds of things they might do at home."[68] Silverman did, however, require that bathhouses post warning notices about AIDS. In his own effort to alert gay men to the risks of unsafe sex in the baths, Shilts attempted throughout 1983 and 1984 to get his articles about the risks of promiscuity and the bathhouses published on Fridays, before gay men headed out for a weekend of fun. As he put it, "I wanted everyone to have the fear of God in them."[69]

As gay activists battled one another over the bathhouses, they demonstrated—as they are wont to do—how little their ideologically driven arguments had to do with the real lives of most gay men. According to the estimate of Sal Accardi, the owner of a large bathhouse in San Jose, attendance at the baths in San Francisco dropped by 65 percent in 1983.[70] Half a dozen of the city's twenty bathhouses closed, including the Caldron, Cornholes, Liberty Baths, Sutro Baths, and Bulldog Baths. The owner of the Hothouse said he closed the bathhouse because his business had been cut in half by the fear of AIDS.[71] It seemed that the gay rank and file were catching on to the idea of safe sex—or were at least having their sex outside the bathhouses.

In February 1984, the CDC's Jim Curran said, "I wish the gay community would officially express concern over the bathhouses. I'd like to see all bathhouses go out of business. I've told bathhouse owners they should diversify and go into something healthy—like become gymnasiums. Gay men need to know that if they're going to have promiscuous sex, they'll have the life expectancy of people in the developing world." Openly gay city supervisor Harry Britt announced plans to meet with doctors and AIDS researchers to organize a campaign to inform gay men that "sexual activity in places like baths or sex clubs should no longer be associated with pleasure—it should be associated with death."[72]

The following month, longtime gay activist Larry Littlejohn—who in 1964 founded San Francisco's pioneering gay group, the Society for Individual Rights—announced that he would move to place a measure on a citywide ballot to prohibit sexual activity in the baths. Many believed the ballot measure would pass. Pressured to move against the baths, but still hoping the gay community itself would act against them, Silverman on April 9, 1984, proposed a ban on sexual activity in the baths, rather than an outright closure as some were hoping.

Coincidentally, the same day, *Time* magazine published a cover story announcing the end of the so-called sexual revolution. In view of the fear of AIDS gripping the nation at that point, and the increasing deaths of gay men, it is nothing short of astounding to note that the 4600-word article never once mentioned the epidemic. And homosexuality—not homosexuals themselves—is mentioned only in one sentence of the final paragraph, together with porn on television and teenage sex, as part of what the magazine called "the gray area."[73] If we were to gauge the nation's awareness of AIDS and gay people from one of its leading news magazines at that point, we would conclude that America simply didn't want to know.

More than a decade later, Silverman recalled that he continued to hope that the gay community itself would take responsibility for dealing with the issue of sex in the bathhouses. "I felt that since it was a situation having to do with sex," he said, "the government never dealt well with those issues." The gay community had dealt effectively with other gay-owned businesses that were in violation of city health or safety codes, and Silverman felt they would do so again. When some gay bars had only one exit, making them a fire hazard, gay people set up pickets and information tables outside. Said Silverman, "It didn't take long for the facilities to change." Silverman pursued people within the gay community, saying, "Why don't you all do what you did with fire hazards? Get out there and really do something to get them to clean up their act."[74]

As controversy swirled around the issue of the bathhouses, Health and Human Services Secretary Margaret Heckler announced on April 23 that government scientists had discovered the cause of AIDS: a retrovirus dubbed HTLV-III (Human T-cell lymphotropic virus type III). A late 1986 compromise between the American (who called it HTLV-III) and the French (LAV, or lymphadenopathy-associated virus) "co-discoverers" of the virus, led to a renaming of the virus as human immunodeficiency virus, or HIV. Besides lauding the efforts of National Cancer Institute researcher Robert Gallo—and giving a passing nod to the Pasteur Institute researchers in Paris who technically had discovered the virus that Gallo was then able to reproduce in large quantities—Heckler promised there would be a blood test within six months and a vaccine inside of two years. Her groundless promise stunned the scientists listening to her. But her words gave hope to a gay community that was reeling from fear, grief, confusion, and its own internecine battles over sex.

The day of Heckler's announcement there were 4,177 reported AIDS cases in forty-five states—including more than sixteen hundred in New York City alone, and more than five hundred in San Francisco.

San Francisco mayor Dianne Feinstein resisted closing down the bathhouses lest such a move be seen as a political, rather than public health, decision. Instead she pressured Silverman to do it. Part of Silverman's reluctance to take action—besides his characteristic style of consensus-seeking—was a fear that closing the baths in San Francisco would be viewed nationally as a move against gay people in the country's most liberal city. As he put it, "If San Francisco, as a bastion of liberalism, closed down the baths, what impact would that have on other communities?" Would it mean gay bars would be closed next? That sodomy laws would be either instituted or acted upon? As Silverman and others grappled with these volatile issues, a group of gay men, clad only in towels, demonstrated at one of the health director's press conferences, carrying placards saying, "Today the tubs, tomorrow your bedrooms" and "Out of the Baths, Into the Ovens."

A proposal by Jim Ferels, head of the K.S./AIDS foundation, to impose a "safe sex code" on all gay sex venues seemed to be headed in the right direction. Ferels' plan, which he had worked out with the gay political clubs, would mandate that the baths and sex clubs give space to posters, literature, condoms, lubricants, public service announcements, minimum lighting standards, and educators from AIDS information groups.[75] But just before the foundation was to announce its plan publicly, Silverman finally took action and closed down the city's remaining bathhouses and sex clubs. Speaking more forcefully than he had up until then, Silverman announced at an October 9 press conference that he had ordered the closure of the city's fourteen remaining bathhouses that "promote and profit from the spread of AIDS." The health chief was blunt. "Make no mistake about it," he said. "These fourteen establishments are not fostering gay liberation. They are fostering disease and death."[76] The baths reopened within hours, and forced the city to take the matter to court. Seven weeks later, the state superior court ruled that the baths could remain open—but only under the conditions that they no longer provide private rooms and have monitors available to prevent high-risk sex.

In other cities, there were debates over bathhouses, often with the same kind of rancor and resistance—also with more outright political, as opposed to public health, justifications—as in San Francisco. New York City and Los Angeles closed down their bathhouses within a year after San Francisco. New York health authorities in November 1985 closed down the Mine Shaft, the bar famous for the raunchy, no-holds-barred sex it allowed. In Miami, Shilts reported that Club Baths owner Jack Campbell "brushed off questions about the baths' role in the epidemic by insisting that most of Florida's AIDS cases were Haitians, and it wasn't a problem for gays."[77] Of course this was specious, as most of the early AIDS cases in Miami—as in the rest of the country—were among sexually active gay men. But Campbell's financial and political clout provided him with an effective shield against criticism by gay leaders. In Chicago, David Ostrow left Howard Brown, which he had helped to found, in part because the agency's leadership—associates of Chuck Renslow, owner of the city's largest bathhouse and several bars—handled the bathhouse issue with kid gloves lest they incur the wrath of their patron. Said Ostrow, "I thought it was inappropriate for the head of the baths to have so much control over the clinic. But of course he had a lot of political clout."

Although Ostrow firmly believes the baths should be allowed to stay open and can be effective venues in which to provide prevention education, he brooks no disagreement on the pivotal role the bathhouses played in widely disseminating HIV among gay men. "Normally," he explained, "people have sex within a social network of a certain race, age, and economic status. In the bathhouses, you had sex with anybody you wanted to have sex with, and they went on to have sex with others. So not only do you spread it rapidly in that bathhouse, but you spread it into all sectors of the community that are in that bathhouse, and they go out and spread it."[78] Even lots of sex within a closed network would keep the virus in check, Ostrow said. But the mingling at the baths literally "amplified" HIV far and wide among American and Western European gay men.

Would the community have resisted less if gay men had been more confident that their basic human rights were not at stake in the debate over sex and bathhouses? Of course it's impossible to know with certainty. The more important, because more fundamental—and still unanswered—question is whether gay men would have attached so much value to sex itself if they had been treated as full human beings, and offered the same rights as heterosexual Americans to enjoy the social and legal approbation of their relationships. Larry Mass's suggestion that promiscuity would diminish if gay relationships were accorded the same recognition, support—and expectations of mutual commitment—as those of heterosexuals continues to make good sense in the late nineties. It also continues to be ignored.

To stem the further spread of AIDS among gay men, the community struggled to figure out, as Callen and Berkowitz's groundbreaking booklet put it, "how to have sex in an epidemic." Too often the struggle was with one another, as anyone who questioned the status quo of the ghetto was derided as a traitor to the "cause" of gay liberation. At the same time that gay men managed to accomplish the most remarkable degrees of behavior change ever seen in the history of medicine, they chafed against the second-rate role they were cast in as the whipping boys and worst nightmares of mainstream America. The old demons of guilt and shame still haunted them, reinforced by the condemnation of the religionists who now slandered all gay men as "disease-carrying deviants."

Before disparaging the way gay men dealt with AIDS in the early years, a bit of perspective is highly recommended. As even Randy Shilts conceded—despite his own antipromiscuity agenda—"The gay response to the bathhouse problem was not a homosexual reaction; it was a human reaction."[79] In the years ahead, gay men would demonstrate a profound humanity as they transcended their own fears, doubts, and outlaw status to care for one another. The darkness of hatred, internal and external, would yield to the brilliant light of love as gay people rallied a true "army of lovers" to fight the viral scourge, bind the wounds of the stricken, and prevent further destruction to their lives and community.

3

RALLYING THE TROOPS

Thou shalt love thy neighbor as thyself.

LEVITICUS 19:18

The personal was never so political as when the personalities of local elected officials, their public health chiefs, and gay activists defined the ways that people with AIDS would be cared for. The degree of visibility, acceptance, and influence of gay people in the nation's hardest-hit cities determined the parameters of caring, funding, and support. Gay people themselves argued over whether to stick to providing palliative care for the stricken or to channel the extraordinary outpouring of community support into the gay civil rights movement. Gay doctors and lawyers used their professional skills to help people with AIDS maneuver through the medical and legal minefields they were forced into by a disease that seemed to underscore their social status as "outsiders." Black gay men who felt like outsiders wherever they were, found that the only thing to do—as it was for their white brothers—was to say "Enough of the charade!" For everyone who cared enough to get involved, the practical love they gave and received among the ruins of lives shattered by illness and death helped to heal their own emotional and spiritual wounds.

In the grand foyer of San Francisco's City Hall is a bronze bust of George R. Moscone, the city's mayor from January 1976 until his assassination, with gay supervisor Harvey Milk, in November 1978. Beneath it is engraved a Moscone quotation about what makes San Francisco unique. As I paused to read it, I understood more clearly why San Francisco was able quickly to mount what became a model of compassionate, coordinated AIDS services. The fallen mayor said, "San Francisco is an extraordinary city, because its people have learned to live together with one another, to respect each other, and to work with each other for the future of their community. That's the strength and the beauty of this city—and it's the reason why the citizens who live here are the luckiest people in the world."

I was at City Hall to interview Margaret Kisliuk, the city's lobby-ist in Sacramento. When Dianne Feinstein became mayor, after Moscone's assassination, Kisliuk was her liaison to the public health department. Her role in Feinstein's office became increasingly impor-tant as AIDS began to strike gay men in the city, and as the mayor sought to balance the demands of public health and the realities of politics. Fortunately for those afflicted by AIDS, Kisliuk explained, the city in the early eighties was enjoying a budget surplus; the mayor was the daughter, wife, and mother of doctors, and so was receptive to the counsel of public health and medical leaders; and the gay community already had enjoyed years of political clout un-known anywhere else in the country. In addition, the city's legislator in Sacramento—Willie Brown, currently San Francisco's mayor—was Speaker of the State Assembly, and could use his considerable power to steer state funding to his hometown.[1]

Peter Nardoza, Kisliuk's coworker in the mayor's office, was Feinstein's unofficial liaison to the gay community. Nardoza con-curred with the reasons that Kisliuk suggested were behind the city's early and effective AIDS response. But he added that perhaps the most important reason Mayor Feinstein was able and willing to view AIDS as a health concern—rather than as the political hot-button issue it became for, say, the federal government—was that she had gay friends. Echoing Armistead Maupin's description of the city in the seventies, Nardoza said, "No matter where you went, gay and straight people meshed in a very comfortable blend." When AIDS appeared, then, the mayor, the public health director, and the board of supervisors were supportive because they all personally knew gay people. As Nardoza said of the mayor, "In her mind, it wasn't a matter of '*they* are dying.' It was '*we* have a problem.'"[2]

San Francisco's ability to deal with AIDS had everything to do with its willingness to muster financial resources and political sup-port, even as other cities and the federal government equivocated as to whether and to what extent they ought to be involved in addressing what they saw as a "gay plague." In New York, the epidemic's East Coast epicenter, gay people certainly were visible. But the gay vote was fractured and not viewed as a serious political force among the city's many competing subcommunities. An outspoken and highly conservative Roman Catholic archbishop watched like a hawk for anything that might threaten his moral authority. And a bachelor mayor who for years had dodged rumors that he was gay couldn't afford to be seen as too supportive of homosexuals.

A city far bigger than San Francisco, New York staggered under the weight of social and infrastructure burdens largely unfamiliar to the city by the bay. According to Stephen C. Joseph, New York City's director of public health from 1986 to 1990, the problems plaguing the city and contributing to its slow response to AIDS included a huge homeless population, an estimated two hundred thousand heroin addicts, a shortage of low- and middle-income housing, a growing prison population, and a federal policy in the Reagan years that abandoned the nation's cities. As Joseph put it in *Dragon Within the Gates,* "In the sea of New York's troubles, AIDS was just one more rock dropped into the waves."[3]

As it is in so many other ways, New York in the AIDS epidemic would prove to be in a class by itself. The city's large numbers of injection drug users meant that from the early years of the epidemic, the sharing of needles was as much a source of infection among its many poor heterosexual blacks and Hispanics as unprotected anal intercourse was among white middle-class gay men. With a relatively small population of users in San Francisco, that city's AIDS epidemic would continue to the present day overwhelmingly to affect gay men. These were the two poles of virtually the entire AIDS pandemic in America: an affliction mainly of injection drug users and their sexual partners in areas where there are many of them, and of gay men virtually everywhere else in the country.

Besides the differences between their respective cities and the epidemic in them, the personal nature of the two cities' public health directors at the start of the epidemic also shaped their responses in important ways. From his 1977 appointment by Mayor Moscone, Mervyn Silverman had directed the health department in San Francisco with the kind of consensus-seeking style he'd developed in the

Peace Corps and the sensitivity to citizen "consumers" he had cultivated as director of consumer affairs for the Food and Drug Administration. In 1982, New York hired David Sencer, the former director
of the Centers for Disease Control, to be its public health director.

During his tenure at CDC, Sencer had presided over two major
public health events in which ineptitude in one case, and intentional
neglect in the other, would echo into the 1980s and beyond in the
AIDS epidemic. Under Sencer's direction, the CDC in 1976 projected an epidemic of swine flu and called for the innoculation of
every American man, woman, and child. This was based on the death
from swine flu of one soldier. After the government spent millions of
dollars on vaccine, fifty-eight people died from a wasting neurological
disease caused by the vaccine itself. The dead soldier remained the
nation's only case of swine flu. Also in the bicentennial year, the
outbreak of a strange bacterial disease among a convention of American Legion members prompted panic and the rapid deployment of
public health forces. This was a sharp contrast to the decades-long
Tuskeegee experiments in which federal government scientists observed poor black men afflicted by syphilis, without offering readily
available and simple treatment, merely to learn the natural history
of the disease. On Sencer's watch, the CDC finally investigated the
matter.

Perhaps Sencer was merely continuing the government's tradi-
tion, established in Tuskeegee, of downplaying the medical catastro-
phes afflicting unpopular groups of people when he repeatedly denied the impact and importance of AIDS. Randy Shilts reported that
Sencer stated in 1983 that AIDS was not a major problem in New
York. In 1985 he again dismissed the suggestion that AIDS was a
"crisis" in the city—despite the fact that by then there already were
three thousand cases in New York alone.[4] In an empty gesture to
the gay community, Sencer in March 1983 created the Office of
Gay and Lesbian Health Concerns, directed by gay physician Roger
Enlow, within the department of public health, to serve as a focal
point for its meager efforts against AIDS. He did so only after gay
community leaders, in a letter to Mayor Koch from the AIDS Network, penned by Larry Kramer, warned that "the gay community is
growing increasingly aroused and concerned and angry."[5] As Dennis
Altman has pointed out, the establishment of the office was "an odd

response to the epidemic in a city where almost a third of the cases are not gay."[6]

For the next couple of years, New York continued to make gestures to show "concern"—a few small grants here and there—but had no systematic response. San Francisco, on the other hand, gave millions of dollars for AIDS services. By mid-1983, the city already had spent more than $3 million for AIDS—at that point more than the entire AIDS extramural research budget of the National Institutes of Health.[7] New York, with the nation's highest number of AIDS cases, left it to the gay community to fend for itself. San Francisco recognized that each of its diverse subcommunities was an essential part of the whole. The responses of cities and towns across the U.S. varied between these two approaches.

Not long after the first cases of AIDS were reported, Larry Kramer wrote in the *New York Native*, "This is our disease and we must take care of each other and ourselves."[8] In August 1981, Kramer hosted a meeting at his home of gay men interested in learning what little was then known about the strange diseases that already had killed some of their friends. The following January, Kramer and five other well-known gay men—Nathan Fain, Larry Mass, Paul Popham, Paul Rapoport, and Edmund White—gathered again at Kramer's apartment. From their meeting came a new organization they called, straightforwardly, Gay Men's Health Crisis, which they created as a means to share information with gay men and raise money for medical research. As with many AIDS organizations that would form in later years, GMHC's first service was a hotline—originally nothing more than the answering service of Rodger McFarlane, Kramer's boyfriend at the time.

GMHC initially was a kind of ad hoc committee of volunteers who contributed time and created services according to their interests and abilities. Larry Kramer recalls, "We almost allowed anybody to do anything if they seemed responsible and passionate about it—whether it was doing an epidemiological study, or wanting to start a buddy system, or translating some stuff into Spanish that we would give out in the bars, or designing a brochure, or putting out a newsletter. We didn't have an office; we met in different people's apartments every week."[9]

By the time of its first anniversary, GMHC had grown from

its original six founders to more than three hundred volunteers. GMHC's board noted in its second newsletter that the group had raised more than $150,000; distributed twenty-five thousand copies of its first, and one hundred thousand copies of its second, newsletter; produced three hundred thousand brochures (in English, Spanish, Creole, and French); fielded almost five thousand hotline calls; formed a network of "buddies" to provide practical support for people with AIDS; provided legal and financial advisers; organized community forums; trained medical professionals; and served as a source of information about AIDS for the news media. All of its services were provided by volunteers and were offered free. Written by Kramer, the board's statement in the newsletter continued, "We have never encountered so much love between men as we have felt at GMHC, and watching this organization grow in response to our community's terrible new needs has been one of the most moving experiences we have ever been privileged to share."[10]

From its inception, Kramer and cofounder Paul Popham, GMHC's first president, disagreed about the organization's mission. Their competing visions would lead within a year of the organization's founding to Kramer's ouster from the board, and years of antipathy that would be resolved only when Popham himself was nearing death from AIDS in 1987. Beyond the personal nature of the disagreement, the two sides represented a split that would remain at the core of GMHC's identity for many years. As Kramer tells it, his own vision "was to spread information, fight and confront the system." On the other hand, he said that Popham, "who was in the closet and who was supported pretty much by the board, felt that we should very quietly take care of ourselves." Another GMHC cofounder, Larry Mass, recalls it somewhat differently. "Paul Popham's thing was to get this organization to work," said Mass. "Larry's thing was not compromising." He added, "We wanted to get a legitimate organization going—something like the American Heart Association, or American Cancer Society. A level of radical protesting was necessary, but not for this organization. It was primarily to be an information and service organization."[11]

Lost in the gulf of anger and hurt feelings that divided GMHC's founders was Kramer's important critique of how the gay community's lack of political clout in New York had forced it to create a parallel health care and social welfare system to educate the gay community and serve those with AIDS. In San Francisco, as Kramer constantly pointed out, the city simply funded existing organizations in the community to provide AIDS services. Said Kramer, "If we quietly take care of ourselves, we are saying not only that the system isn't *going* to help us, but we're not *making* the system help us. We're paying twice for the services—what we're paying for the city and state to provide from our taxes, and what we're also giving GMHC contributions to do."[12]

Kramer dramatized the situation in his play *The Normal Heart.* In it, the playwright's alter ego, Ned Weeks—portrayed by Brad Davis, who died of AIDS in 1991—complains about GMHC (unnamed in the play, but clearly the subject), "Now they've decided they only want to take care of patients—crisis counseling, support groups, home attendants. . . . I know that's important, too. But I thought I was starting with a bunch of Ralph Naders and Green Berets, and the first instant they have to take a stand on a political issue and fight, almost in front of my eyes they turn into a bunch of nurses' aides." When the play opened at New York's Public Theater, on April 21, 1985, the whitewashed plywood walls of the set were painted with facts, figures, and names relevant to the burgeoning AIDS crisis. Among them were these: "MAYOR KOCH: $75,000—MAYOR FEINSTEIN: $16,000,000," a reference to the wide disparity between the commitments of New York and San Francisco for public education and community services.[13]

When Marcus Conant arrived in San Francisco in 1965, the young dermatologist volunteered to work one night a week at the Haight Ashbury Free Clinic. While he was there, he observed some of the country's earliest cases of genital herpes, then beginning to run rampant among the free love crowd. "Those kids in the late sixties were sleeping with whoever was available," said Conant. He formed a clinic at the University of California–San Francisco to study the disease. In early July 1981, Conant organized another multidisciplinary clinic at the university; this time, the patients were gay men, like Conant himself. His phone conversations earlier in the year with his friend and fellow herpes expert Alfred Friedman-Kien, convinced Conant that San Francisco needed to brace itself for what he expected would be an onslaught of Kaposi's sarcoma cases. The

K.S. Clinic solicited patients from the city's physicians, who were only too glad to refer them because, as Conant explained, "They knew it was a fatal disease; they were scared of it; they didn't know anything about it; and they couldn't offer the patient anything."

The following May, Conant realized that his clinic would have no end of patients if something wasn't done to try to prevent them from becoming sick in the first place. He said to himself, "Wait a minute. It's not enough to sit up here in your ivory tower and diagnose them, you've got to get out there and stop it."[14] Recognizing that he needed political support in the community to form an organization to provide information about the new disease, Conant contacted Cleve Jones, then an aide to city supervisor (and future mayor) Art Agnos. Jones recalls, "Marcus said he wanted to start a foundation, and I said I would help him. I had the political knowledge and connections. He brought Frank Jacobson, who has since died, and Paul Volberding, from the General [hospital]. We also got Bob Ross, who is the publisher of the *BAR* [*Bay Area Reporter*], the gay paper. And we set up the Kaposi Sarcoma Research and Education Foundation."

The group had little information to give out, so little was known about AIDS then. "We rented this one room on Castro Street, and had one phone line," recalls Jones. "That phone started ringing—and it never stopped." Young men began showing up with purple spots on their feet. There were no services available at the time, nowhere for these men to go except the K.S. Foundation. Said Jones, "People would call and all we could really say was 'we care,' and 'give us your name and number.'"

Like Kramer, Jones recognized that the community's response to AIDS had enormous political implications. "It was the beginning of this incredible grassroots movement," he says. In the foundation's first year, Jones would go down onto Castro Street and wait for someone he knew to walk by. He recalls, "I'd say 'You! How would you like to serve your people? Come up here and answer my phone, would you?'" Those young gay men were the first class of recruits in the fight against AIDS. Says Jones, "Many of them now hold high administrative positions. Many are dead."[15]

In addition to the K.S. Foundation, a second organization in San Francisco found new life in providing support services to men facing certain death from AIDS. Psychologist Charles Garfield in 1975 founded the Shanti Project in Berkeley, across the bay from San Francisco, after he was asked to monitor the psychosocial needs of patients in the cancer institute where he was working at the time. Shanti put out word that the project needed volunteers, who would be trained to provide emotional and practical support services to terminally ill cancer patients and their survivors. As far back as five years before the first reported cases of AIDS, Garfield recalls, something odd seemed to be happening at Shanti. "As early as 1976," he said, "we started getting calls from the gay community that seemed out of proportion to the population. I had a feeling that it doesn't make sense for there to be a 'gay cancer.' How does cancer differentiate between gay and non-gay?"[16]

Efficient management was never Shanti's strong suit, and by the time K.S.—which gay men themselves dubbed "gay cancer"—was first reported officially in 1981, the organization was languishing. But after relocating to San Francisco, and an infusion of cash from the city government, Shanti (whose name in Sanskrit means "the peace that surpasses all understanding") volunteers began to serve gay men with AIDS. Within a few years, the Shanti model of AIDS services became famous and widely emulated throughout the country.

Helen Schietinger became the nurse coordinator of Marc Conant's K.S. Clinic shortly after its formation in 1981. "I thought, 'Good Lord, why are gay men getting cancer?'" Schietinger recalls. "It doesn't make sense. But it sure sounds like a place where I, as a lesbian, could be useful." The counseling degree Schietinger had earned to augment her nursing skills soon led her to take more than a research interest in the gay men coming into the clinic. "I was providing emotional support to them as they were getting worked up by these doctors," she said, "and then trying to find ways for them to get support in the community." After eighteen months at the clinic, Schietinger realized that she was mainly interested in trying to ensure that "people who were being told that they had this scary cancer" found support. The only place in the city for them was Shanti, which had begun to offer support groups. Schietinger realized that Shanti would be the best place for her to work with men affected by the new disease, so she went over to Shanti to put together a new AIDS housing program. "It was wonderful to become part of a community-based organization and make something happen that needed to happen," she said.[17]

Like Shanti, gay health clinics across the country—created in the 1970s to treat gay men for the sexually transmitted diseases raging among them like wildfire—expanded into providing AIDS services as a natural extension of the work they already were doing in the community. They had certain advantages over the newly formed AIDS service organizations, such as GMHC and the K.S. Foundation, in that they already had visibility in the community, organizational infrastructures, and valuable connections with the medical and research communities going back to the hepatitis B studies of the late seventies. Even in the seventies, the clinics had dispensed both penicillin and politics as they became important institutions in the gay community. In the AIDS epidemic, their roots in the feminist and lesbian health movements showed as they readily grasped the inherently political nature of the epidemic and the government's faltering response to it. Experienced in treating STDs, though, even these seasoned organizations learned quickly that a fatal STD, which gradually undermined an individual's health, required a whole new way of thinking about gay health issues.

At Whitman-Walker Clinic, in Washington, D.C., John Hannay became the first full-time employee when he was hired to manage the clinic's brand-new AIDS program in September 1983. Hannay's only experience with AIDS—far more than most people's at that point—was as a member of a small group of friends who were helping another friend, who had AIDS, when the man came from New York for weekly screenings at the National Institutes of Health, just outside of Washington. When he started at the clinic, said Hannay, there were maybe a dozen AIDS cases in D.C., and even fewer in the surrounding areas in Maryland and Virginia. "It took a while to realize it would be a serious problem," he recalls. "It was perceived as being concentrated in gay megacenters of the country, and D.C. was not perceived that way. There was a lot of difficulty getting people to see this was something urgent." The clinic tried futilely to draw attention to AIDS in newspaper ads. Finally, said Hannay, "When people began getting sick and dying, that got a lot more people to think."[18]

Whitman-Walker sponsored the first community AIDS forum in Washington, on April 4, 1983. "We ran a few ads in the *Blade*," recalls Jim Graham, the clinic's board president at the time and its director from 1984 to 1998. "We had no idea whether or not people would be interested." By December of that year, the clinic's AIDS Evaluation Unit began to see patients. "There was no pretense of any treatment," said Graham, "and I wouldn't say it was a full diagnosis because there was no test." As if to underscore the fact that the fight against AIDS was a losing battle in those early years, he added, "We *did* have the ability to know what was a K.S. lesion."[19] At a time when even medical diagnoses of AIDS were vague at best, no one could be precise about what, exactly, AIDS services ought to be.

Certainly the District government didn't know at the time. Jane Silver, who was the AIDS adviser to D.C.'s public health commission in 1983 and later the first director of the District's AIDS office, said that Whitman-Walker took the lead in providing services to people with AIDS even as the city tried to figure out what hit it. Silver, now the policy director for the American Foundation for AIDS Research, added, "I wish the government had taken more responsibility early on for requiring that the government services be on a par with Whitman-Walker Clinic."[20] But as New York did with GMHC, the District of Columbia mostly left it to the gay community to address AIDS on its own. The outcome was too many horrific and heartbreaking stories like one Caitlin Ryan told me. Their theme was always the same: AIDS is gay people's problem, not their elected leaders'.

Ryan, who was the first director of Whitman-Walker's AIDS program, recalls a phone call from the local prison telling her that a young man with AIDS was on his way to the clinic. She said, "This guy was probably twenty-two years old, very scared, his eyes were big as saucers, he had huge swollen lymph glands—serious lymphadenopathy. They assumed because he was gay that he had AIDS. He thought he had AIDS. All of his possessions were in a paper bag. They put him in a taxi and gave him cab fare. He showed up at the doorstep and just sat there with the stuff in a paper bag, with these huge tears rolling down his cheeks. He was just terrified. Of course later we found out that he didn't have AIDS; he had lymphadenopathy, and got treatment and care."[21] Like its federal overseers, the District government figured that any health problem of a gay person was a problem for gay people alone.

Established one year after Whitman-Walker, Chicago's Howard Brown Health Center also added AIDS services with the first appearances of AIDS in the city. Continuing its involvement in medical research that began with the hepatitis B studies in the seventies, Howard Brown in 1983 was chosen by the National Institutes of Health to participate in the Multicenter AIDS Cohort Study (MACS), the largest government-sponsored epidemiological study of how gay men's sexual practices might relate to the spread of AIDS. "I thought we were in a very good position at Howard Brown, since we had just completed the hepatitis B study, had a cohort, and blood stored away," said David Ostrow, who became the MACS principal investigator at Howard Brown. "So the whole idea of the MACS was that if anybody had an idea what the vector was, we could go back to these blood samples and figure out the early curve of this in Chicago."[22]

In other cities, gay health clinics organized AIDS services as freestanding agencies. Boston's premier AIDS service organization, for example, literally started out as a board committee of the Fenway Community Health Center, which was formed in 1971. Card-shop owner and longtime social activist Larry Kessler was a member of the committee from its first meeting, at the popular Back Bay gay bar, Buddies, in January 1983. In September of that year, Kessler was appointed as coordinator of the committee. Like most other AIDS service organizations, AIDS Action Committee saw its first function as educating the community, offering what little information was available about the disease at the time. To raise money and awareness, the committee held its first community fundraiser on March 29, 1983, a thirty-five-dollar-per-person dance at another gay bar off Copley Square called Chaps. AIDS patients were referred to Fenway for medical care. And as it became clear that people with AIDS would need services, the committee created them. Kessler recalls, "There was a perceived need for a lot of specialized services, and a perceived need that unless we did it, nobody else would."[23]

The Gay and Lesbian Community Services Center in Los Angeles emerged in 1971 from the gay liberation movement that had begun to blossom in L.A. as early as the fifties, when pioneering activist Harry Hay formed the Mattachine Society there. Eric Rofes, who became the director of the community center in the mideighties, explained, "It was founded by a group of people, including Morris Kite and Don Hill Heffner, who said they were trying to do political organizing among people who had been damaged by societal homophobia. They needed a place to bring people to heal while doing that work." By the time Rofes took charge, in 1985, the community center had become the largest gay social service organization in the world, with a $15 million budget, a staff of sixty, and a large building it owned. Among its many activities, the center ran an STD clinic, provided legal services, job training, and services for youth. "When the epidemic hit," said Rofes, "the center stood in a frontline position."[24]

The community center opened a hotline in its health clinic to provide information about AIDS to Los Angelenos. Soon enough, disagreement about how to run the hotline led the small group of people working on it to split from the center and form AIDS Project Los Angeles, today the second-largest AIDS service organization in the country. Bill Meisenheimer took advantage of a program offered by his employer, Xerox, to become a paid "volunteer" at APLA throughout 1983. He officially joined the staff on January 1, 1984, and within a month became the acting director of the fledgling agency. "I was not involved in the gay community, not in political organizing," Meisenheimer told me. "I was just somebody driven by my fear." He recalls that, although there was a groundswell of support from the community (even before it had the capacity to coordinate them, well over one thousand volunteers had come forward to help APLA), the political environment in Los Angeles was "a disaster." Said Meisenheimer, "The county board of supervisors were worthless. They didn't care about anything because of who [AIDS] was affecting. I would go and testify, and they would get up and walk out."[25]

Meisenheimer's successor as director of APLA was Paula Van Ness, who, as he had done, joined the organization as a volunteer. "I got a call from United Way," recalls Van Ness, "and they said we have an organization that needs some help." She was running a family-planning agency at the time. "Because you're in the sex business," they told her, "we thought of you." They said it was an AIDS organization—not exactly a group most heterosexuals would have wanted to be associated with in 1985. As Van Ness recalls, "They were having a hard time getting the straight community involved. I said if they asked me to serve, I would serve on the board as a hetero-sexual woman. They said okay."

So Van Ness joined the board, became its treasurer, and then was appointed executive director in 1985—just after APLA's first "AIDS Walk," and just before its first "Commitment to Life" event, which brought out Hollywood stars for one of their rare early appearances on behalf of AIDS. Both events benefited from the July 25, 1985, announcement that Rock Hudson had AIDS. APLA would certainly benefit from the cash and cachet of Tinseltown as the agency grew prolifically in the coming years. When Van Ness went to APLA, the organization had a $700,000 budget and seventeen staff members. By the time she left, only a year and a half later, APLA had exploded into a $7 million organization with a full-time staff of eighty-two. "It really was on a very fast climb," she said, "and quite remarkable that we did as well as we did to build the organization, expand services to deal with what then felt like a crush of new cases, and meanwhile build the board. It was a pretty remarkable time."[26]

Like its counterparts in New York, San Francisco, Boston, Chicago, and Washington, APLA's growth and success made it a source of "how-to" information for those in other areas of the country who were interested in starting an organization to serve their own increasing numbers of people with AIDS. In October 1985, Van Ness and the directors of the country's biggest AIDS service organizations at the time decided to form a national association of community-based AIDS providers. Based in Washington, D.C., the National AIDS Network was created to be a kind of clearinghouse of technical assistance for new AIDS organizations across the country, a centralized conduit for sharing information on a national level.

The sharing of information was a lifeline sustaining the new AIDS organizations in the early years of the epidemic. They compared notes with one another, and contrasted their own experiences to those of mainstream organizations that operated with widespread support and the good will of their communities. The social stigma attached to AIDS might have held back people more sensitive to it than the long-stigmatized gay men and lesbians who formed the early AIDS organizations. But the fact that they often were the only ones willing to provide care and services to people with AIDS meant that as the epidemic grew, the organizations they created to address it had to grow as well.

Because AIDS service organizations felt they had to create a parallel system of health care and social services specifically for gay men, the most heavily affected group at the time, they tended to look to one another for direction, rather than to mainstream social service agencies that had experience they might extrapolate to AIDS. The frequent result was programs, and whole organizations, cobbled together by people with far more passion than managerial acumen, and services that were devised more on the basis of hunches than on hard data that could permit the evaluation of their success or failure in traditional terms. At Whitman-Walker Clinic, Jim Graham said, "Everything we've learned, we've learned on the run. And we have learned it largely in isolation from mainstream models." When the clinic wanted to create a housing program in 1984, for example, it sent people to the Shanti Project in San Francisco, rather than looking at housing programs in D.C. itself.[27]

After conferring with the "established" AIDS organizations in the early epicenter cities of New York, San Francisco, and Los Angeles, representatives from cities and towns where AIDS hadn't yet become a major problem picked up useful ideas for services, as well as images of how the epidemic might soon look in their own hometowns. Jim Holm, a cofounder of Seattle's Northwest AIDS Foundation, described the lessons that he and others in the city's gay community took from the "tutors" they brought to Seattle from New York and San Francisco. He said they provided "a snapshot of what faced us just months behind them." Like San Francisco, Seattle's gay community enjoyed an amiable relationship with the city government that would prove invaluable in shaping the city's well-coordinated response to the epidemic. As Holm put it, "Cooperation here between health officials in government and community members was rich and very productive. It was hard, but both sides stayed at the table."[28]

One of the people at the table from the beginning was Bob Wood, a physician long active in Seattle gay politics and a member, in 1983, of the Northwest AIDS Foundation's first board of directors. Wood recalls that gay AIDS groups in other cities, New York in particular, were seeking contributions around the country to support their efforts to provide AIDS services at a time when they had no financial support from any level of government. But the "snapshots" of the epidemic in New York and San Francisco convinced the community in Seattle that it was best to focus its attention and resources locally. Wood recalls, "People put two and two together, and said 'Why should we give money to New York, when it's probably going to hit us, too? We need to develop our own response mechanism for it.'" By the middle of 1983, not only had gay people formed the Northwest AIDS Foundation, but they were also working with the public health department to lobby the Seattle-King County council for a project within the health department to focus on AIDS. Wood became—and remains—the director of that program.[29]

When Bea Kalleigh was hired in August 1985 to be the Northwest AIDS Foundation's first executive director, the organization had a budget of $28,000. During Kalleigh's four year tenure, that budget increased more than fifty times to $1.5 million. After leaving the foundation, she took a year-long, mid-career sabbatical at Harvard Business School. In a leadership class, Kalleigh recalls studying a case that examined the reasons companies go under. Without a forward-looking plan and with too-rapid growth, an organization risked imploding. Said Kalleigh, "I remember thinking that we grew at the AIDS foundation way more than the rate of growth they were talking about, because of the urgency in the community that people brought to it. We ended up starting new services, and the need actually grew faster than we did. There were always new people delivering new services—and the community always wanted more."[30]

During her year-long stint as the Clinton administration's first AIDS "czar," Kristine Gebbie from 1993 to 1994 visited AIDS organizations throughout the country. Gebbie told me she observed a kind of delay in the way the AIDS epidemic manifested itself on the coasts and in the heartland, and in the mobilization of local communities to deal with it. "The middle-of-the-country gay groups are today where the coastal groups were in 1985 to 1987," she said. "I traveled quite a bit in my year, and when I went to Montana, for example, I thought I was in a time warp. I experienced the same thing in the Midwest and parts of the South. This drove home to me over and over again how many little epidemics we're really fighting, and that to think that all gay groups are like the coastal groups is a real error."[31]

To get a picture of the "time warp" Gebbie described, I talked to two gay men involved in AIDS services in America's middle states. Since AIDS first appeared in Oklahoma City, in 1983, psychiatrist Larry Prater has been stirring up controversy with the state government over his safe-sex posters and a large billboard towering over the small AIDS service organization he helped to found. One side of the billboard said, "Masturbation education: Do your homework" (in response to the flap over Surgeon General Joycelyn Elders' comments on the subject), while the other side encouraged condom use. Said Prater, "I'm sure that's the first time the words 'masturbation' and 'condoms' were seen in public—let alone in eighteen-inch-tall letters!" When not shaking things up, Prater is one of the few openly gay physicians in the conservative state to provide AIDS services to the gay men in the area who account for virtually all the local AIDS cases. I visited him in early 1993 at the Triangle Club, a converted automobile showroom located on the same small strip as the city's gay bars and bookstore. Triangle has offered HIV antibody testing since it first became available in 1985. It also runs a food bank, operates a certified day treatment center for substance abuse, and provides limited HIV treatment services—"a big, big money loser," said Prater.

Prater told me in a later interview that in an area like Oklahoma, the Triangle Club's anonymous HIV testing policy and confidential treatment has been essential to bring in people at risk for testing, and to provide treatment to the infected. "For many, many gays in Oklahoma, their families do not know about them," said Prater. "If anything, having HIV is an even touchier issue for a lot of these guys than being gay, and they're not going to tell their families that they have HIV if they haven't told them that they're gay." He added, "Some families in Oklahoma would rather have no child at all than have a gay or lesbian child." Other families simply disown the gay children they do have, and often in rural areas where there are few gay community resources they wind up at an AIDS organization like the Triangle Club.

To illustrate, Prater recounted a recent example. "Last Monday night," he said, "we had this cute young couple, male and female, come in for testing. It turned out they were brother and sister, from Idaho. I asked them how they wound up in Oklahoma City, because more people leave Oklahoma than come there. They left because their family banished them to the hinterlands. These were the only two children of the family, and one's gay and the other is lesbian. I think this was more than the family could handle—they're very religious—and they just sent them away. They said they have each other. They were each about twenty-five, and had been in Oklahoma about three years."[32]

Arkansas native Ron Thompson's first encounter with the epidemic was when one of his best friends from college called to tell him he had AIDS. "I went 'Wow!'" he says. "This is real." The young man was someone Thompson "had done a lot of running around with, and took a couple of boyfriends from." Thompson hooked up with local efforts in his hometown of Little Rock. After volunteering and serving on various boards, he began to use his training as a social worker to provide AIDS education to mental health clinicians and laypeople alike throughout the state. I asked Thompson to describe the people in President Clinton's own home state who had gotten involved with organizing local service groups. "A good chunk of them are gay people," he said. "But a lot of families and parents started stuff because their gay son is dying or has died." As it was throughout most of America, Thompson said that in Arkansas, "In most cases it is gay individuals who started AIDS organizations." But, he added, "You find a lot of little old ladies saying, 'Wake up world!'"[33]

It isn't hard to understand how small towns and rural areas could ignore the epidemic until AIDS turned up in their own backyards. They simply figured it was a problem for city folks. It was more difficult to understand why the early AIDS organizations in hard-hit cities often ignored gay people of color affected by the disease living in their own city. George Bellinger, Jr., a longtime black gay activist, was an early volunteer at D.C.'s Whitman-Walker Clinic in 1983, when it began to provide AIDS education and services. Despite his own presence, he recalls, no one seemed to want to know about the black gay men who were becoming infected and developing AIDS even early in the epidemic.

But this was nothing Bellinger hadn't already encountered in gay bars. An assumption on the part of many white gay men that gayness implies membership in the Caucasian race (and the male sex), meant that they didn't consider a shared sexual orientation to be grounds enough for equal representation in the community institutions they created. Said Bellinger, "When I went to a bar, I didn't see myself reflected." Likewise, he added, the messages put out by early AIDS organizations "were always geared to white gay men who went to the gym, or lived in the gay ghettos. They did not talk to us."[34]

Many white gay men emigrate to the nation's big cities from the small towns in which so many of them grow up because they feel they can live more comfortably in a more tolerant and diverse urban environment. Gay ghettos have flourished in places like New York's Greenwich Village (more recently, Chelsea), San Francisco's Castro district, Capital Hill in Seattle, Houston's Montrose neighborhood, the West Hollywood section of Los Angeles, Chicago's New Town, the South End of Boston, and Washington, D.C.'s Dupont Circle. Not surprisingly, these neighborhoods were the first and hardest hit by AIDS, as well as the locations of the earliest AIDS organizations.

In contrast, most black, Hispanic, and Asian gay men don't uproot themselves from the neighborhoods in which they grow up. As a result, they frequently lead double lives: ostensibly heterosexual while among their families and neighbors, possibly even married to women—but engaging in sex with other men in furtive encounters, or even ongoing same-sex relationships. Because homosexuality is so harshly condemned among many people of color, these men feel driven to hide their sexual orientation at home. But the gay community—most visibly comprised of white men and women—reflects the racial insensitivities and imbalances of the broader society. Unfortunately, this means that gay people of color often don't find a welcoming embrace in that quarter, either. The result is a dual membership in the individual's racial or ethnic community and the gay community, and loyalties often sharply divided between the two.

It wasn't just the white gay community that overlooked the AIDS concerns of people of color. In the hardest-hit black community, for example, the early attitude towards AIDS was, "It's a white gay thing." They saw homosexuality as a "disease" of white people, and since AIDS was viewed by just about everyone as a gay disease, even black gay men at first dismissed it as irrelevant. They were unaware in the early years of how disproportionately hard AIDS was hitting their own. As astonishing as it seems, people in the black community as recently as 1996 were still saying, as did an op-ed article by African-American *Washington Post* columnist William Raspberry, "AIDS is becoming a black disease."[35] Unfortunately for far too many in the community, it had become a disease heavily affecting blacks at least a decade before Raspberry's epiphany.

Fortunately for all people of color, gay and straight, there were gay people willing to speak out about AIDS in their communities. Like their white gay brothers, these people realized that lives were on the line, and they decided that the tacit agreement which kept them hidden conveniently away in the community's closets was no longer binding. The added weight of the fear and grief they were carrying, as they saw friends getting sick and dying amid the denials and outright lies about the real nature of their illness, made the masks they'd hidden behind far too heavy to hold up. Stepping out of their closets and casting off their shame, "black gay men were the leaders in bringing this disease to the attention of the black leadership," as Gil Gerald put it.[36]

Reverend Carl Bean was one of the first to speak out. A successful gospel singer who had become a minister and founded a Christian denomination chiefly for black gay men and women, Bean became known nationally for bearing witness to the impact that AIDS was having on people of color, particularly gay men. When he began traversing the city of Los Angeles by bus and subway to minister to black men with AIDS in the city's hospitals, Bean said, "Even with the virus and T-cell counts, what I was hearing most was 'Would you tell my family that I'm homosexual, or would you be here with me when I tell them?' The other big part of it was 'Am I going to hell?'"

It was clear to Bean that if black gay men with AIDS were going to get the care they needed, something had to be done to disperse the cloud of denial and opprobrium around homosexuality and AIDS that had enveloped the black community. He recalls that he used to open his speeches to black church groups by saying, "Now, you all *know* who we are. You all *know* who's on the piano. You all *know* who's at the organ. Everybody here *knows* who's leading that song on Sunday that makes you happy." He added, "The room would always fall apart with laughter, and it would always take the tension out of the room and everyone would relax and they'd start asking real questions."

Bean realized that his work needed to include starting an AIDS organization in the black community. "I always knew I had to go home," he said. In 1985, Bean formed the Minority AIDS Project as an outreach ministry of his Unity Fellowship Church in South Central Los Angeles—an area that in the early nineties would symbolize the country's festering racial wounds when riots broke out there after the acquittal of city police accused of beating black motorist Rodney King. "Being black and gay," said Bean, "and having been black and gay in the community, I also knew the only voice that was going to deal with the issue was going to be a black homosexual who had in fact had the experience of being very openly homosexual in the community."

Other black gay men told Bean it couldn't be done. He recalls, "Blacks said no, you can't do it." As for Bean's idea that the Minority AIDS Project would be part of his church's ministry, he said the others' reaction was "Jesus and gay and black and church? No!" Bean persisted. "I said yes, it will happen, because all of that is alive in me, and I'm real. I am black, I am Christian, I am gay, and I'm a part of the black church." The other men were intransigent. Bean recalls them saying, "No way, honey. You'd better look for a piece of property up there on Santa Monica Boulevard." Bean held fast. "I said no. To be openly gay on Santa Monica, and you're black, is not openly gay. Until you're openly gay on Crenshaw, in South Central, you are not openly gay. That's how I feel about that. You're really not open until you're open in the 'hood."

Carl Bean's simple belief in the power of integrity would go a long way toward winning the black community's confidence in the Minority Aids Project. When the Brotherhood Crusade, a project of the Black United Front of L.A., made the first-ever donation to Minority AIDS Project, Bean recalls the group's leader saying to him, "You know, my wife and I have gay friends. We go to their house for Christmas, and they never say they're homosexual, they never say they're lovers. Everyone knows they are." The man added, "We'll gladly give you money, but you're the first homosexual black who's stood here in the community and said you're homosexual. Yes, we'll help you with this AIDS thing."[37]

When gay men spoke out honestly, and little old ladies said "Wake up, world!" others also came forward because they knew that, as Patti Austin's AIDS anthem puts it, "We're all in this together."

*

The AIDS epidemic broke out not long after Ernesto Hinojos finished a degree in public health. As a gay man, Hinojos wanted to become involved with AIDS because the disease was striking his own community. Marc Conant offered Hinojos a position in his new K.S. Clinic. Years of AIDS work later and a continent away, Hinojos recalled in an interview in New York his first experience of seeing a K.S. patient at the clinic in San Francisco. "This was such a disfiguring disease," he said. "I just cried and cried. But that was out of my own fear, my own sense that that's a brother, and that's somebody who's depending on me as his only link. So I rubbed my eyes and walked back into the room. I said if you'd like, I could walk you over to the radiation unit, and I'll sit with you if you'd like. If you don't have anybody here, I don't mind doing that."

Of course the young man had no one there with him. Likely his family were far from San Francisco, that he'd been one of the thousands of homosexuals who'd fled a small hometown and flooded the city in the seventies. But in the early years, even gay men were wary of other gay men with AIDS because of the lack of information about the disease's cause, downright fear, and the self-protective belief that somehow those men had brought it on themselves. Gay friends too often fell away when AIDS was diagnosed. So here was this young man, with a confounding and hideous disease, alone in a medical clinic—in the city where he thought, as had so many other men like him, he would find freedom, his very own pot of gold. It's highly unlikely that he expected to find a horrific and lonely death at the end of his particular rainbow.

"That would be really nice," said the young man. "I'd really like that."[38]

As Hinojos had been to this early AIDS patient, gay people and organizations throughout the country were one another's only link to information about the epidemic, the government's faltering response to it, and the political implications of it all. The social and political contacts established in the gay community nationally during the seventies now became invaluable connections as everyone puzzled out what was happening and how to respond. Telephone lines burned up with inquiries and news from city to city, coast to coast, as the newly formed AIDS organizations—typically with a handful of underpaid staff, a group of volunteers offering their energy, and no one on staff capable of fully channeling it—shared information with one another. Many of those leading the groups had been local gay political activists in the seventies. Few of them had the kind of management and fundraising skills that would be needed in the coming years as the service organizations grew in tandem with the burgeoning epidemic.

As would be proven repeatedly and in a variety of contexts in the AIDS epidemic, information truly was power. And a community painfully aware of its own history of powerlessness insisted upon receiving scientific information as it became available. The nascent AIDS organizations assumed the role of translators, frequently through the volunteered services of gay physicians and other medical professionals, digesting and disseminating the latest scientific information to others in the community. This information sharing would serve as the catalyst for the community's ability to mount a political response to the epidemic in coming years.

It was only natural that an information hotline would be the first AIDS service ever created, as it was at GMHC and many other AIDS service organizations. Rodger McFarlane's personal answering service that became GMHC's first hotline; the single phone line at the K.S. Foundation that Cleve Jones said "never stopped ringing"; the hotline at the Gay and Lesbian Community Services Center in Los Angeles that became AIDS Project Los Angeles—each of them, like so many others in cities and small towns across America, represented an effort to provide information, prevent panic, and promote a feeling of "connection" to the community. They provided life-links for individuals diagnosed with or at risk for AIDS, and they became the nerve centers for a gay community fearful of the medical and political uncertainties of AIDS.

Today GMHC's hotline receives an average of three to four thousand calls a month. When AIDS is in the news, the number increases. When Magic Johnson announced in 1991 that he was HIV-positive, for example, the GMHC hotline logged 7,800 calls within a month. Before leaving GMHC in late 1997 to pursue a counseling career, Bruce Patterson was director of the agency's hotline for nearly twelve years—the longest-serving staff member at the world's oldest AIDS organization. Patterson was volunteering at GMHC before leaving his job in the film business to become the assistant to GMHC's hotline coordinator in February 1986. He was offered, and happily accepted, a salary that was half of what he gave up. "I had to go back to living again like a poor student—spaghetti every night," Patterson recalls. "Plus I was trying to support a lover who had AIDS and wasn't working. I don't know how I did it!" Patterson is clear, though, about why he did it. He said, "I think one of the reasons I got involved in this work was that it was a way to help the community, which really needed help because no one else was helping us back then."[39]

When the federal government finally decided to create a national hotline to make AIDS information widely available, the CDC sent representatives to the National Gay Task Force, then based in New York City. Ginny Apuzzo, the task force director at the time, recalls that GMHC in 1983 had given the group money to create a hotline. Apuzzo turned the task force's violence crisis-line into the very first national AIDS hotline in this country. She recalls, "When PHS [Public Health Service] finally agreed to establish a national hotline out of New York, they came to NGTF's offices in New York, on Fifth Avenue, and sat there and watched the way we did the job."[40]

Most other AIDS services were created because having the disease typically meant the loss of a job and the ability to live independently. Psychologist Lewis Katoff, who worked for years at GMHC until his own death from AIDS, explained in a *Primary Care* article that most community-based AIDS services attempted to address a limitation or problem—whether physical, social, or psychological—that has resulted from the illness. He noted that the mix of volunteers and professionally trained staff used in providing AIDS services had several advantages, including cost effectiveness, empowerment, flexibility, quality of attention, accessibility, and cultural sensitivity.[41] The main goal of all AIDS services was always to keep people out of the hospital and functioning as independently and for as long as possible. But because AIDS was a progressively debilitating disease, the particular types of services needed varied over the course of the illness.

Bea Kalleigh said that people organizing services recognized early on that "health care was extremely necessary, but health care alone was not the whole story in a healthy life." She explained, "With AIDS, people's physical as well as financial and emotional situation changed, sometimes regularly and precipitously." Supportive services that had been designed for other groups of people—the elderly or the chronically mentally ill, for example—weren't intended for young gay men with a disease that could fluctuate wildly, sometimes incapacitating them, and other times making hardly a mark in their day-to-day functioning.

The earliest services for people with AIDS were designed to assist with the bare necessities of life—shelter and food. In December 1982, the Shanti Project contracted with the San Francisco Department of Public Health to create the world's first housing program for people with AIDS, which was to be replicated throughout the country. Helen Schietinger, the program's first director, explained that Shanti rented houses and apartments, furnished them through volunteer donations, and then rented rooms to people who were screened to keep out those who were active drug users or acutely ill. She noted how novel the program was, created because young gay men with AIDS were not seen as viable residents of geriatric nursing homes. "We were making things up as we went along," said Schietinger.[42] As it had been for Washington's Whitman-Walker Clinic, the Shanti program served as a model for a number of other AIDS service organizations across the country.

When Ruth Brinker's next-door neighbor in San Francisco, a gay man, developed AIDS in 1984, the widowed lady was startled to learn that because he was too weak to prepare his own meals, and friends were too busy to help, the man often went without food. A volunteer with Meals on Wheels, Brinker realized that "there was absolutely no way that people with AIDS could have meals brought to them unless they were over sixty years old—usually not the case for PWAs—and could qualify for Meals on Wheels." In the fall of 1985, Brinker decided that "no one who was ill should have to go through anything like that." After putting in a full day at Meals on Wheels, she began cooking up stews, pot roasts, and fish for seven people with AIDS. With the help of a few volunteers, she delivered the meals, often going into the city's Tenderloin district, where people with AIDS who had lost everything because of their illness were forced to live in seedy hotels.

Brinker talked Trinity Episcopal Church into letting her use its kitchen. Without funding, infrastructure, or fanfare, Project Open Hand was born. When word about the project got out, volunteers by the score came in to help. Within three years, Project Open Hand was serving 450 people with AIDS two meals a day through the efforts of a part-time staff of seventeen, scores of volunteers to deliver the meals, and even well-known chefs who would occasionally take a turn in the kitchen. When Open Hand began delivering meals, Brinker noted that many people, suffering from both AIDS and malnutrition, could barely walk to the door to let in the volunteers bringing their food. Thanks to Open Hand, that happened less often. Brinker said, "I use only fresh produce, the best ingredients I can find, and no preservatives. I believe that giving really good, wholesome food to people *before* they are debilitated helps them stay healthier longer and enjoy life more."

By 1988, Brinker was using her own energy to help other communities around the country begin food programs like Project Open Hand. In 1989, the project published *The Open Hand Cookbook*, a collection of complete menus prepared by prominent California chefs. In keeping with the neighborly spirit that led Ruth Brinker to begin cooking for people with AIDS, the book is subtitled, "Great Chefs Cook for Friends." When she started Project Open Hand, Brinker said, "I just wanted to feed a few people." Asked at the time whether preparing 900 meals a day for 450 people with AIDS was an overwhelming task, Brinker said, "Not when you think of the number of PWAs Washington tells us we're *going* to be serving."[43] When Ruth Brinker began Project Open Hand in 1985, "only"

22,996 Americans had been diagnosed with AIDS. Within a decade, well over half a million people in this country alone had been diagnosed with or already died from AIDS.[44]

After the basics of shelter and food were satisfied, the psychological well-being of people with AIDS was made a high priority. The physical insult of this disease, added to a lifetime of psychological injury, made gay men with AIDS extremely susceptible to major depression and even suicide. Volunteers from the Shanti Project, trained in working with death, dying, and bereavement, were the first to offer support groups to people diagnosed with AIDS. Support groups soon became a standard part of the treatment of people with AIDS throughout the country. San Francisco psychologist Steve Morin noted in a 1984 *American Psychologist* article on the subject, "The physical contact in support groups is of great importance to people with AIDS, who may not get much physical comfort elsewhere due to people's unjustified and ill-informed fears of casual contagion. The group also helps people express their anger and resentment as a result of having lost friends, lovers, and homes, and at being asked to leave bars, restaurants, and even juries."[45]

To help people with AIDS take control of their lives and function as normally as possible, Shanti created another novel service, the volunteer buddy program. "Buddies" helped out with practical matters, such as grocery shopping, cleaning, and cooking. Typically they weren't expected to provide emotional support, an area that belonged to other volunteers. But it is probably impossible to come as a stranger into someone's home, help him in his efforts to retain his dignity and functioning, and not become a friend. In many cases, gay men literally had no one to count on. Families were often far away, possibly alienated. Good-time friends stopped calling. Fortunately, there were many "buddies" in the community—people who, though probably also living far from their own families and perhaps their pasts, understood the importance of connection to others who cared.

In addition to pulling together a group of doctors and community activists to advise the city on how to handle AIDS, Boston's liaison to the gay community, Brian McNaught, wrote a regular column for the local gay newspaper, called "A Disturbed Peace." He authored a book of the same name, in which he explored the experience of being a believing but disillusioned Catholic. And he trained to become an AIDS buddy. "For a lot of us," said McNaught, "being a buddy was completely consistent with our image of what it meant to be a person of faith. The Gospel said 'I was naked and you clothed me. I was sick, and you visited me.' Francis of Assisi talked about 'Make me an instrument of your peace,' and 'Where there is despair let me bring hope.' All of that plays heavily into my feeling about our responsibility to each other."[46]

"All of that" figured prominently in the belief of many gay people and those who cared about them that, as W. H. Auden put it, "We must love one another or die."[47]

*

For Peter Lee, a job that seemed "abstract" and a growing awareness of AIDS led him in 1984 to volunteer as a buddy at Whitman-Walker Clinic. He says he had been "transformed" by working with an AIDS patient at the National Institutes of Health. "The immediacy of AIDS in terms of my personal life swamped anything else I could do," Lee told me. "So I began looking around for anything else I might do directly in relationship to AIDS." Which is what took Lee to HERO, the Health Education Resources Organization, an AIDS service group established by Baltimore's gay community. From there he moved to a position with the National AIDS Network, the Washington-based "trade association" of local AIDS organizations. Through his volunteer and then-compensated work on AIDS, Lee, like many others, was truly transformed into what became known as an AIDS professional, one whose full-time work revolves around some aspect of AIDS. Today Lee, a lawyer in Los Angeles, continues to work with AIDS issues.[48]

Others came into AIDS services as professionals whose particular skills were important to meeting the various needs of people with AIDS. In the early years especially, before there was an Americans with Disabilities Act to protect them, people with AIDS often were fired from jobs, evicted from their homes, discriminated against, and abused in countless ways. Houston lawyer John Paul Barnich was someone who put his considerable legal skills to good use on behalf of people with AIDS. When Barnich was studying comparative religion in India on the Fulbright grant he'd won halfway through law school, he visited one of Mother Teresa's homes for the poor. "I had what I guess is as close to a religious experience as I ever hope to have," recalls Barnich. "On the wall, someone had painted, 'God is love in action.' I said, 'This is a concept of God I can deal with—translating caring into some sort of action.'" Not long after the former schoolteacher finished law school, what Barnich calls "the great plague" hit, and, with it, "a great opportunity to get involved and do things."

Barnich joined the board of AIDS Foundation Houston in 1984, two years after the organization's founding. "I was present the night we became a social service foundation," he recalls. "This PWA showed up, didn't have money, and no place to stay. We chipped in and gave him money, and found him a place." Barnich's usual role with the foundation and its clients was as a legal protector of people with AIDS in Houston. Having lost his own lover to AIDS in 1994, Barnich said, "It's very, very personal to me, the fight against AIDS. I tend to react to people being discriminated against based on their HIV status like a wounded mother grizzly protecting her cubs. I have no mercy if people choose to be intentionally discriminatory. I see my job as making it as costly as possible for them."

In fact, Barnich has been involved in several prominent AIDS discrimination cases, including a highly publicized one involving unethical behavior by television reporters who fomented a sensational AIDS story so they could cover it. With the colorful storytelling characteristic of his adopted state, Barnich regaled me with one case after another. The case of Fabian Bridges stands out. Bridges was a thirty-year-old black gay man with full-blown AIDS, who came to Houston, and into Barnich's life, in late 1985. After a couple of public TV reporters talked to the board of AIDS Foundation Houston about doing a "humane" story on AIDS, they reappeared with Bridges. They were actually following him around the country. Barnich explained, "Every place Fabian went they would report to health departments that there was this young male prostitute with AIDS who was having sex." Barnich said that Bridges told him the reporters had given him money to eat and stay in shabby hotels while they reported on the "story."

When they landed in Houston, Barnich and a local gay activist met with Bridges in a gay coffeeshop. "The media were like sharks circling the coffeeshop," Barnich recalls. S. R. Andrews, an officer from the vice division of Houston's police department told Barnich he had orders from the health department to get Bridges off the street. Barnich had other plans. "I suggested to Officer Andrews that he not waste his time, that I'd be down there with a writ of habeas corpus, or the guy's bail, before they even got him arrested." Bridges agreed—initially—to commit himself to one of the county hospitals. After a few days, though, he became restless and wanted out. Eluding the assembled news media by leaving the hospital through underground tunnels, Barnich says he "snatched up" and "stashed" Bridges at his own house.[49]

Most people who have provided AIDS services have had far less dramatic experiences than Barnich's involvement with Fabian Bridges. They have quietly gone about the business of helping people with HIV and AIDS however they needed to be helped. Although AIDS services, like the epidemic itself, typically have included the same basic features, communities across the country have shaded them with local color to meet their particular needs. The case of Provincetown, Massachusetts, is one example.

Alice Foley remembers vividly when AIDS hit P-town. When a man asked her in 1981 to visit a sick friend, Foley was shocked at what she found. "I still remember walking in and seeing the young man," she says. "He was covered in what I know now to be Kaposi's. I never saw anything like that in my life. It looked like someone took a paintbrush and shook purple paint at him." Foley had just begun to hear about "gay cancer," but she was unprepared for this. "He was dehydrated," she recalls. "He was very, very sick. He didn't have any help, and died within a week. That really sent up a flag that this was a serious situation."

The next AIDS case in P-town was a referral from Massachusetts General Hospital, in Boston. A young gay man had driven to Boston from his home in Colorado, because the city's many hospitals and three major medical schools give it the reputation of being a medical "mecca." After being diagnosed with an AIDS-related infection, and having everything stolen from his car during the two weeks he spent in the hospital, the man was referred by a social worker to P-town because there was a visible gay community there. "This was in November, which is a terrible time to come here if you have no work," said Foley. She got him on the senior Meals on Wheels program.

After Foley bumped into Preston Babbit, a fellow Business Guild board member, as they both sneaked into the winter apartment where the young man was staying, the two pulled together a group of about five people—including a realtor, a guesthouse owner, and a bartender—to discuss the situation and figure out how to deal with it. When AIDS finally had a formal name, the group took a name as well: the Provincetown AIDS Support Group. At the time, P-town had only two or three people who were sick.

Because P-town is isolated, particularly in winter, and many year-round residents have little money and few have cars, transportation was the first, because most-needed, AIDS service there—as it has been in rural areas throughout the country. The AIDS Support Group enlisted volunteers with cars who could help drive clients to doctors and hospitals in Boston, more than two hours away. Volunteer drivers rented cars because none of them had a car deemed safe enough. The $480 from a fundraiser at Alice's Cafe—"We thought we were very, very wealthy," said Foley—didn't go far. At ninety dollars per trip, the group realized the service wouldn't work. It wasn't until 1986, four years after the group formed, that they finally had a Ford Escort station wagon donated.

The second service created in Provincetown was home care. If the goal of AIDS services everywhere was to keep people out of the hospital as long as possible, in P-town it was simply a necessity because of the town's remote location. Said Foley, "From here, if you were in the hospital in Boston, friends couldn't really visit you because of transportation. They'd have to get there on the bus." More than a decade after she led the formation of the P-town AIDS Support Group, and a few months after her departure as its only director to that point, Foley looked back with hard-won pride on the group's success. "From the beginning we were fortunate in having a tremendous sense of volunteerism in the community," she said. By the time of our interview, nearly four hundred people already had died from AIDS in the small community. But Foley emphasized that only a dozen of them had died in the hospital, while "the rest died at home."[50] As the hometown of choice for growing numbers of gay men and lesbians who truly feel free in Provincetown, "death at home" has had more than usual significance.

In Provincetown I also interviewed a physician who had just moved there from another small New England town—my own hometown, Norwich, Connecticut. I first saw Larry Millhofer's name in a front-page article about him in the *Norwich Bulletin* in late 1994. The article described Millhofer's experience as a gay physician (actually a gerontologist) in Norwich, and mentioned his role in organizing the local AIDS group. I was intrigued to know about his experiences in Norwich, where Millhofer had practiced since completing his medical residency in San Francisco in 1978.

"It was fairly known in the community I was a gay physician," says Millhofer. "But a lot of gay men didn't come to me for fear of being labeled gay." Millhofer's first AIDS patient was John, an elementary school janitor. Despite AIDS-related memory problems and wasting syndrome, John was supporting his mother, lover, and grandfather, who lived with him in a duplex house. After the landlord began to suspect that something was going on, Millhofer got a call from a *Bulletin* reporter. Millhofer had put on John's death certificate "AIDS dementia complex," and it was, technically, a matter of public record. The reporter was planning to write an article about the situation—until Millhofer threatened to sue the paper. The good doctor says, "Even though this man was just the janitor, I think his working in the elementary school had the potential for it to be blown out of proportion." Noting that public hysteria was common at the time, Millhofer added, "I think this was after the Rays were burned out in Florida," referring to the family whose home was torched because their hemophiliac boys were infected with HIV.[51]

In the early years of the epidemic, most people with AIDS were cared for by a small number of gay doctors like Millhofer. Some of them, like David Ostrow, had already been involved with gay health issues for years. Others became AIDS specialists because so many of their gay male patients were showing up with exotic HIV-related problems. Still other doctors, who were not gay, refused to treat gay men, with or without AIDS. As Millhofer puts it, "A lot of physicians actively avoided learning about how to treat AIDS-related illnesses so they could say they were ignorant about it. A lot of people avoided becoming involved."[52]

Considering the way so many physicians avoided AIDS, it's interesting to note that all the gay doctors interviewed for this book have said they still would have become involved with caring for AIDS patients even if the patients weren't gay men. Ken Mayer, for example, said, "It's actually easier for those of us who have a professional calling, because if AIDS wasn't a gay problem tomorrow, I'd still be interested because my interest is social medicine. I wouldn't be totally dispassionate even if I was only taking care of women"[53]

Don Abrams says he went "kicking and screaming" from his job at Marc Conant's K.S. Clinic to the AIDS clinic at San Francisco General Hospital. As one of the handful of physicians who were "in the right place at the right time" when AIDS appeared, Abrams was recruited by Paul Volberding, the clinic's director, who was in charge of caring for patients with K.S. and malignancies. Volberding and Abrams specialized in the pre-AIDS stage of illness formerly called AIDS-Related Complex (ARC), and Connie Wofsy was in charge of treating opportunistic infections. Wofsy died of breast cancer in June 1996. The decaying hospital with graffiti-sprayed elevators was not the ideal of either Abrams or his gay patients. Said Abrams, "My patients were all educated, well-to-do, with insurance and high socioeconomic status. I didn't appreciate that they had to be transferred across the city for treatment at the county hospital."[54] But even the K.S. Clinic, like physicians around the city, had begun to send patients to San Francisco General for treatment. Soon the hospital's reputation for excellent AIDS care would spread worldwide.

Before the AIDS epidemic, "you were hard-pressed to find a gay man in San Francisco who wanted to be caught dead at San Francisco General Hospital," says Cliff Morrison, a clinical nurse specialist and former head of nursing at the hospital. That changed significantly after Morrison created the hospital's AIDS unit in July 1983. "I couldn't understand why all of a sudden there was this group of patients and nobody wanted to deal with them," he said. For Morrison, it only made sense that if gay men with AIDS had nowhere else to go, they should be able—like anyone else in dire medical straits—to count on the General. Suddenly, middle-class gay men, many of them destitute because of AIDS, were literally dying to get into Ward 5A.

The ward's operating philosophy was to provide the services that patients wanted. One of its unique components was a strong emphasis on mental health, considered a high priority by patients. Another was the ward's policy to respect gay relationships. Patients chose a "significant other" who would be involved in medical decisions, and visiting hours were abolished so friends and family were welcome twenty-four hours a day. (In 1990, the San Francisco Health Commission extended this policy in a measure encouraging the city's hospitals to give visitation rights to the unmarried partners of gay AIDS patients.)[55] This "client-centered" approach to medical care was a radical departure from what Morrison calls the "we know best, you come to us and we don't go out to you" model that prevailed at the time. As many health care providers and AIDS researchers were to learn in the coming years, gay men were not ordinary patients. Said Morrison, "For the first time, health care found itself in the position where there were highly motivated, informed patients who said, 'We need your assistance, but we're not going to roll over and do everything you say to do.'"[56]

Ward 5A became famous for the compassionate, holistic care it provided to AIDS patients, and was emulated by dozens of specialized AIDS units in hospitals around the country. It hosted many visitors, including former Surgeon General C. Everett Koop and world-renowned bereavement expert Elisabeth Kübler-Ross. The staff were surprised and pleased by the media attention they received because it meant others would learn about the model of services they had created at the General. Said Morrison, "The only spotlight we thought we were going to get was negative, so when we had all this positive attention, I was very surprised." All the nurses who staffed the ward were volunteers. Half of them were openly gay. A number of them eventually died of AIDS themselves. In addition to the nurses, the ward had a psychiatrist, a medical social worker, consulting psychiatrists and psychologists, and five full-time counselors from the Shanti Project.

Oddly enough, Morrison notes, initial support for the ward "did not come from gay men, particularly within the health care establishment itself." At a time when public debates over gay bathhouses were heating up, there was hesitation about drawing attention to gay men's sexuality by singling out AIDS patients for special treatment. Doing so, some feared, would add to the stigma of those with the disease. While many gay men were reluctant to support the AIDS ward, straight women and lesbians didn't hesitate one moment. As Morrison put it, "Our sisters really stepped to the forefront and said to hell with everybody else, we'll do what we have to do."[57]

For many lesbians who got involved, politics—and sometimes the opinion of other lesbians—had little to do with their involvement. During her years at GMHC, in the early eighties, New York therapist Sandi Feinblum ran up against the misogyny of many gay men. She described the frustration of dealing simultaneously with the bigoted and fearful attitudes of the public toward AIDS, and the "women-less existence" preferred by some gay men. "Here you have this pressure cooker and all these terrible things happening," said Feinblum. "In those days it was not unusual for us to go to someone's apartment and scrape shit off the floor, call an ambulance, then fight with the ambulance to take the person. And then you had a lot of gay men who never dealt with women, who constructed their lives not to deal with women. I met lots and lots of men who had no women friends, and except for on the job, they really eliminated women out of their lives."

Despite the lack of women in their lives, Feinblum said these gay men still felt it their due as men that women should help them in their moment of need. "As in the rest of the world," she said, "women helped men, and men expected them to help." As GMHC's first deputy director, Feinblum recalls, "People used to say to me all the time, 'Why do you work with AIDS and GMHC? They wouldn't work for breast cancer.'" Underscoring the nonpolitical motives that spurred her own AIDS work, she said, "That's partly true—but what did it have to do with the fact that all my friends were dying?"[58]

For many heterosexual women who joined the fight against AIDS, the only thing that mattered was that people—regardless of their sexual orientation—were suffering injustice. A self-described maverick social services administrator with the Dade County government, Catherine Lynch had worked for years with hurt people on issues ranging from domestic violence to rape counseling to bereavement, and her bilingual ability gave her an added glimpse into those issues within Miami's large Hispanic community. One incident among all she had seen in her career pushed her to the point she knew she wanted to focus on AIDS.

Lynch was trying to track a young Hispanic man who had been approved for placement at Jackson Memorial Hospital, Miami's primary public hospital, but then just disappeared. After finding his number in the computer, Lynch called the man's house. She spoke in Spanish with his mother, who started crying. Lynch recalls, "She started talking about how her son was dying of AIDS, and excuse her for crying but there was no one she could talk to about it. Whenever she tried to talk to her husband, he didn't want to hear about it." After a long and difficult conversation, Lynch said, "I hung up the phone and I thought, 'There is something so wrong in the world where I found this woman because I was an administrator who was bothered by a dangling loose end.' If I had not been trained as a crisis counselor, if I was not bilingual, there would be no one to help this woman."

When Lynch took over as director of Miami's Health Crisis Network, in 1988, she had no reservations about working with an organization rooted in the gay community. "It wasn't a risk for me to go to a gay-identified organization, possibly because I was married," Lynch said. "I trust my gut. My gut said these are good folks, decent, honorable, caring folks." During the interview process, Lynch was asked what she would do if someone snubbed her at a social event because of her affiliation with an AIDS organization. She said, "If you are a relatively assertive, intelligent woman in this world, a good number of people hate you because you don't do what you're expected to do. The people who would stigmatize me for working in a gay organization are the people who would have stigmatized me for being me anyway."

How did Lynch find AIDS work in comparison with the other troubling issues she'd worked on in the past? "I did not have any understanding of some of the things I was getting into," she said. "You don't until you experience loss after loss after loss of wonderful people. I had not understood that I was going to face this once a week, and once every month or two with someone I knew well enough to care about, to feel that it wasn't just a loss for me but it was a tremendous loss for the community."[59]

The awareness of their loss motivated many to get involved by showing they cared through direct action of one sort or another. Most amazingly, people with HIV and AIDS themselves refused to accept the role of victim, and frequently volunteered to help others in the same situation. Shanti Project founder Charles Garfield borrows Swiss psychiatrist Carl Jung's concept of the "wounded healer" to describe the phenomenon of caregivers who are themselves living with, at risk for, or bereaved by AIDS. Garfield writes, "The wounded healer recognizes himself or herself in the patient, and the patient recognizes his or her reflection in the healer." Particularly when both the care provider and recipient are living with HIV, the "wounded" one and the healer are interchangeable roles. "Both caregiver and patient step through the looking glass, in a manner of speaking, and into the territory of the other," Garfield says. "Ancient healers, shamans, believed that this ability to 'move between the worlds' of health and sickness was the source of their powers to heal."[60]

Robert Washington was thirty-six years old in 1984. Although the HIV antibody test was not available at the time, the Washington, D.C., psychologist said he "knew" he was positive even though his doctor dismissed his symptoms as hypochondriacal, induced by being around people with AIDS. Subsequent testing revealed that in fact Washington was infected with HIV. Comfortable in his various identities—black man, mental health care provider, father—it took time to become comfortable revealing other aspects of himself: gay, HIV-positive. But when Washington, then living in Chicago, got involved with the Cook County buddy program in October 1984, the experience changed his life by forcing him to learn to be comfortable with far graver matters than others' perceptions of his sexuality.

"My first buddy was a hustler," Washington told me, "a young African-American man who was twenty, uneducated, and absolutely gorgeous." The clinic staff assigned him to Washington because they felt he had the professional expertise to handle the case. "This young man was quite distraught, angry, upset—all the things you might expect," said Washington. "But more than anything else, he was quite afraid he was going to be damned to hell, something I didn't believe." Long phone calls taught Washington the "power of presence," simply being there for someone. He said, "Nothing I could say would take away the feeling, but I could sit on the other end of the phone and just be there for him."

Washington's buddy lived for nine months, during which time they became almost constant companions. Washington says, "It was the first time that I was a witness, an intimate witness, to the dying of somebody. And it changed me." Although he is a psychologist, Washington had no formal training in work with death and the dying at that point, so he went from the gut. He recalls, "When it became clear he was going to die, he called me and told me. I picked him up—literally, I had to pick him up and carry him down the stairs—and took him to the Cook County Hospital, where he was put in the intensive care unit. He died peacefully. He died young—a couple months after his twenty-first birthday."[61]

Describing voluntary efforts to care for people with AIDS, Philip M. Kayal writes, "AIDS is such a shattering human event that it is only possible to capture its horror in a direct face-to-face encounter—by living in a relationship with a PWA." Like Robert Washington, gay and nongay people alike who have been involved in providing care are changed by the experience. For individuals who have the virus themselves, the experience can be empowering as they support and encourage others' efforts to survive and thrive with AIDS. It can also be a sobering glimpse of what may lie ahead. No matter who it is and what their HIV status, volunteering and providing AIDS services are profoundly political acts. As Kayal puts it, AIDS voluntarism provides "the prime opportunity for both intimately knowing AIDS and understanding its political dimensions."[62]

Gay men, lesbians, and others involved in AIDS-related services and political work often speak of the AIDS "movement." By this they mean the broad community of people—including both gay and nongay people, men and women, and all races—who seek a rational response to the epidemic; medical and social services that treat people with AIDS with skill and compassion; a voice for clients in how and what services are provided; and, ultimately, accessible and affordable treatment for people in general who are afflicted by life-threatening illness. People caring for their own formed the core of what became a broad community of concerned, caring people who, despite their many social and demographic differences, shared one belief: People with AIDS deserve kindness, care, and effective services merely because they are fellow human beings. AIDS service organizations were created essentially to channel and coordinate the community's outpouring of caring.

Suzanne Ouelette, a graduate psychology professor at City University of New York, for years has studied the role of volunteers in providing AIDS services, particularly at GMHC, the organization that pioneered so many of them. Ouelette described to me a survey of five hundred GMHC volunteers, conducted in the late eighties, in which the question was asked: What should happen to GMHC if a cure for AIDS were found tomorrow?

Of course there were what Ouelette calls the "pragmatists," who said the agency should celebrate and close its doors, its mission at last accomplished. But 75 percent of the volunteers said that GMHC should remain in operation. One group said the agency should shift its focus to other pressing gay community issues, such as antigay violence and lesbian health concerns. Another group went even farther. Said Ouelette, "They saw GMHC as a place that could fix just about anything that was wrong with society. There would always be social problems, and the special kind of helping that went on at GMHC would have to continue." She noted that many people have been drawn to organizations like GMHC precisely because of the specialness of their work. "GMHC represents a very important kind of community in which help and caring and sharing goes on," she said. "A lot of straight folks get drawn to that, too." Ouelette added that while GMHC plays an important role in the gay community, "if there's any hope for us, it's establishing our identity but then being able to find some larger way that we're linked."[63]

AIDS caregiving has forged linkages among many who, had it not been for their concern about people with AIDS, were unlikely to have met—let alone worked, struggled, and wept together. The result has been a level of solidarity that, before AIDS, gay people never had with one another, let alone with heterosexuals. Their involvement in caring for people with AIDS politically galvanized many bereaved parents, concerned coworkers, and huge numbers of gay men and lesbians. They saw firsthand the correlation between the hostility of antigay politicians and the struggle to provide compassionate care for people with AIDS. Demagogues like Senator Jesse Helms continued to retch out one diatribe after another against the "deliberate, disgusting, revolting conduct" Helms said led to AIDS, typically doing so in the name of their twisted versions of morality and a vengeful god.

AIDS caregivers, on the other hand, offered love. Not the mushy, sentimental kind glamorized in fairy tales and soap operas, but love based on an understanding of shared humanity, that seeks through acts of mercy to cushion the blow of mortality that eventually strikes us all down. Beginning with those who have HIV or AIDS themselves, and radiating outward to include lovers, friends, family members, neighbors, and coworkers, the "troops" of caring Americans who have worked and volunteered to provide AIDS services in communities across the country have supported the dignity and prolonged the lives of those with the disease. In doing so, these "wounded healers" have discovered a richness of life that can't be bought and that not even bigots like Helms can steal.

While those caring for people with AIDS found new richness in their lives, others working to help gay men adopt safer behaviors faced an even more daunting challenge than right-wing bigotry: helping gay men to love and respect themselves and one another enough to prevent AIDS from spreading in the community. Not even the "love in action" of AIDS volunteers would be sufficient to prevent many men from endangering themselves and others in risky behavior. Gay men would ultimately have to find their own way of being safe and sexual at the same time. In doing so, they would find themselves engaged in some of the fiercest battles—psychological, social, and political—ever to be waged in the war against AIDS.

4

SAFETY DANCE

One moment of passion, one lapse of concentration, a second out of consciousness, an instant of ecstasy and it's done.

HARVEY FIERSTEIN, *SAFE SEX*

The devotion to sexual "freedom" of the seventies refused to die even as AIDS killed increasing numbers of gay men in the eighties. As gay America was devastated, gay men looked to the new AIDS organizations for direction, trusting them to filter information from government scientists through a gay-friendly screen. "Safe sex" became a kind of religion, and prevention educators its "priests," arbiters of gay community values and molders of gay men's psyches and sex drives. Decreeing safe sex to be the new community "norm," and shaming those who strayed from it, educators believed they could stop the epidemic. Astonishing numbers of gay men changed their behavior, and the rate of new HIV infections slowed in the community. The U.S. Public Health Service could claim little credit for the change, mired as its own prevention efforts were in conservative Republican politics that viewed helping gay men survive as "promoting" homosexuality.

When news surfaced that some gay men, weary of being told how to have sex and now able to know whether or not they were infected, were having unprotected sex, they were once again condemned as sexual outlaws—by other gay men. Fortunately, a few people were willing to cut through the bombast to point out that, just maybe, gay men would have safe sex when they themselves felt safe, and, just maybe, homophobic bigots and useless federal prevention programs should be the target of the community's rage—not other gay men.

In the spring of 1983, Edmund White was fresh from a book tour promoting his latest novel, *A Boy's Own Story,* the tale of a troubled adolescent coming to grips with his homosexuality. Perhaps it was his absorption in the character he'd created that led White, in a June 1983 essay in *Mother Jones,* to celebrate the "adolescence" of "contemporary big-city gay life." He likened this gay subculture to the ancient royal courts of Japan and Versailles, where "participants can afford to behave as they please," and the wealthy enjoyed "the rapid succession of affairs, the scheming and intrigue, the scrambling after popularity, the dismissal of the solid future in favor of the shimmering present."

For White, like many other big-city white gay men, the guilt-free slide in and out of sexual liaisons, the assumption that all gay relationships are "open," and a seemingly innate ability to distinguish sex and love were what separated gay men from heterosexuals—as well as from "mere" homosexuals "whose lives follow straight conventions," as White dismissively put it in the essay. To the man who had surveyed the landscape of late nineteen-seventies gay life in *States of Desire* and was a cofounder of Gay Men's Health Crisis, the casual couplings that he and other affluent white gay men in New York and elsewhere drifted in and out of were just some of the trappings of a privileged life they took for granted. "Gays," wrote White, "not only consume expensive vacations, memberships in gyms and discos, cars, elegant furnishings, clothes, haircuts, theater tickets and records, they also consume each other." What's more, he asserted, "a uniform gay culture is being created: a standard look, with its emphasis on macho clothes and the heavily muscled body; and a uniform set of values, cheerfully hedonistic though recently imbued with a sense of responsibility to less fortunate members of the gay community."[1]

The title of White's essay, "Paradise Found," seemed, even at the time it was published, to redefine the word "irony" with its "let them eat cake" attitude toward the presumably less enlightened who might value something like commitment and fidelity—even as the latter-day guillotine was dropping on so many men like White. In fact, the irony of White's words in 1983 was palpable when a photograph of him appeared in the *New York Times Magazine* a decade later with the caption, "I'm HIV positive. I need your help." Was it the gay culture's cheerful hedonism or its sense of responsibility to less fortunate members to which he now appealed?

Looking to ancient history to rationalize modern promiscuity, White overlooked the best-known example of approved homosexual love: ancient Greece. But he had to ignore the Greeks because, as Gabriel Rotello notes in *Sexual Ecology,* "The Greeks may have accepted homosexuality, but they hardly condoned promiscuity. Immoderation and lack of restraint were among their chief horrors."[2]

Not all gay men in 1983 agreed with White that being gay implied being promiscuous. Many were in coupled relationships, and many of those relationships were monogamous as well. Others questioned the status quo of the urban gay ghetto, where promiscuity was an expected fact of gay life—and where casual sex with multiple partners was referred to as anything else but promiscuity because the word itself was viewed as tacky and "politically incorrect" among men such as White. Still others had already awakened to the fact that there was a fatal sexually transmitted disease epidemic underway, and that it had serious sexual and political ramifications.

In Boston the same month that White's essay was published, gay psychiatrist Marshall Forstein was one of a panel of speakers addressing several hundred gay people who had gathered at historic Faneuil Hall on June 16 for the city's first-ever forum on AIDS. Thirty Bostonians had been diagnosed with AIDS to that point; half were dead. Forstein recalls telling the audience that although sex should remain an important part of the lives of gay people, "we needed to use condoms, which we knew would protect us from viruses because it works with hepatitis and other STDs, and we also needed to make every effort not to curtail having sex, but change how we had sex." Then Forstein hit the group directly in the status quo. "For years we were giving each other diseases and saying it's no big deal," he told them. "But in fact people have died from these diseases. People with gonorrhea have lost use of their joints. People with syphilis have gone crazy. People with hepatitis have died at a rate of about 10 percent of those who get it."

Underlying Forstein's remarks was a fundamental question about the degree to which gay men's "internalized homophobia" affected their sexual relationships with other men. Was it love they were making, or an unconscious desire to harm? He wondered, "How much of our anger towards our position in the world was being acted out through our anger towards each other as men—so when we fucked somebody, we were experiencing rage as well as lust?" He says he wasn't saying gay people shouldn't be sexual and play by their own rules, "but that we needed to think about how we were going to handle the next few years—or some of us might live to see the devastation in our community that we would have brought on ourselves."[3]

While many gay men, like Edmund White, had transplanted themselves to the relative openness of the big cities to escape small towns and small minds, they often struggled between their own desire for love and acceptance by a special partner and the availability of guilt-free sex with any number of randy partners to be had virtually any time and any place. In *Decade*, his one-man play about the effects of the AIDS epidemic on ten different men, Bruce Ward movingly captures the ambivalence that so many men felt in the urban gay world at the dawning of the epidemic—torn between its free love and the enslaving loneliness that drove many of them to test their mortal limits in unchecked drug use and sexual abandon.

Ward's first character, Melvin, echoes White's own words, though he is more forthright about the ambivalence of an existence of one-night stands strung end to end. With Donna Summer's disco hit "I Feel Love" throbbing behind him to set the scene, Melvin says, "Sometimes that's all I want, just to lie there with a warm body next to mine." Equivocating about the man actually lying in bed next to him, Melvin continues, "We'll get dressed and maybe exchange numbers . . . but maybe not . . . and we'll say goodbye and maybe see each other again. But maybe not. And it'll be worth it. It'll all be worth it. 'Cause I am young and free and gay, and life is a fabulous ride into the unknown and I know I'll 'never pass this way again!' And maybe someday, someday soon, I'll want that body next to me to be the same one every night, to be there to come home to and to grow old together. But not now . . . 'Cuz there's time. Lots of time."[4]

But by mid-1983, the clock was already ticking on the community's—and the nation's—ability to stem the spread of AIDS. Many gay men were themselves like time bombs set to go off at some unknowable point in an explosion of horrific infections related to the mysterious new disease.

The same month that White's essay appeared, and that Boston held its first AIDS forum, gay health and political activists gathered in Denver for the Fifth National Lesbian and Gay Health Conference, with a second national forum on AIDS. Ginny Apuzzo and Pat Norman led a workshop that looked at blood banking, future relationships between public and private agencies, and the implications of AIDS being labeled a disease of the gay community and other disenfranchised groups. Other sessions in the AIDS forum considered such topics as the epidemiology of AIDS; the emotional impact on patients, care providers, and society at large; and a report on what would become known as the San Francisco "model" of coordinated AIDS services. Tim Westmoreland, chief counsel to the House Subcommittee on Health and the Environment, and gay health-care activist Lawrence "Bopper" Deyton were given "Health Pioneering in the Eighties" awards "for their lobbying and political research efforts in facilitating AIDS appropriations."

Now that basic support services were in place through the newly established AIDS organizations, gay people's attention turned increasingly to developing more systematic prevention efforts to replace the earlier ad hoc delivery of information (and conjecture) as it dribbled down from doctors and scientists. To that end, another workshop at the forum featured gay medical and mental health professionals from San Francisco, looking at "Creating Positive Changes in Sexual Mores." The conference program promised a session in which "Positive aspects of the gay male sexual revolution will be examined with implications of healthy sexual behavior in the context of the current AIDS/sexually transmitted disease crisis." Overall, the program's objective was "to initiate positive change towards attainable, safe and satisfying sexual behaviors for gay men."[5] Psychologist Steve Morin was one of the panelists for the "sexual mores" workshop in Denver.

Morin recalls how he and other gay health professionals in San Francisco developed the city's—and the nation's—first real "safe sex" guidelines for gay men. In 1982, Morin joined fellow psychologist Leon McKusick, who has since died from AIDS, in gathering data through questionnaires given to people coming out of bars, initially in the Castro and then some other sites. People responded to ads in newspapers, bathhouses, dance clubs, and by being "nominated" through networks of couples. The goal was to determine how people were changing or reacting to news as it became available.

Around the same time, the K.S. Foundation began to formulate its official "message." Morin, who participated in discussions at the foundation and the city's public health department, says, "We had a somewhat different view, I think, in San Francisco than in a lot of other places in the country, at least among the gay community leadership. We were more willing to put out there to people that this was probably an infectious disease and that you could get it with one sexual contact."[6] Morin helped to develop safe sex materials for distribution by the Bay Area Physicians for Human Rights (BAPHR) and the K.S. Foundation.

Operating on the assumption that whatever caused AIDS was likely to be spread in the same ways as hepatitis B, Morin and BAPHR officials Rob Bolan and Tom Smith categorized sexual activities into safe, possibly safe, and unsafe practices. As defined by BAPHR—"safe sex" includes mutual masturbation, social kissing, body massage and hugging, body-to-body rubbing, "light S&M activities," and using one's own sex toys. "Possibly safe" practices include anal intercourse with a condom, "fellatio interruptus," mouth-to-mouth kissing, urine contact, vaginal intercourse with a condom, and oral-vaginal contact. "Unsafe sex" practices include receptive and insertive anal intercourse without a condom, "manual-anal" intercourse, fellatio, oral-anal contact, and vaginal intercourse without a condom.[7]

In New York, GMHC persisted in telling gay men simply to limit their number of sexual partners and make sure their partners were "healthy"—a message the K.S. Foundation also had issued in 1982, before the BAPHR guidelines. GMHC didn't want to offend gay men by presuming to tell them anything about specific sexual practices. While San Franciscans had moved on to the soon-to-be-proven assumption that the cause of AIDS was probably an infectious agent, New Yorkers took the attitude that, unless they could present irrefutable evidence, they couldn't expect gay men to listen. Rodger McFarlane, who became GMHC's executive director in the same month as the Denver conference was held, told me, "We were all taking the same fucking drugs, sitting in the same bathhouses, sprayed by the same mosquito sprays in the same resorts. How dare you suggest we knew it was infectious." Without that certain knowledge, McFarlane argued that GMHC couldn't have done prevention programs any earlier. But his memory blurred and his argument faltered when he downplayed GMHC's leading role in the community. "I defy you to suggest that GMHC was as influential or responsible as the CDC," he said.[8]

McFarlane failed to mention that gay men *did* look to GMHC, and to the gay press, for information about AIDS. In fact, one of the main reasons for GMHC's formation—as it was for the San Francisco AIDS Foundation and the other earliest AIDS organizations formed by gay people—was to disseminate information to the gay community. As Larry Kramer put it, "[GMHC] was not founded to help those who are ill. It was founded to protect the living, to help the living go on living, to help those who are still healthy to stay healthy, to help gay men stay alive."[9] Gay men looked to these organizations for the "truth" about AIDS. The CDC, like the rest of the government and medical establishment, was seen as just another oppressor. In fact, in the earliest years of the epidemic, gay and AIDS groups throughout the country—and in other countries—looked particularly to GMHC and the San Francisco AIDS Foundation for guidance on how to approach the AIDS crisis. The AIDS educational materials developed by the two groups were widely circulated and highly influential in gay communities across the nation and, literally, around the world.

Like the disagreement between the New Yorkers and San Franciscans over what, exactly, was safe sex, the gay community's earliest efforts to translate scientific information about AIDS into educational messages for gay men were pulled in two directions. Some believed that whatever was said had to be couched in "sex-positive" language, while others believed that the only way that gay men would change their behavior was if they were scared enough to do so. In late 1983, the San Francisco AIDS Foundation produced a poster depicting two naked men embracing, with the caption "You Can Have Fun and Be Safe Too." Respectful of gay men who had heard all their lives that they were "sick" for loving other men, the poster was explicit and positive, yet subtle, in its message—and caused an uproar among nongay San Franciscans.[10]

Another group in San Francisco believed that a fear-based campaign was needed to discourage gay men from having sex at all. Their materials depicted an hourglass with blood-colored sand pouring into the bottom, with the slogan "Time Is Running Out." One of the earliest AIDS posters in San Francisco was nothing more than a blown-up color photograph of the Kaposi's sarcoma lesions on the foot of early AIDS patient Bobbi Campbell. It was simple and bone-chilling in its directness and horror.

Ultimately, the AIDS Foundation took a middle course, adopting the slogan "The Best Defense Against AIDS Is Information."[11] Give men enough information, it reasoned, and they would make not merely well-informed, but life-saving decisions. Still, the public health and marketing professionals working with the foundation to design its first prevention campaigns faced a daunting challenge in a community whose members largely thought the best defense against AIDS was the denial of its reality.

A November 1983 survey of 650 gay men in San Francisco found that even men who were well informed about the relative risks of various sexual activities "displayed discrepancies between what they believed about AIDS and their sexual behavior." The survey found an increase in the rate of unprotected receptive anal intercourse, despite its being considered, even at the time, to have the highest risk. Sixty-nine percent of the men surveyed who had three or more sexual partners in the previous month agreed with the statement, "It is hard to change my sexual behavior because being gay means doing what I want sexually." On the other hand, 43 percent of those reporting two or fewer partners agreed with the statement, "I can recall seeing a victim in the advanced stages of AIDS." Clearly, firsthand experience with AIDS was highly effective in making men change their sexual habits to protect themselves. Leon McCusick and his fellow researchers concluded that other motivational strategies would be needed beyond merely providing information. "Sexual behavior," they wrote, "may be comparable to other high-risk behaviors such as tobacco smoking, obesity, non-seat belt use, and alcohol consumption, where knowledge alone is not sufficient to change behavior."[12]

Not long after the discovery of the AIDS virus was announced in the spring of 1984, the AIDS Foundation developed the first plan anywhere for a systematic strategy to assess and, it hoped, alter the high-risk sexual behavior of gay men on a large scale in San Francisco. The Comprehensive AIDS Education and Prevention Plan, written by consultant Sam Puckett, aimed to raise awareness of the close relationship between alcohol, drug abuse, and unsafe sex; the decrease in unsafe sex practices; and the continuing drop in the city's rate of rectal gonorrhea—considered a proxy for AIDS risk. With a view toward the future, the plan also sought to provide research data on which to base future AIDS prevention campaigns. The plan committed the AIDS Foundation to being sex-positive, promising to operate "on the conviction (despite some evidence from the past to the contrary) that gay and bisexual men fundamentally want to be healthy and productive, want to live, and want to deal responsibly with the AIDS issue as rational, intelligent adults."

The cornerstone of the plan, which was funded by the San Francisco Department of Public Health, was a city-wide random sample telephone survey of five hundred gay and bisexual men. Besides providing the city's first-ever demographic profile of gay male residents, the thirty-minute telephone interviews were intended to assess the men's risk behaviors and the attitudes that influenced those behaviors. A follow-up survey would measure behavior change. In addition, the AIDS Foundation conducted four small focus groups that sampled the attitudes about AIDS and sexual activities of forty randomly chosen gay men. Largely because of these early focus groups in San Francisco, the involvement of community members in the design of prevention campaigns would become another central tenet of prevention efforts nationwide.

Focus group participants reported reductions in the number of their sex partners along with attempts to select partners who were perceived as healthy and not promiscuous—just as they'd been advised to do by the AIDS Foundation. They said that they relied on the gay press and other community sources for information about the AIDS crisis. Although the men had considerable awareness of what was thought to be safe and unsafe, most of them were willing to eliminate the unsafe practices that didn't interest them—but were not willing to give up their own favorite sexual activity, even if it was considered unsafe. In addition to a high level of concern about the political implications of the AIDS crisis for the gay community, the men also felt that AIDS could have the unexpected positive effect of improving the quality of gay relationships by fostering more monogamy, intimacy, and closeness in sexual relationships.[13]

Armed with an unprecedented knowledge of gay men and their sexual behavior, the AIDS Foundation used a multifaceted "hybrid" strategy to saturate the city of San Francisco with information about AIDS and how to avoid it. Jackson Peyton, the foundation's director of education from 1984 to 1987, calls this period the "golden age of prevention."[14] Innovative programs were created, and Peyton was given a fairly large budget with which to provide AIDS education to gay men. The AIDS hotline provided callers with information and referrals. A People with AIDS Switchboard offered recently diagnosed individuals a place to talk with others in the same situation. Ads in the initially resistant gay press told gay men, "Let's stop making excuses. Let's stop the spread of AIDS." Brochures were designed to reach various subsections of the community. Condoms were distributed. Educational events, from small gatherings of a few men to large public forums, were routinely held. And the AIDS Foundation and other AIDS-related organizations established a presence at the city's street fairs and the annual Lesbian and Gay Freedom Day Parade.

While the AIDS Foundation's focus groups originally were intended simply to provide a marketing research base for the agency's education program, the men who participated in them got a great deal out of them as well. For many of them, this was the first time they'd had a chance to talk with other gay men about the growing epidemic, to feel they weren't alone in facing its horrors or in their struggles to change their sexual behavior. The Stop AIDS Project emerged in 1984 from the original AIDS Foundation focus groups and the interest of gay men in having additional programs. Stop AIDS recruited gay men throughout the city to participate in one-time, four-hour meetings in which they discussed everything from what AIDS meant for them personally, to the challenges of safe sex, to what kind of gay community they envisioned in the future and how they could help make it a reality. Finally, the men were asked to pledge themselves—and to support one another—to practicing safe sex as their contribution toward stopping the AIDS epidemic.

Researchers in 1984 in other cities also began to gather information about gay men and their sexual habits that had never before been available. In New York, for example, psychologist John Martin and his research partner Laura Dean, began studying the impact of AIDS on gay men's sexual behavior. Bruce Ward was living in New York at the time and worked with Martin and Dean as they interviewed 745 gay men. Ward recalls, "The first summer was really draining because people were freaking out. I was taking that in as an interviewer, and it was really affecting me."[15] The interviews revealed that kissing had declined by 48 percent, oral sex by more than 60 percent. Anal intercourse of any kind had declined by more than 75 percent. They also found that the men seemed to be having more sex, but with fewer partners—and more often at home than in places like bathhouses or backroom bars.[16]

As with the focus groups in San Francisco, one of the unexpected effects of recruiting gay men for research studies was that the men who participated in them discovered a heightened political awareness of what it meant to be gay in America at a time when their own government seemed to be doing all it could to ignore the growing epidemic. Beginning in 1984, the Multicenter AIDS Cohort Study (MACS) recruited gay men in Baltimore, Chicago, Los Angeles, and Pittsburgh to participate in the largest (4,950 men) longitudinal study of gay men in the AIDS epidemic. MACS was a biomedical study of the natural history of AIDS, funded by the National Institute of Allergy and Infectious Diseases. Men were recruited through gay publications, clinics, college campuses, gay organizations, and in bars.

When Curt Decker was asked by a doctor from Johns Hopkins University to help recruit twelve hundred gay men for the MACS in Baltimore, Decker, a well-known member of the Baltimore community, recalls saying, "I don't even know if there are twelve hundred gay men in Baltimore! But no way are we going to get twelve hundred men in this blue collar, closeted city to come forward and pour out all their most intimate details about sex, drugs, and alcohol use." Decker described his efforts to recruit gay men for the MACS at the Hippo, a popular dance bar, asking them to stop the music so he could talk to the crowd. "We were practically stoned," he said. "People said, 'Don't bring us down, we're out here having a good time, don't talk about AIDS.'" The next step was to offer door prizes if participants would commit to making all the required visits to the clinic each year for the expected four years of the study.

As it turned out, the prizes and other enticements weren't needed, and the study continued for more than a decade afterward. Decker, who is a lobbyist in Washington, said, "What I discovered is that as we got people to show up, it was a very politicizing kind of experience. One thing I liked about the MACS study so much—apart from my involvement in research—is that I thought it was a very political statement."[17]

At first, men would go into the clinic for their MACS visit and give blood, feces, urine, semen—and toenails, because the epidemiologist felt that a lot of the body's minerals end up in the toenails, making them a good source of "information" about someone's health. When an antibody test finally became available, in March 1985, there was no further need for toenails or bodily fluids other than blood. In fact, the MACS already had three blood samples from each man in the study. Now it was possible to know who was and was not infected, and who had seroconverted since the beginning of the study. Thirty-one percent of the participants in Baltimore were already HIV-positive. Altogether in the four MACS cities, 1,809 men of the original 4,954—nearly one in three—were HIV-positive at "baseline."[18]

The Enzyme-Linked Immunosorbent Assay (ELISA), the first antibody test, initially was intended to screen the blood supply, rather than to be used as a diagnostic test for individuals. While it provided information about whether or not someone had been exposed to the virus, no one knew what, exactly, exposure to the virus and the presence of antibodies meant. Moreover, no one knew how the information provided by the test might be used. Fearing yet further—and even more consequential—"bad blood" stigma, gay rights and AIDS groups warned gay men not to be tested. No one knew at the time whether a positive test meant that one would actually develop AIDS, or that he was already immune. There were no real treatments even if a positive test did prove to mean an ongoing infection. And there was the very real chance that an already hysterical public would insist that draconian measures be taken against those with antibodies in their blood.

At the first international AIDS conference, in Atlanta in April 1985, a small but vocal minority of researchers advocated mass testing of at-risk individuals as an educational technique. Former CDC official Don Francis says that he personally thought it was inevitable that mass testing would become part of the total AIDS prevention picture. Breaking ranks with other gay leaders, former National Gay Task Force codirector Bruce Voeller also advocated mass testing as part of the educational program for gay men at risk for AIDS. From his own experience, he claimed that gay men would change their sexual behavior if confronted with a positive test.[19] "Take the Test!," he urged gay men in the *Advocate*.[20] Despite the warnings of gay leaders, many people did take the test. The *Washington Post* noted that at the Whitman-Walker Clinic in the late summer of 1985, "since recent publicity about AIDS, including the news that actor Rock Hudson has the disease, the clinic's Wednesday night screening sessions have been filled to their fifty-person capacity."

But in San Francisco, where homosexuals had long understood the inextricable link between the personal and political aspects of their lives, gay men by and large avoided the test. Although they had expressed interest in a hypothetical test, Steve Morin said at the time, "As the test became a reality, the psychological conflicts became more real."[21] That no one knew the real meaning or significance of the test, and that the AIDS Foundation warned not to take it, were reasons enough for many gay men in the gayest city in the country to ignore it—thus delaying the day of reckoning for the nearly 50 percent of all gay men in San Francisco alone who would eventually learn they were infected with the virus.[22]

As the gay community sounded alarms over the potential uses and abuses of the antibody test, the Defense Department on October 24, 1985, ordered the beginning of what would be the largest AIDS screening program in the world. All recruits were to be tested, and positives would be refused entry to the armed services. Those already in the military who tested positive on the mandatory periodic tests would be discharged.[23] A military long obsessed with ousting homosexuals from its ranks seemed, to some anyway, to have found the kind of marker for homosexuality that had never been found among the gay men who had served in the U.S. military since there was a military to serve in—these men were mostly undetected because they were, for all intents and purposes, indistinguishable from everyone else.

It wouldn't be until 1989, four years after the test became available, that GMHC finally advocated HIV testing and many more gay men learned their antibody status. But by 1987, researchers were reporting vast reductions in the number of new HIV infections among gay men in the hardest-hit cities. In New York, the rate of rectal gonorrhea dropped by nearly 80 percent between 1983 and 1986.[24] And in San Francisco, the rate of HIV infection among gay men remained stable at about 50 percent. But new infections had decreased from an estimated 18.4 percent per year between 1982 and 1984, to only 4.2 percent by the first six months of 1986. The number of reported cases of rectal gonorrhea in the city had plunged from nearly three hundred in 1982 to less than fifty.[25] The CDC noted that these declines coincided "with the period of heightened awareness and concern about the incidence of acquired immune deficiency syndrome among homosexual males."[26]

It was described as the greatest behavior change ever seen in public health. "Education has been a dazzling success with homosexuals," proclaimed *U.S. News & World Report.*[27] It seemed the gay community had managed to get AIDS under control, gay men had modified their high-risk behavior to avoid transmission of the virus, and the community could get back to the business of gay liberation. Riding this wave of optimism, San Francisco's Stop AIDS Project closed its doors in 1987. It seemed gay men "got it," that they knew what they needed to do and not do in order to protect themselves and one another. Not only were the STD rates down and gay men reporting less risk behavior overall, but they seemed in general to be having less sex. Prevention educators congratulated themselves for stemming the tide of infection and reshaping gay community sexual norms.

But safe sex wasn't the only reason for the drop in HIV and other STD infections. Some men became celibate because of a consuming fear of AIDS bordering on pathology. "Jack," for example, described in a *Newsweek* article in early 1986 as "a twenty-nine-year-old gay artist in Chicago," told the magazine that he had practically become a recluse. An experience with another man, who had AIDS but didn't tell him, left him frightened and cynical. "I told him it was the end of my innocence because from now on I'm not going to trust anybody," said Jack. Now he stayed home, night after night. "Basically," he said, "I make love to my VCR a lot."[28]

Despite the reports from the hard-hit cities, it is safe to say that most gay men at this point were indeed still having sex, a good deal of it unsafe. If big-city homosexuals had changed their behavior, it could be attributed to their having access to the messages put out by AIDS organizations and a strong chance of personally knowing someone who had the disease. This was not the case for their brothers in smaller towns and rural areas. The first of the many so-called "second waves" of the AIDS epidemic was already rolling in to shore as gay men outside the major coastal cities ignored the epidemic and partied on. In New Mexico, for example, a 1987 study reported that 20 percent of a group of 166 gay men were already HIV-positive. Seventy percent of them reported practicing receptive anal intercourse in the past twelve months, and only 13 percent used condoms. A history of having had sexual partners outside of New Mexico was correlated to an increased risk for seropositivity.[29]

The intermingling of gay men in the major cities—men from small towns frequently visit or move to cities like New York or San Francisco—meant it was inevitable that HIV would spread from the coastal cities, where it first appeared, to the heartlands. In the major coastal cities themselves constant influxes of gay men—many of them becoming sexually active for the first time—meant that community efforts to create social norms that supported safe sex were undermined by the very mobility that brought so many gay men to the cities in the first place. As Daniel Wohlfeiler, the Stop AIDS Project's education director, put it, "In 1987, the day the Project shut, there was a community norm that favored safe sex. But that norm is only as durable as the community is static." As he pointed out, San Francisco is anything but static: In 1987, upwards of a third of the gay men in the city had lived there less than two years. Said Wohlfeiler, "The norm is obviously not going to withstand that kind of transience."[30]

Clearly it was going to take more than brochures, posters, and workshops to make gay men alter their entrenched sexual habits. As Leon McCusick had pointed out in 1983, knowledge alone isn't enough to make people change behavior they enjoy, even if they know its potential risks. By the time Stop AIDS closed, Jackson Peyton was gone from his three-year stint as education director for the AIDS Foundation. What he called the "golden age" of prevention ended with the realization that safe sex had not become quite as "normal" as educators believed and that the epidemic was not going to end in the foreseeable future. Said Peyton, "I truly don't believe that anybody thought this was going to be a 'rest of our lives' kind of thing until about 1990."

That's the year the Stop AIDS Project reopened, this time with no set closing date.

*

In 1984, CDC teams surveyed the AIDS prevention efforts in nine different cities: Atlanta, Chicago, Houston, Los Angeles, Miami, Newark, N.J., New York, San Francisco, and Washington, D.C. They found that San Francisco alone had the kind of collaboration between the public health department and community-based AIDS groups that was deemed essential if prevention education was to succeed. The teams concluded that the "translation" of scientific information into usable, understandable prevention messages required "graphic language to provide explicit advice about sexual behaviors or needle sharing." They added that to be successful in reaching a particular population, prevention efforts "must be appropriate for and responsive to the lifestyle, language, and environment of the members of that population."[31]

Despite the recommendations, a 1985 report by the congressional Office of Technology Assessment faulted the federal government's inadequate attention to AIDS prevention education. The OTA noted that it had been mostly left to those at greatest risk—gay men and injection drug users—to educate themselves. This made a certain amount of sense, until one realized that those groups, particularly drug users, had neither the financial nor scientific resources on their own to conduct the kind of massive national prevention campaigns it would take to prevent the spread of AIDS. The OTA report said that the government had shirked its responsibility at least partly because providing advice on preventive sex practices might be viewed as "condoning the lifestyles" of homosexuals.[32]

Conservative Reaganites weren't the only ones in the government obstructing efforts to do anything useful to prevent the spread of AIDS. Dr. David Sundwall, described in *Mother Jones* as "a clean-cut Mormon physician," was the physician adviser to the Senate Committee on Labor and Human Resources before becoming the administrator of the Health Resources and Services Administration. In early 1985, Sundwall described memos that had been issued from some Republican committee members' offices. "I don't want to name names," he said, "but I can tell you that the most blatant kind of homophobia possible is indicated in these memos. Very judgmental, very negative statements questioning whether the government should play any role whatsoever in [stopping the disease]—it's probably God's wrath and so be it."[33]

To avoid scrutiny of its prevention funding by the radical right and its supporters in the White House and on Capitol Hill, CDC in 1985 funneled seed money to community-based organizations through the U.S. Conference of Mayors. The USCM at the time represented about 860 cities, which accounted for 90 percent of the nation's reported AIDS cases. The organizations funded by USCM were required to collaborate with state and local public health departments, and to generate community cooperation and support for AIDS prevention activities—a dubious prospect for prevention efforts targeting gay men, in view of the antigay attitudes even among the nation's elected leaders.

Alan Gambrell, who in January 1985 became the first full-time staffer in USCM's AIDS program, recalls that one early prevention effort supported by USCM with CDC funds was a safe-sex brochure developed by AID Atlanta, a gay community-based AIDS organization in the CDC's own hometown. When an article about the brochure appeared in USCM's newsletter, Gambrell said there was "some negative feedback from a small number of mayors," including the resignation from USCM of one mayor of a small Texas city. Gambrell also noted that there were already "rumblings" from anti-gay North Carolina Senator Jesse Helms about the content of educational materials directed at gay men.[34]

From June 4 to 6, 1986, some eighty-five clinicians, epidemiologists, public health policy-makers, and basic research scientists gathered at the Coolfont Conference Center in Berkeley Springs, West

Virginia. Convened by the Public Health Service, their task was to review the government's plan for preventing the spread of AIDS by the year 2000. At that point, there were already 20,517 AIDS cases reported in the United States. By the end of 1991, the group estimated, upwards of 30 percent of the one million to one-and-a-half million Americans believed to be infected with HIV would develop AIDS, bringing the cumulative death toll to more than 179,000. More than 70 percent of the cases would be diagnosed among gay and bisexual men, they predicted, though increases in AIDS among heterosexuals were "likely." They didn't expect a possible vaccine for at least a decade, despite HHS Secretary Margaret Heckler's promise two years earlier of a vaccine within two years.

"In the absence of a vaccine and therapy," noted the Coolfont Report, "prevention and control of HTLV–III/LAV infection depends largely upon effective approaches to decrease sexual transmission, transmission among IV drug users, and perinatal transmission from infected mothers." The report went on to say, "National information and education campaigns on AIDS and HTLV–III/LAV infection should be targeted to individuals and groups whose behavior places them at high risk for AIDS, other sexually active adults, adolescents, preadolescents, and health care providers." Further, it recommended, "With the assistance of appropriate organizations, programs should be implemented to provide culturally sensitive, meaningful information and education to blacks and Hispanics, including homosexuals."[35]

The news from Coolfont was overshadowed by a Justice Department legal opinion on June 23, 1986. Attorney General Edwin Meese determined that an employer could legally fire employees with AIDS—or even those perceived as having the disease—if other employees feared "catching" it. A week after Justice's decision, the Supreme Court issued a crushing blow to the gay civil rights movement in the landmark case *Bowers v. Hardwick.* In a five-to-four majority, the Court ruled that gay people were not constitutionally entitled to privacy and could be prosecuted for making love in their own bedrooms. As Lisa Keen noted in the *Washington Blade* on the tenth anniversary of the decision, "The *Hardwick* decision was used to impeach every gay person's character, whether they engaged in sodomy or not and in areas that had nothing to do with oral and anal sex at all. Its impact, like that of sodomy laws themselves, delivered both a powerful quake and a more devastating series of aftershocks."[36]

In New York, the Justice Department and Supreme Court decisions couldn't have come at a more ironic time. In March, fifteen years after it was introduced, the New York City Council finally passed an ordinance to protect gay people against discrimination in jobs and housing. Mayor Koch told reporters, "The sky is not going to fall. There isn't going to be any dramatic change in the life of this city."[37] For gay New Yorkers, though, merely knowing they had legal recourse in the event they were discriminated against was a tremendous change and a great improvement in the city's quality of life.

Arnie Kantrowitz celebrated the adoption of the new ordinance he and other members of Gay Activists Alliance first lobbied for in 1971. Kantrowitz thought the measure's passage by a vote of 21 to 14 was due to the growing awareness of the public and politicians of who gay people really were as they rallied in response to, and died in incredible numbers from, AIDS. Kantrowitz observed, "Possibly some of the attacks on the ailing gay community had generated enough sympathy to gather the required votes, but most of it was politics."[38]

Two major reports in late 1986 echoed the recommendations from Coolfont. In his unexpectedly forthright report, Surgeon General C. Everett Koop said, "We can no longer afford to sidestep frank, open discussions about sexual practices—homosexual and heterosexual."[39] And the prestigious Institute of Medicine, part of the National Academy of Sciences, noted in its own report, *Confronting AIDS*, "The present level of AIDS-related education is woefully inadequate." The panel of prominent researchers and clinicians who developed the report observed that "in general the only efforts with any claim to success have been those conducted by homosexuals through voluntary activist organizations."[40]

In October, the federal government mailed a brochure called *Understanding AIDS* to every American household, offering less explicit information about AIDS and how to prevent it than Americans could get from their daily newspapers at that point. Meanwhile, President Reagan that month suggested at a White House meeting that Libyan dictator Moamar Gadhafi, rumored to enjoy dressing in drag, should be sent to San Francisco because "he likes to dress up so much." Secretary of State George Shultz diplomatically added, "Why don't we give him AIDS?" As fear gripped the nation, and although thousands of Americans were dead from AIDS, the epidemic was treated as a sick joke at the White House.[41]

Despite the recommendations of the nation's leading medical and public health experts in the three major reports in 1986, the CDC that very year went berserk after Gay Men's Health Crisis allegedly used federal funding to produce a video that presented explicit gay sex—albeit with condoms—as part of the agency's prevention program. GMHC considered the video to be precisely the kind of "targeted, explicit" educational tool it needed, and that CDC would support, to reach gay men. Gay men presumably would understand the safe-sex message the video conveyed, and emulate what it depicted in their own sex lives. Its use of familiar language provided a safe-sex vocabulary that GMHC hoped would prove useful in real-life sexual negotiations. As social worker Michael Shernoff put it, "For safer sex education to go on, you have to have it happen in a context that's recognizable to the people who are involved. People are more likely to talk about 'dicks' and 'cum,' as opposed to 'penis' and 'semen.' I don't know anyone who thinks about sex as 'anal intercourse' except the doctor—and he's not the one getting fucked."[42]

CDC prohibited the further development of explicit, "offensive" materials, and required that anyone getting funding to produce HIV prevention materials had to establish local review panels to screen the materials.[43] This requirement was precisely what the Institute of Medicine advised against when it said it was "concerned about the Centers for Disease Control directive that empanels local review boards to determine whether materials developed for AIDS education are too explicit and in violation of local community standards"—what it called "the 'dirty words' issue."[44] Such oversight panels meant that prevention targeted at gay men would have to pass muster with the nongay people who would participate in these review panels. It didn't take genius to see the direction this would take.

Despite the gutting of anything like effective prevention, Health and Human Services Secretary Otis Bowen said he would be "disappointed" if public education efforts were not effective within a year.

As *Newsweek* noted, "The bottom line: the Reagan administration, like most Americans, is betting on a scientific breakthrough to deliver America from the epidemic."[45] But Reagan's sentimental rhetoric about its being "morning in America" aside, his pandering to the far right, combined with his evisceration of the nation's health and scientific research institutions meant that even America's world-renowned scientists couldn't prevent the encroaching darkness as the shadow of AIDS moved across the land.

"Federal prevention programs have been in almost total disarray the last few years," said AIDS Action Council director Gary Mac-Donald, in a lengthy *U.S. News & World Report* article in January 1987. While the Institute of Medicine report had recommended that the federal government increase its AIDS funding by five times—to $2 billion in fiscal 1990, with money divided equally between education and research—less than one-quarter of the government's funds went to prevention at the time of the report's release. The Reagan administration saw no need to increase its funding for prevention for this particular disease. Ken South, then the director of AID Atlanta, the group that had received $12,500 from the CDC through the U.S. Conference of Mayors, noted that the meager amount of funding the agency received had come with a mandate "to change the most intimate behavior of one hundred thousand people at risk." As South put it, "We're trying to put out a forest fire with a water pistol."[46]

At the CDC itself, Don Francis was thwarted at every turn in his efforts to get the government to provide serious prevention education. His requests for additional funding were repeatedly turned down. Francis told me, "I was in Atlanta, sandwiched between CDC's philosophy of aggressive public health and the Reagan Administration. And I was literally told, when I made the first plan for HIV prevention for the U.S., for $37 million—a small amount of money—that we couldn't afford that, and to 'look like you're doing something, but we can't get into that prevention stuff for this disease.'"[47]

Even in the mid-nineties, Francis's blood still boiled the way it did when he testified before a congressional committee on March 16, 1987, saying, "Much of the HIV/AIDS epidemic was and continues to be preventable. But because of active obstruction of logical policy, active resistance to essential funding, and active interference with scientifically designed programs, the executive branch of this country has caused untold hardship, misery, and expense to the American public. Its effort with AIDS will stand as a huge scar in American history, a shame to our nation and an international disgrace."[48]

As if to underscore Francis's point, President Reagan finally delivered his first speech on AIDS two months after that hearing—six years into the epidemic. He called for "routine" HIV testing of certain groups, including immigrants, federal prisoners, and applicants for marriage licenses. Despite the recommendations from Coolfont, the Institute of Medicine, and his own surgeon general, Reagan saw widespread testing as the answer to the nation's utter lack of a concerted AIDS prevention program. The *New York Times* said, "Mr. Reagan's Administration has been slow to respond to the AIDS epidemic, yet its first thought is to compel testing. That is inconsistent with what public health officials advise and with the compassion evident in Mr. Reagan's words."[49]

Compassion was not a quality usually associated with the Reagan administration when it came to AIDS (or much else). It would prove to be in even shorter supply—with rational thinking scarcer still—when Republican Senator Jesse Helms delivered a diatribe that will go down in history as one of the most hate-filled, yet amazingly persuasive, speeches ever delivered in the U.S. Senate. A mere three days after an estimated 650,000 gay people and their supporters participated in the second National March on Washington for Gay and Lesbian Rights, and the premiere display of the AIDS Memorial Quilt, Helms took to the Senate floor on October 14, 1987, waving a copy of GMHC's "Safe Sex Comix." He threatened to "throw up" after viewing the booklets and video, which illustrated safe-sex techniques for gay men. GMHC had developed the materials based on a study of eight hundred gay men, which found that frank, explicit prevention information worked best for gay men—just as the CDC and all those official reports had recommended.

But Helms, never one to miss an opportunity to show his bigoted ignorance, claimed the materials had been funded by taxpayer dollars, and condemned them as "pornographic." Rather than protecting the lives of gay men, as the materials were intended to do, the senator said they merely promoted "safe sodomy." Helms succeeded in convincing ninety-eight of the Senate's one hundred members to support his amendment to the Labor, Health and Human Services and Education Appropriation Bill. The amendment prohibited the use of federal funds for any AIDS educational materials that "promote or encourage, directly or indirectly, homosexual sexual activities."

Senators Ted Kennedy and Alan Cranston were the only ones to oppose Helms. Kennedy successfully reworded the amendment in committee so it would disallow the promotion of sexuality in general, rather than homosexuality in particular. But the damage was already done. For Helms, talking about homosexuality was tantamount to promoting it. Gay activists naturally dubbed the Helms amendment "No Promo Homo." But how could anyone possibly talk about protection against a deadly sexually transmitted disease without talking about sex? About a disease largely affecting homosexuals without talking about homosexual sex?

As if it hadn't been made all too clear all too many times in the epidemic, the fallout from the Helms amendment meant that if gay men were going to be educated about protecting themselves, the gay community would have to do the job itself. Although homosexual Americans pay taxes like everyone else, it became apparent in 1987 that they would also have to pay for their own AIDS education if they hoped to stem the tide of new HIV infections among the nation's hardest-hit group. That is to say that a subcommunity, totaling at best 10 percent of the population, would be expected to carry the burden of fighting the greatest health threat of the century in the wealthiest, most medically sophisticated nation on earth.

*

Still hoping to look as though it had the AIDS epidemic under control, the CDC, through the U.S. Conference of Mayors, began in 1987 to award HIV education and prevention funds almost exclusively to community-based racial and ethnic minority organizations.[50] In what would define CDC's skewed approach to AIDS education for people of color, a report on the new efforts targeting minorities said, "Although homosexual and bisexual contact is a major mode of HIV transmission among blacks and Hispanics, intravenous drug use and heterosexual contact are more prevalent modes of transmission for them than for whites."[51] While it noted correctly that "70 percent of heterosexuals, and 70 percent of women, and 75 percent of children [with AIDS] are black or Hispanic," the report failed to mention that the number of gay and bisexual men with AIDS in the country's minority communities far surpassed the number of heterosexuals, women, and children with the disease.

There was an odd assumption on everyone's part that somehow intravenous drug users were all black or Hispanic, and that all homosexuals were white. By not challenging this assumption, countless gay men of color were sacrificed in order to placate the homophobes—only this time the skin color of those homophobes was darker than that of Jesse Helms.

At a 1988 conference organized by the Department of Health and Human Services to shape a prevention agenda for minority communities, black, Hispanic, Native American, and Asian/Pacific Islander caucuses defined what they felt were the major considerations for prevention education in their respective communities. The report from the black caucus in particular was permeated with fear that African-Americans would be "blamed" for the AIDS epidemic because of its suspected origins in Africa, and by the paranoid belief that blacks had been targeted for genocide by research scientists who "have exposed the race to a deadly 'Andromeda Strain.'" Of course gay men had their own conspiracy theories early in the epidemic. Reading the caucus report, though, one wouldn't know that homosexuality even existed in the black community—or that black gay and bisexual men accounted for most of the community's AIDS cases—as neither fact is ever mentioned.

The caucus said "the black community" was resolved "to look to our black clergy and church for absolute assurance that CDC national AIDS testing and counseling initiatives are not just another Tuskegee tragedy being perpetrated on the black race." The group feared, not altogether irrationally, a repeat of the infamous government-sponsored syphilis studies that, in a page from the Nazis' own playbook, had allowed black men in Alabama to remain untreated as a means of observing the course of the disease. As for prevention, they said, "We not only categorically reject, but also deem offensive, all AIDS literature and advice that teach and promote sexual practices and behaviors that offend the cultural integrity of the black race and go against the teachings of our church and religious beliefs."[52] Strangely enough, the black caucus included several well-known black gay activists whose voices, one charitably assumes, were not heard by the rest of the group.

Overlooked by CDC and the white gay community, and ignored by their own community, it was clear that black gay men and other men of color—like their white gay brothers—would have to educate themselves. Fortunately, black gay men had a bold and visionary leader in Reggie Williams, who recognized early on that the only way gay men of color would survive the epidemic was to mount their own educational campaigns. In 1984, Williams was a member of the San Francisco chapter of Black and White Men Together (BWMT), a nationwide network of social support and advocacy organizations. After a presentation at a BWMT meeting by representatives of several AIDS organizations serving people of color, Williams offered to host another meeting in his home the following week for anyone inter-ested in talking about the AIDS-related concerns of gay men of color. This would be the first meeting of what became the AIDS task force of BWMT/San Francisco, a group dedicated to advocating on behalf of gay men of color for services in the city.

Pulling together the AIDS efforts of other BWMT chapters un-der the auspices of the National Association of Black and White Men Together, Williams in 1988 won a contract from the CDC to pro-vide AIDS prevention to gay men of color. Reflecting on those years in a telephone interview from his home in Amsterdam, where he was living with both his German lover and AIDS, Williams recalled saying to himself, "If they're not going to do it [prevention for gay men of color], then goddamn it, we can do it for ourselves. We're not crippled! We have power. That's why we created the National Task Force on AIDS Prevention—to do it for ourselves."

From its inception, the task force brought together gay men of color—including African-Americans, Hispanics, Native Americans, and Asian/Pacific Islanders—to advocate on their own behalf and devise ways to reach other gay men like themselves who felt they were not being served adequately by either gay or "mainstream" orga-nizations in their communities. The group believed strongly that for gay men of color to be receptive to AIDS prevention messages, they would need to get those messages from other men who "looked like" them. As Williams put it, "The messenger is just as important as the message."

For Williams, "doing for ourselves" began with honesty about one's identity—in terms of race, sexual orientation, and even HIV antibody status. He described the liberation he felt personally because of such frankness. "I was able to walk up to the podium and say, 'I'm Reggie Williams, a black gay man with HIV,' instead of saying, 'I'm Reggie Williams, executive director of the National Task Force on AIDS Prevention.'" And it always had an effect on the audience, says Williams, "whether hetero, gay, white, or black." He explained, "I didn't look like most people's idea of a person with HIV/AIDS since I wasn't dragged in or wheeled out to the podium."[53]

Besides promoting a sense of gay pride, the task force realized that prevention education targeted to gay men of color had to build upon and support a man's sense of cultural identity—including loyalty to his family, racial or ethnic community, and religious faith. The organization understood that gay men of color face what Williams calls a "double-edged sword"—torn as they often are between their sense of belonging to the largely white gay community and their racial or ethnic community and not fully accepted in either. For that reason the task force viewed its role as largely that of building self-esteem so that gay men of color would be motivated to protect themselves against HIV. As Randy Miller, Williams's successor at the National Task Force, explained, the key to the agency's unique workshops and media campaigns was to use the community and family loyalty of gay men of color as a jumping-off point, "tying a sense of cultural survival to individual survival."[54] The operating philosophy of the organization, which until its 1998 closing because of fiscal mismanagement was the nation's largest prevention and advocacy agency working specifically on behalf of gay men of color, was handed down directly from the life of its founder. As Williams said, "I know what it is to have low self-esteem and not feel like your life has value; I've been there. I grew up in the ghetto, so I know what it's like."[55]

Beginning in the late eighties, there was constant talk about "the changing face" of the AIDS epidemic. In 1987, *Time* magazine put it this way: "The face of AIDS in America is changing; it is getting younger, darker, more feminine."[56] But the rates of AIDS and HIV infection in the northeast have skewed the national figures on the epidemic because the region has the nation's highest prevalence of injection drug use, with a correspondingly high incidence of HIV and AIDS among female sexual partners and their children. Outside the northeast, particularly New York and northern New Jersey, the "main epidemic" (there are several different epidemics in the U.S., including, for example, a rising epidemic among black women in the South) is still among gay and bisexual men.[57]

What's more, gay and bisexual men of color account for both the largest proportion of cases among racial and ethnic minorities as well as a growing percentage of the cases among gay and bisexual men in general. By 1993 in Chicago, for example, 69 percent of the AIDS cases among African-American men were among gay and bisexual men, some of whom were also injection drug users. In Los Angeles, 76 percent of the AIDS cases among African-American men, 80 percent among Hispanic men, and 86 percent among Asian and Pacific Islander men involved homosexual contact.[58]

In spite of the large numbers of gay men of color affected by AIDS—a third of the cumulative total of AIDS cases among those whom the CDC calls "men who have sex with men"—funding for prevention programs targeting them ranged from a paltry 1 to 13 percent of the total city and county prevention funds in five major cities described in a report by the U.S. Conference of Mayors.[59] As the National Commission on AIDS noted in its own report, *The Challenges of HIV/AIDS in Communities of Color,* "Serious questions have been raised as to whether the populations most at risk for AIDS within communities of color are being appropriately targeted." The commission noted that although half of African-American and Hispanic male adults with AIDS at the time were men who have sex with men, services in communities of color are often not designed to reach them. Because the same could be said of predominantly white gay organizations, the commission concluded, "gay men of color are frequently left in limbo."[60]

As a result, the number of AIDS cases among black and Hispanic gay men continued to rise from the late eighties through the nineties. By the middle of 1997, there had been 612,078 AIDS cases reported in the United States. Of these, 298,699 were among men who were infected with HIV through sex with another man; an additional 38,923 men had sex with men and injected drugs. Together, these two groups accounted for well over half of all the nation's AIDS cases. Of them, 214,427 were white, 74,140 black, and 44,680 Hispanic.

Contrasting these numbers to the rates of AIDS among women and children provides a study in the politics of prevention. Men with no other risk factor than sex with another man *alone* accounted for more than three times the total number of women with AIDS— and nearly thirty-eight times the total number of children with AIDS.[61] Yet, in the state of California, for example, a study of funding for HIV prevention found that although gay men comprised 88 percent of the state's AIDS cases, prevention efforts targeting gay men accounted for a mere 5 percent of the state's prevention money.[62] The Gay and Lesbian Medical Association estimates that less than 5 percent of all prevention funding in this country targets gay men.[63] The belief obviously persists that gay men can and should take care of themselves, fund their own prevention efforts, and not expect a share of public prevention dollars commensurate with their rates of infection and disease.

When the surgeon general's report on AIDS was updated in 1993, gay men were described—and dismissed—on page 1 like this: "In this second decade of the AIDS epidemic, *gay men still account for the majority of AIDS cases reported each year* [my italics] and continue to suffer an enormous burden. However, AIDS is becoming more prominent in the young and in heterosexual men and women." After that "however," gay men are never again mentioned in the next twenty-five pages of the report. Instead, it focuses exclusively on heterosexuals, women, children, and teenagers—without even acknowledging the fact that two-thirds of male adolescents with AIDS are infected through homosexual behavior.[64] A CDC catalog of HIV and AIDS education and prevention materials produced the same year doesn't mention gay men even once.[65] In the private sector, the table of contents for the on-line service AEGIS (AIDS Education Global Information Network), which bills itself as "the largest HIV/AIDS database in the world," never mentions gay men. It does, however, include women, children, and "other," a category that encompasses the visually impaired, the deaf, the developmentally disabled, and racial minorities.[66]

CDC's longstanding "offensiveness" standard—going back to its 1986 crackdown on explicit prevention materials targeting gay men—was overturned by a federal district court in May 1992. GMHC was vindicated in its claim that the "Safe Sex Comix" that so upset Jesse Helms was not paid for with public funding. "But," noted a congressional report on federal prevention efforts, "CDC, not to be outdone, the following month, issued new requirements that order program review panels to ensure that CDC funds are not used for prevention materials considered to be 'obscene.'" As a reminder of the "chilling effect" lingering from the Helms amendment, the report continued, "The CDC's directive continues to require the review panels to ensure that prevention materials do not 'promote or encourage directly homosexual or heterosexual activity or intravenous substance abuse.'"[67]

Throughout the nineties, CDC continued to be told that it needed to target AIDS prevention education to those who needed it most. According to its own epidemiological reports, that largely should have meant gay and bisexual men, intravenous drug users and their partners. In 1993, an eight-month investigation of CDC's HIV prevention program—representing about 85 percent of its $539 million AIDS budget at the time—recommended, yet again, that the government's public education should offer explicit information on how HIV is transmitted and on the value of condoms in disease prevention.[68] Scientists also were urging that prevention education focus on people at the highest risk in the nation's hardest-hit areas—some twenty-five to thirty neighborhoods altogether in cities that included Camden, N.J., Houston, Los Angeles, Miami, Newark, N.J., New York City, and San Francisco. In a front page *New York Times* story, Dr. John Gagnon, a sociologist at the State University of New York at Stony Brook, was quoted as saying, "We've got to put the money where the problem is, instead of spreading it around in a Johnny Appleseed way."[69]

Did the government listen? Had it ever, really? Instead of targeted, explicit prevention education that might actually work to save the lives of Americans by telling them forthrightly how to protect themselves against HIV, the government continued its scattershot approach—targeting everyone in general, no one in particular, and offering only emotional appeals aimed at "raising awareness." Of course most Americans already were quite aware of AIDS, though not all of them viewed their own behavior as risky because the government's vaguely worded educational programs gave them multiple opportunities to deny their own risk.

Although they already had been widely criticized as too vague and ineffectual, CDC in 1992 launched yet another round of its "America Responds to AIDS" print and broadcast ads. Announcing the new ads at a press conference, Assistant Secretary for Health James Mason denied that political pressure had forced the government to produce conservative ads. Yet he stunned the audience when he said, "There are certain areas [in] which, when the goals of science collide with moral and ethical judgment, science has to take a time out."[70] It seemed science had been given a permanent hiatus by the nation's leading disease prevention institution.

The latest round of "America Responds to AIDS" ads maintained the government's unswerving commitment to avoid controversy at all costs. But besides the hundreds of millions of taxpayer dollars wasted on efforts considered by experts to be useless, the costs of delaying an effective educational program included the very lives of those who would become infected with HIV because politically beholden bureaucrats refused to allow frank discussion of sexuality and drug use. Instead of useful messages, we got more pabulum. For instance, after an "America Responds to AIDS" message designed, as Mason put it, to "convey personal meaning about the tragedy of AIDS," viewers were told they could "find out how you can prevent HIV" by calling the CDC's AIDS hotline.[71] The ad never once told viewers how, exactly, to protect themselves. In fact, condoms are never once mentioned in the ads. Instead "abstinence" remained the sine qua non of the government's prevention message: If you want to protect yourself from getting AIDS, don't have sex or shoot drugs. It's as simple—and simplistic—as that. If you do have sex or shoot drugs, you're on your own. Jeff Levi said of the ads, "You don't sell things by stating an eight hundred number. If you're selling laundry detergent, you don't say, 'Are you concerned about dirty laundry? Call 1-800-DETERGENT.'"[72]

Why has the government been so singularly spineless in its efforts to prevent the spread of AIDS? Quite simply, because all these years and nearly two-thirds of a million AIDS cases after the start of the AIDS epidemic, the government remains hobbled by its fear of upsetting Jesse Helms and his antisex, antigay compatriots at the outer fringe of the right wing. Instead of forthright discussion of the behaviors that put an individual at risk, and the explicit, targeted messages recommended by every scientist and medical expert working on AIDS in this country, what the *New York Times* called a "deathly silence" about sexuality continues to reverberate throughout the government's prevention programs.[73] As politicians continue to placate religious bigots, gay men—as well as women, adolescents, and injection drug users—continue to become infected and die.

*

The Stop AIDS Project reopened in 1990 because of the rising incidence of unprotected sex and new HIV infections among gay men in San Francisco. When the project closed three years earlier, its efforts to quickly change the way gay men had sex by making safe sex the norm seemed to have paid off, as the rate of new HIV infections and reports of unsafe sex declined. Everyone celebrated, prematurely as it turned out, what they believed was the community's adoption of safe sex—including the "normalization" of condoms. It seemed the gay community had accomplished a feat never before seen in the history of public health: Through their own efforts, gay men on a wide scale seemed to have heeded the warnings about AIDS and modified their behaviors accordingly.

But as the years passed and the epidemic wore on, fear alone didn't suffice to prevent some men from having unsafe sex. Researchers puzzled over what was driving them to do it, despite the gay community's high awareness of AIDS and what is and isn't safe. In the same way as serious scientists wondered in the earliest years of the epidemic what unique quality in gay men made them particularly susceptible to AIDS, they now wondered why some gay men, a decade after the epidemic began, were returning to the sexual behavior they had practiced before safe sex allegedly became the "norm." Among the reasons suggested, one study said that a "high subjective gratification derived from past risky sexual practices" was a major predictor of unsafe activity.[74] Put simply, those who enjoyed the kind of sex they practiced before the epidemic—or at least until they presumably began to practice safe sex—were "at risk" for engaging in sexual behavior, now proscribed, which they obviously enjoyed and that was natural for them. If ever a commonsense observation had been gussied up as science, this was it.

A 1993 article in the *New York Times* shocked both San Francisco and the nation when it reported that a "second wave of AIDS" was feared and forecast in San Francisco. One out of every fifty gay men in the city was becoming infected each year—twice that number among men under twenty-five. Although the rate was a considerable drop from 1982, when eighteen gay men in a hundred were infected annually, it was climbing again from its 1985 nadir.[75] Researchers, many gay men, and heterosexuals alike wondered: Why did these men put themselves at such risk? Didn't they know better? Did they have a death wish?

As everyone argued and finger-pointed their way to an answer, San Francisco therapist Tom Moon pointed out something so obvious as to have eluded everyone: prevention isn't simply a matter of knowing how to have safe sex. "People have emotional lives," said Moon. "They're not just information-processing machines."[76]

Moon was on to something no one had taken into account as they planned and launched campaigns aimed at changing the way gay men think about and engage in sex. After a decade of an epidemic that was expected to have ended years before (and still no cure in sight), thousands of deaths, countless hours spent at hospital bedsides and memorial services, it finally began to dawn on prevention professionals that years of loss, grief, and self-denial were eating away at the resolve of gay men to protect themselves in order to survive the epidemic. Stop AIDS Project's Daniel Wohlfeiler said, "What happens when survival becomes a very iffy concept? When five of your boyfriends have died? When fifty of your closest friends have died? When people you used to see walk down the street—the baker, the banker, the people you do business with every day, the people you dance with, all the people you wanted to survive with—aren't there anymore? It wears down the resolve so that when push comes to shove, the decision of whether to put the condom on or not is not so clear-cut anymore."[77]

Researchers recommended that prevention efforts shift from focusing only on getting men to have safe sex, to a longer-term strategy that emphasized the maintenance of safe sex—assuming, of course, that it had been adopted in the first place. Finally, prevention educators were beginning to realize that knowledge alone isn't enough to make people protect themselves. Only now were researchers noting, forebodingly, that studies on other behaviors—smoking cessation, alcohol abstinence, and dieting—had shown that it is extremely difficult to maintain healthy behaviors over time. At the national gay and lesbian health conference in 1993, held that year in Houston, David Ostrow said, "Information alone is not going to be enough to maintain safer sexual behavior. People have a tendency to go back to learned, pleasurable behaviors."[78] Leon McCusick made the same point a decade earlier. Had anyone listened?

But gay men are hardly unique in this regard. When it comes to sex, most people are hedonistic by nature, and the sternest of warnings will not suffice to deter everyone from pleasurable activities all the time, particularly in an emotionally intimate relationship. As Abraham Verghese, a heterosexual AIDS doctor, puts it, "No cerebral abstraction involving sex—whether it was the need for contraception, proscriptions against adultery, or the need for safe sex—had ever in human history fared well in the face of raw lust."[79]

Lust and the irrational desires and needs that drive most of us sexually were not really taken into account when educators conceived of prevention programs for gay men in the eighties. They figured that if the men knew about AIDS and how to protect themselves from getting HIV, they'd naturally do so—100 percent of the time. But no one in 1986 expected the epidemic to last as long as it has done, or to practice safe sex longer than absolutely necessary. By the nineties, gay men were tired of AIDS, worn down by grief, and questioning the authority of prevention educators. When had they become such "authorities," anyway? Rather than directing people to information they could use to make their own choices, educators had anointed themselves as the sole mediators of scientific knowledge about AIDS, doling it out in sound bites and slogans that did little to address the underlying reasons why men have sex at all—to say nothing of the reasons, some quite legitimate, they might choose to have unprotected sex.

Educators who may have had no formal credentials in the relevant areas of public health or the behavioral sciences, were accorded a certain authority in the community. Whatever professional credibility they lacked they simply assumed for themselves in their visible roles. The granting or withholding of "permission" for particular activities by people in positions of authority meant that a high-risk activity like unprotected anal intercourse, became "frowned upon," or stigmatized, in the community. Those who engaged in the forbidden behavior were seen as "sinners," betrayers of the gay community, shamed into silence. Of course this meant that when men did have unsafe sex, no one would talk about it for fear of being condemned by these authority figures. As Eric Rofes puts it, "It became clear very rapidly which subjects were appropriate to discuss and which ones, under the constraints of safe sex guidelines, had become heretical."[80] To admit one had engaged in unprotected anal intercourse— irrespective of the fact that it might well have been a conscious choice because both partners were either HIV-negative or positive, so there was no chance of new HIV infection—was certainly seen as heretical, a falling away from the faith. In fact, to prevention educators it was viewed as no less than blasphemy itself against the god of safe sex we had created as our talisman against AIDS.

Prevention educators continued using social marketing techniques to try to make gay men "want" to use condoms. Referring to them as "lifeguards" and calling them by other euphemistic and sexy names, they tried to make safe sex appealing by making it "fashionable": If you practiced it, you were part of the "in" crowd; if you didn't, you weren't. The problem with this approach is that it once again reduced and simplified complex emotions and behavior. As Rofes puts it, "Gay men appear as consumers to be pitched specific messages, as if their erotic desires have much in common with consumer urges for Pepsi Cola, a Big Mac, or a Jeep Cherokee."[81]

One of the actual consumer products in which safe sex is literally "packaged" and sold to gay men—even if not everyone bought into it—is gay pornography. Porn videos, like telephone sex, blossomed in popularity in the AIDS epidemic as men sought ways to have sex as safely as possible. Some activists viewed porn-watching as a golden opportunity to influence gay men to have safe sex. They insisted that gay erotica portray only safe sex, that condoms be visible at all times during videotaped anal intercourse. Most filmmakers for the first years of the epidemic weren't insisting on condoms because they thought them unerotic. No one insisted on condoms for oral sex—which was surprising in view of the conviction with which so many educators vilified the practice if done without a condom.

Chuck Holmes is the president of Falcon Studios, the largest producer of gay male erotica in the country. Holmes has served on the boards of several national gay political organizations, including the Human Rights Campaign and the Victory Fund. Shortly before our interview, Falcon had produced its one hundredth video. It had an additional seventy titles on its "Jocks" label, more than forty on its "Mustang" label, and its seventh international video was under production in Eastern Europe. Holmes described Falcon's corporate philosophy as being "proudly, openly gay." He said that Falcon in the mid-eighties began to use condoms and nonoxynol-based lubricants in its videos, as recommended by prevention educators. He noted, however, that other producers didn't immediately do likewise, and that even today a condom-free film occasionally will slip into the market. Emphasizing that safe sex had become the norm in gay erotica, Holmes said, "No responsible gay erotica producers would ever make a decision [not to use condoms]. They'd be drummed out of the business because the models wouldn't talk to them, the distributors wouldn't touch it." He added, however, "Anybody who can get two nickels together can get a high-eight camera and produce gay videos. But the usual distribution channels wouldn't be available to them, and a hue and cry would be raised against them."[82]

Boston's AIDS Action Committee attempted, in the late eighties, to produce a safe sex film featuring porn star Al Parker. Cindy Patton, who worked on the project, notes that the group's goal for the video wasn't to "eroticize" safe sex, but rather "to retrieve already and always safe activities," such as mutual masturbation, licking, and all the other sexual things gay men might do together that seemed to have been lost in the shuffle as everyone focused so singlemindedly on eliminating unprotected anal sex. Ultimately, said Patton, the project was shelved because the group couldn't agree on what constituted safe sex. But in the process, they learned a valuable lesson. As she put it, "Porn videos are useful if they suggest positive attitudes about gay male sexuality because that helps create and sustain a social environment in which safe sex is practiced *because* it is viewed as a positive aspect of gay male sexuality."[83] The group reasoned that gay men would practice safe sex if they were persuaded to view it as something positive rather than as a kind of punishment for being homosexual—as too many men had come to see it.

To reach this point, naturally, discussion would be needed to try to find answers to important questions: Why were men still having unsafe sex? What value did it have for them? Could they learn to value and enjoy a different activity—or, less onerously, continue the ones they already enjoyed but practice them safely? Unfortunately, this discussion wasn't allowed to happen for several years after it became apparent that some gay men were either not practicing safe sex at all, or were doing so only some of the time. To acknowledge publicly that gay men were flouting supposed community norms meant prevention education wasn't working, and that prevention educators weren't quite as influential as they thought they were.

Some feared that if word about gay men having unsafe sex a decade into the epidemic got out to the public, the long-awaited backlash against gay people would happen. AIDS service organizations feared that if politicians found out that prevention wasn't working 100 percent of the time, their funding would be cut. So they did their best to suppress the information, to keep it under wraps within the community. As in the early years of the epidemic, the view was that the community's "dirty laundry" shouldn't be aired in public. But not everyone agreed that this was a good policy. David Ostrow, for one, said, "To me, one of the biggest mistakes in the history of the whole AIDS movement was when, for political reasons, we decided that we would tell the public and the politicians that gay men had stopped having unsafe sex around 1987 or [19]88. I was against it then, and I'm still against it."

It was a political decision to say that gay men stopped having sex without condoms. But, as numerous studies showed, that was never the case anywhere. If the threat of negative pressure was going to be used to motivate gay men to give up their favorite sexual activities, there was bound to be relapse. "That's the way behavior works," says Ostrow. "When you ask people to give up something, and you don't give them something else to replace it that provides the same form of intimacy and pleasure, you're going to have high rates of relapse."[84]

The debate over unsafe sex within the gay community reached a fever pitch in 1995. On Easter Sunday, the *New York Times* reported that New York authorities had closed two gay theaters and a sex club. "Places like this facilitate multiple, anonymous sexual contacts, and the risk of transmission is so much greater there," said Doron Gopstein, an attorney for the city who had handled similar cases going back to the 1985 closing of the Mine Shaft. The *Times* noted that the closures may have been little more than a "quick political fix" to the troubling, unanswered question of whether sex in public places was any riskier than sex at home. The situation wasn't helped by the state sanitary law used to close the establishments, which inaccurately described any oral, anal, or vaginal sex in these places as "high-risk," whether or not a condom was used and regardless of the HIV status of those involved. In the city's convoluted definition, illegal equaled high risk, only further confusing an already difficult issue.

The day after the *Times* report, the *Washington Post* raised its own chagrined voice to note in a front-page article, "A gay men's social club where the lights are low and patrons must leave their clothes in lockers has opened near downtown Washington, reviving a dispute over public health and civil rights in the era of AIDS." The *Post* observed that similar clubs in other cities had become the settings for "proselytizing" AIDS educators "who once condemned such places." The article mentioned—and quickly dispatched—the fact that elsewhere in the city a bathhouse and other establishments catering to those who wanted anonymous sex had remained open throughout the years of the epidemic. In a follow-up editorial, the *Post* called the new Crew Club "the Washington area's latest AIDS breeding ground" and "a site that fosters deadly behavior." Whitman-Walker Clinic director Jim Graham was quoted as saying, "In the midst of an epidemic, I am disappointed this is part of the landscape of this city."[85]

Perhaps if the *Post* had done a more thorough job of reporting the situation, it would have focused on specific sexual acts performed on the premises, before lambasting the Crew Club in sweeping and harsh terms. It also would have noted that the new club was only a few blocks from its own offices. Graham's own disappointment might have stemmed from the club's proximity to Whitman-Walker, only a couple of blocks away on the same street. Why hadn't the newspaper and the clinic been concerned about the city's other existing sexual establishments? Could it have been that they were simply on the other side of the city, rather than in their own "backyard"? Out of sight, out of mind?

For the rest of the year, the issue of what was being called "permissible sex" dominated the gay press. It seemed that some, including former prominent members of ACT UP/New York, had finally realized that, while the AIDS treatments they advocated certainly are important, there are considerably more gay men at risk for contracting HIV than there are those already infected with it. Activists had never given prevention the same priority as treatment. Suddenly, and with both the zealotry and "religion" of new converts, the self-styled "prevention activists" in 1995 tried to rally the community to pay attention to what they asserted was a huge new upswing in unsafe sex. Some had personally observed unprotected sex in the clubs, and then apparently looked for data to support their assumption that gay men everywhere had "relapsed." With arguments harkening back to the bathhouse controversies of the early eighties, some went so far as to call upon public health and legal authorities to police, or even close down, sexual establishments.

In New York, small groups of prevention activists formed in 1995 in response to reports of unsafe activity in the clubs, each with its own "solution" to the "problem" of unsafe sex. Two of the groups, Community AIDS Prevention Activists (CAPA), and the AIDS Prevention Action League (APAL), viewed AIDS prevention as an issue to be solved within the gay community itself. The two groups were founded by HIV-positive men who feared that a quick fix, like closing sex clubs and bathhouses, would simply drive unsafe sex back to the parks and piers—where, incidentally, as I have personally observed, it has never ceased or abated in spite of the availability of indoor spaces catering to men seeking it. Carlos Cordero, founder of CAPA, said, "If you want behavioral change, then you have to give people support at every level, not condemnation or vilification. There's such a hunger to talk about stuff, but people really need to feel safe to talk."[86] Stephen Gendin, APAL's founder, wrote an open letter to the community in which he said, "Do not demonize gay men because of where we choose to have sex. Do not take away our ability to make choices for ourselves. Do not characterize gay men as victims who have no ability to control ourselves. Do not polarize the discussion before it even begins."[87]

Unfortunately, the reasonable voices of these two men were virtually drowned by the flood of outraged op-ed pieces and articles of the media-savvy handful of members of a third group called Gay and Lesbian HIV Prevention Activists (GALHPA). Led by gay journalists Duncan Osborne, Gabriel Rotello, and Michelangelo Signorile—"along with a handful of other skilled propagandists," as *POZ* magazine described them[88]—the group demanded, in the pages of the city's mainstream newspapers, that the city close down establishments that allowed their patrons to have unsafe sex. Acknowledging that they had patronized such establishments themselves—presumably to have sex like the other men there—GALHPA activists didn't see a contradiction between their own activity and their call for closure by a city government that considered *any* sex in such places to be illegal and, therefore, "high-risk." *Out* magazine quoted Gabriel Rotello as saying, "HIV transmission must stop. And a moderate restriction in civil liberties, if that's going to make the difference between salvation and catastrophe, then that's something we have to accept."[89]

Such views were roundly condemned by many other gay men, weary of being viewed as criminals merely because of their sexual orientation. Ben Stilip, director of communications for New York's Lesbian and Gay Community Services Center, said, "Why would we invite the very institutions that in so many ways ignore and hurt and neglect us to police our lives? It's like inviting Mata Hari over to baby-sit your kids."[90] The singleminded focus of Rotello and his fellow GALHPA members on sexual establishments ignored the fact that prevention researchers had been saying for years that most of the unsafe sex transmitting HIV takes place in the privacy of the bedroom, not in public places. In his regular *Out* column, GALHPA member Signorile quoted Columbia University AIDS researcher Martina Morris as saying, "Public sex is not the problem. Unsafe sex is the problem."[91]

Bob Warfel, a professional health educator in Washington, D.C., responded to the flap over the city's Crew Club in the kind of thoughtful and reasoned fashion that eluded New York's GALHPA and, it seemed, most everyone else. In a letter to the editor published in the *Washington Blade*, Warfel wrote, "There is no reasonable—or realistic—argument for prohibition. And there shouldn't be as long as the majority of people are self-aware and capable of making personal decisions or choices. For those who cannot—because they are impaired by alcohol, or drugs, or low self-esteem—there are much more effective things our community could do for our brothers than shutting down a club. Like, perhaps, talking about why so many men find anonymous sex—or getting trashed, or getting stoned, or putting each other down—so appealing or necessary in the first place."[92]

A discussion of self-esteem and mental health issues during the first-ever national summit on HIV prevention, sponsored by the Gay and Lesbian Medical Association and held in Dallas in July 1994, revealed the paucity of attention these issues had received in the community's prevention efforts. In a workshop led by Tom Moon, issues of isolation, alienation, a sense of not belonging, loss, and absence of family were among the reasons cited for many gay men's ongoing risky behavior. The group concluded that to be effective, prevention education should address issues of wellness, self-esteem, self-love, and the affirmation of love. One major obstacle to achieving these goals, said Moon, is society's treatment of gay men as outlaws. As he put it, "Until we have our civil rights, self-esteem is going to be very difficult to attain." In the meantime, the group urged community advocates to speak publicly about gay mental health issues "without apology or fear of backlash or airing 'dirty laundry.'"[93]

One speaker at the Dallas summit who generated considerable debate was Berkeley, California, psychologist Walt Odets. With his sharp criticism of what he viewed as outmoded prevention efforts, Odets became a lightning rod for prevention educators loath to let go of the slogans and strategies they had used in one form or another since the early years of the epidemic. Of the community's efforts to "hide" unsafe sex, Odets says, "This apologist approach that says we should keep our problems under our hat because people won't like us, that we have to fight for our right to be human beings, to have foibles and complexity—it hasn't accomplished anything. We're never going to get anything by being good; we never have, they're not interested in us. We're not going to make them less interested by revealing that we're human beings."

Odets believes that the incidence of unprotected anal sex among gay men is much higher than reported in the literature, and certainly higher than gay men report to one another, because they, like most everyone, underreport all stigmatized behaviors. And, as he stressed, unprotected anal sex, regardless of the partners' HIV status, has indeed become highly stigmatized. "A man who seroconverts now has a lot of explaining to do," said Odets. "He explains it by saying 'I just suck guys off; I never had anal sex in my life.'" As he does frequently in his writing and talks, Odets offered an illustrative anecdote from his mostly gay psychotherapy practice.

A couple he was seeing in therapy had an arrangement that allowed each man to have sex with others outside the relationship as long as it was safe. One of the men got infected with HIV, but denied having had unprotected sex. After six months of individual therapy with the HIV-positive man after the couple broke up over the issue, he finally admitted the truth. He told Odets, "Dan and I had a fight one night and I went to the baths and I let a guy fuck me without a condom." To show how much shame this man felt about his behavior—instilled by prevention educators—Odets contrasted it with another experience in the man's past. "One of the first things he told me in therapy," said Odets, "is that he'd grown up fucking the family collie! He didn't mind telling me *that*. He spent his whole childhood fucking the collie, but he couldn't tell me about anal sex."

Acknowledging and discussing unsafe sex are even harder when people perceived as community leaders harshly condemn such behavior, and go so far as to call for draconian measures to suppress it. As Odets put it, "A lot of people don't trust their own impulses and want external control—like the bathhouse thing in New York. It seems to me to be a lot of anxious people who want external controls to deal with their own impulses about things."[94]

As prevention researchers explored the workings of the gay male psyche in the second decade of the epidemic, trying to learn why some men will have unprotected sex despite its potential risks, they also began to look at what we might call situational co-factors that contribute to unsafe sex. Topping the list of circumstantial enablers are alcohol and drug use. "Substance abuse is one of the principal risk factors for getting infected," says Tom Coates, a psychologist and the director of the AIDS Research Institute at the University of California–San Francisco. "We have terrible epidemics of substance abuse in the gay community—a lot more than in the general heterosexual population—alcoholism, cocaine, and amphetamine use." He noted that the central role of bars in the social lives of many gay people fosters the overconsumption of alcohol and the accompanying inability to make healthful choices.[95]

In early 1995, psychiatrist Bob Cabaj had recently left his position as director of the substance abuse and HIV program at San Francisco General Hospital, and was the president of the Gay and Lesbian Medical Association. A noted expert on issues around substance abuse in the gay community, Cabaj told me, "I have seen tremendous numbers of gay men who abuse substances." He described a pattern of drug use among a fairly large number of gay men in San Francisco and elsewhere along the West Coast that, he said, even shocked him. "I did not see a single gay male patient with HIV at the General for the three years I was there who was not also an IV-injecting speed user."

Methamphetamine, commonly known as "crystal meth" or speed, is the drug of choice among many gay clubgoers from Los Angeles up to Seattle. "It's so addicting," Cabaj explained. "Your tolerance goes up so high that you don't get anything after a while from snorting, so you have to start injecting." Are gay men who are injecting the drug sharing needles? I asked. "Yes," he answered. "Of course everyone starts out with the best intentions. But once you're high from the first shot, you're not going to worry about the next one." Of course you're also unlikely to worry about whether the sex you have is protected or not. And men on "crystal" tend to have a lot of sex because one of the drug's effects is to make one "hypersexual," capable of multiple episodes over the course of a strung-out, sleepless "trip."

This information was astonishing given the presumably high level of knowledge among middle-class gay men, particularly in San Francisco, about the most basic ways to protect themselves against HIV infection—foremost among them, not to share needles. I pursued the questioning further. "Does their sharing needles have something to do with the fact that they don't see themselves as junkies because they're not poor, don't have ragged clothes, or dark skin?" Cabaj answered, "Exactly."[96]

Recalling Reggie Williams' description of the "double-edged sword" that gay men of color face—not fully at home in either the white gay community because of their race, or in their racial or ethnic community because of their sexual orientation—it's not surprising to learn that black gay men are especially susceptible to substance abuse and its attendant HIV-related risks. But even prevention efforts targeting minority gay men typically have viewed them as either substance abusers or homosexual, as though the two are mutually exclusive identities rather than behaviors that often go hand-in-hand. Thirty-five percent of the clients at San Francisco's Eighteenth Street Services, a highly regarded substance abuse treatment program in the heart of the Castro district, are black gay or bisexual men. The agency's outreach director, Bert Bloom, said that for black gay men, like white gay men—and people in general—"If everybody is telling you that you are worthless and you feel like shit, why not get high?"[97]

That at least will help to keep you from dealing with yourself, even if it also prevents you from taking precautions against HIV. As Bob Cabaj puts it, "Unless you can generate a sense of confidence, or a sense that you're okay with who you are, you don't do much to protect yourself in life." For Cabaj, coming to terms with being gay is the starting point for self-esteem—and, by extension, for HIV prevention. "Drugs and alcohol have a tremendous impact in helping us to dissociate and deny," he said. "So some people can have gay sex after they get drunk. They don't think about it, but substance abuse is woven very tightly into the gay community in promoting disconnection and denial."[98]

Bars and nightclubs are typically major ports of entry for young gay people coming out into the community. From the beginning of their gay "career," many young gay men are exposed to situations that aren't necessarily the most conducive to their health and well-being. Unfortunately it's not terribly surprising that there are frequent lapses in safe sex among many younger gay men, often under the influence of alcohol or drugs, and at least partly because they haven't had firsthand experience of seeing their friends get sick and die. A 1996 report by the Office of National AIDS Policy indicated that of the estimated forty thousand to eighty thousand Americans infected with HIV each year—between 110 and 220 a day—from twenty-seven to fifty-four of the daily infections are among young people under the age of twenty.[99]

After an interview I had with Patsy Fleming, then director of the Office of National AIDS Policy, Fleming called me because, she said, she wanted to make a couple of points about young gay men. The mother of a young gay man herself, Fleming softly (and, I thought, sadly) told me that she has met young men who actually *want* to become infected with HIV. "I run into young gay people," she said, "who say they are negative, but go into an AIDS organization and say they are positive so they will get attention."[100]

The rising rate of new infection among young gay men has certainly gotten attention. A 1993 survey by the San Francisco Health Commission found that nearly 12 percent of twenty- to twenty-two-year-old gay men in the city were already HIV-positive, as were 4 percent of seventeen- to nineteen-year-olds. "If those figures are not reversed," noted the *Advocate*, "the current population of young urban gay men"—what the magazine already was calling the "lost generation"—"will have as high an infection rate by the time they reach their mid-thirties as middle-aged gay men are thought to have today—close to 50 percent."[101]

Gay youth remain at particularly high risk for HIV infection, and not merely because they tend, like all adolescents, to engage in risky behavior. Pediatrician Gary Remafedi, a nationally known expert on gay adolescents at the University of Minnesota, told me that his research on young gay males has found certain predictors of risk that make them especially vulnerable. These include substance abuse; being in a steady relationship (they "trust that their partner is not going to do anything to hurt them," said Remafedi); academic underachievement; having a lot of gay friends, which provides more opportunities to meet others and engage in unsafe sex; and, perhaps most alarming, he said, "risky behavior is associated with the belief that they are likely to get HIV." With a sense that HIV infection is inevitable, these young people give up on safe sex before they've even had the chance to discover behavior that can be both healthy and satisfying. Remafedi explained, "Young people who are well-instructed have grown up to think of safe sex as sex, period. On the other hand, when young people come out they hear from adults, 'You're going to get AIDS and die.' Young people who have to deal with the possibility that they have been exposed are often fearful to find out whether they have HIV because it fulfills the parent's prophecy."[102]

A study of 149 young gay men in New York, including ten who were HIV-positive, found that those who had partners over the age of twenty-five tended most often to have unprotected anal sex, the highest possible sexual risk behavior. They were described as "the leading edge of infection" for their age group. "It is clear that young gay men are now standing on the brink of a second wave of the AIDS epidemic in their community," the Columbia University researchers concluded.[103] A companion study reported that in 1990–91, 62 of the 149 young men in the study—nearly half—had engaged in unprotected receptive anal intercourse, mainly at home. Compared to the men who didn't do it, more men who engaged in receptive anal sex knew the HIV status of their partner. (In a significant oversight, the report doesn't note whether or not the men knew beforehand if their insertive partners were HIV-negative or positive).

The study drew a very disturbing conclusion reminiscent of the sometimes rancorous arguments in the gay community over issues like sex clubs and bathhouses. It found that for the young gay men studied, higher levels of sexual risk-taking correlated to their involvement in the gay community. This would seem counterintuitive to the prevention educators and activists who claim the gay community has become a "safe sex culture." But the researchers noted, "This suggests that a strong community consensus may have adverse effects by forming the impression that risky behavior is extremely rare, and by creating taboos that inhibit open discussion of sexual behavior."[104] What's more, for young gay men coming out in the urban ghettos where there are high rates of HIV infection, being HIV-positive can too easily seem not only inevitable but "normal." Walt Odets says, "In this social and psychological climate, we are now also seeing younger gay men who are often unable to make any distinction at all between being gay and being at risk for, or actually contracting HIV."[105]

Is this what gay liberation and the community's awesome response to AIDS had come to? A perverse state of affairs in which the words "gay" and "plague" had become synonymous? As gay men in the late nineties continued to become infected with HIV and die of AIDS in staggering numbers, the community still struggled to address the troubling issue of unsafe sex, too often in harsh, condemnatory terms. Gay men who had risky sex felt they couldn't bring up the subject with gay friends because no one was willing to risk censure by talking about it. So they didn't talk about it. Yet they continued to do it, fearful and furtive lest their friends find out and upbraid them for being so "stupid." They felt they couldn't talk with AIDS educators about it, either, because that risked being criticized for violating a supposed "community norm" which said, in effect, unprotected sex is "abnormal." So they accepted the risk of HIV infection as simply a kind of occupational hazard in the business of being gay.

Are they fools? They're hardly ignorant. Do they have a death wish? A deep-seated desire to end a lifetime of pain caused by being considered sick, criminal, and second-class? "They don't," said Tom Coates. "They have a love wish."[106] Used to rejection and condemnation simply for having a different sexual orientation than that of most people, gay men want to be loved. Like virtually everyone with a beating and breakable heart, gay men can be, and often are, fools for love. But is heaping yet more scorn on them the way to make them want to protect themselves and one another from HIV? Or is there a better solution in creating prevention efforts that will begin by making gay men feel so loved, so cared for, and so respected that they will treat themselves and each other the same way? The answer seems obvious in light of the failure of the former approach. Of course the latter requires a great deal of work—and a considerable amount of heart. Surely the lives of gay men are worth the effort.

And surely if anyone ever doubts the ability of gay men to effect change, all they have to do is look at the way gay men with AIDS effected unprecedented changes in American medical research and in how medical consumers are treated. Insisting that their voices be heard and their needs considered, they challenged the system to become better than itself. The rage of an oppressed, distressed people, aimed at appropriate "targets" and not at one another, yielding to reason once they were listened to, could change the world. That is precisely what gay people with AIDS did.

THE MAKING OF SOLDIERS

To skies that knit their heartstrings right,
To fields that bred them brave,
The saviours come not home to-night:
Themselves they could not save.

A. E. HOUSMAN, *A SHROPSHIRE LAD* (1887)

Gay men "came out" as having AIDS the way they had come out as being gay. Their years spent "convalescing" had given these men a confidence that their lives had value. By again challenging the medical establishment—as they'd challenged the American Psychiatric Association a decade earlier—gay people subverted the power of those who masked their antigay politics in the guise of "science." Activists in the eighties presaged the national debate over health care in the nineties by arguing that, with a new disease like AIDS, the testing of experimental treatments was tantamount to health care and so should not be denied to anyone. Activists gained access to the highest levels of the nation's medical research institutions. In the process, though, some of them strangely started to sound like the very scientists they had condemned. But even in compromising the gay community's important critique of medical research and health care, these amateur scientists emulated their courageous predecessors in their desire to survive. That was the point, after all.

When he wasn't in the nurse's uniform he wore for his job, Bobbi Campbell often slipped into the habit of his alter ego, Sister Florence Nightmare, one of San Francisco's famous Sisters of Perpetual Indulgence. After he was diagnosed with Kaposi's sarcoma in September 1981, Campbell's willingness to stand out from the crowd led him to stand up and be counted as the first person with AIDS ever to go public about his disease. Proclaiming himself the "K.S. Poster Boy," Campbell in early 1982 began to write a regular column for the San Francisco *Sentinel,* in which he explained what he was experiencing and offered suggestions to others. Besides the K.S. lesions on his foot, Campbell sported a button that captured in one word the singular objective he and everyone else ever diagnosed with AIDS hoped and worked for. "Survive," it said.

In February 1982, Marc Conant suggested that Dan Turner get together with Campbell to share experiences, after Turner was diagnosed with K.S. Their meeting at Turner's house planted the seed for what in a few years would be a nationwide movement of people with AIDS committed to their own and one another's survival. Conant and his colleague Paul Volberding invited Turner and Campbell to attend what turned out to be the founding meeting of the K.S./ AIDS Foundation. Their early involvement with the foundation showed them firsthand the vital roles that people with AIDS could play in AIDS service organizations as advisers, and often as actual service providers themselves, if they were well enough. Together with a few other people, the two men cofounded a group that became People With AIDS–San Francisco, the first organization anywhere of and for people with AIDS.

Across the continent, Michael Callen and Richard Berkowitz followed up their November 1982 article "We Know Who We Are" by organizing a support group called, simply, Gay Men With AIDS. The two met other people with AIDS at the first peer-led emotional support group in New York for those diagnosed with the disease, offered by Beth Israel Medical Center psychiatrist Stuart Nichols. Callen borrowed a page from Alcoholics Anonymous and other twelve-step support groups in defining the goal of Gay Men With AIDS as supporting each other by "sharing our personal experiences, strength, and our hope."

Some people with AIDS in New York had heard of Bobbi Campbell and were torn between thinking him either courageous or foolish for his willingness to publicly identify himself as a gay man with AIDS. Word reached New York in the spring of 1983 that Campbell was urging the fledgling AIDS service organizations in various cities to pay the expenses of gay men with AIDS to attend the upcoming Second National AIDS Forum, in Denver, to be held in conjunction with the annual lesbian and gay health conference. Michael Callen recalled, "The idea struck like a bolt of lightning. Until then, it simply hadn't occurred to those of us in New York who were diagnosed that we could be anything more than passive recipients of the genuine care and concern of those who hadn't (yet) been diagnosed." But gay San Franciscans were long used to taking an active role in the life of their city, and naturally expected the city to commit its political and financial resources to help save the lives of its residents who contracted AIDS.

Calling attention to the epidemic and commemorating those who already had been lost, people with AIDS carried a banner during the first AIDS Candlelight March, in San Francisco, on May 2, 1983. "Fighting For Our Lives," it said. The following month, Bobbi Campbell and Dan Turner took the banner to the AIDS forum in Denver, where its message of hopeful determination was adopted as the motto for people with AIDS. A dozen people with AIDS met together in a hospitality suite during the conference to talk about how they might organize themselves. Bobbi Campbell took charge of the room, articulating plans for a coalition of political groups in all the cities with large AIDS populations, and proposing that the local groups join one another in forming a national group.

Campbell also conveyed the wish of his fellow San Franciscan, Mark Feldman, who had succumbed to AIDS just before the conference, that terms like "patient" and "victim" should be rejected because they were disempowering. After some skepticism about the significance of what is in a name, the New York contingent joined the group from California to insist that those with the disease be known simply as "people with AIDS," or "PWAs."

The PWAs who met in Denver realized they shared the same frustration with not being listened to by health care providers—or even, too often, by those who were providing services to them in the new AIDS service organizations. They drafted a manifesto known as the "Denver Principles," a series of rights and recommendations for health care providers, AIDS service organizations, and people with AIDS themselves. The Denver Principles became the charter of the movement for PWA self-empowerment. Among them was the recommendation that people with AIDS "be involved at every level" of AIDS service organizations, and that they retain the right "to full explanations of all medical procedures and risks, to choose or refuse their treatment modalities, to refuse to participate in research without jeopardizing their treatment, and to make informed decisions about their lives."

Above all, the group was determined to arm themselves with as much information—at times the only ammunition they had, and always a key source of firepower in this war—as they could lay their hands on, girding for the medical and political battles that lay ahead. These people with AIDS were not a passive lot, to put it mildly. As middle-class white American men, they felt a strong sense of entitlement to support and health care services that all middle-class people in this country take for granted. As they put it in the preamble of the Denver Principles, "We condemn attempts to label us as 'victims,' a term that implies defeat, and we are only occasionally 'patients,' a term that implies passivity, helplessness, and dependence upon the care of others. We are 'People With AIDS.'"[1] PWAs hoped that by seizing the word "victim," challenging its meaning, even eschewing it altogether, their roles in the epidemic might be changed from being mere casualties to active participants in the fight against it—the fight of their lives, for their lives.

After the Denver meeting, Callen, Berkowitz, and former newspaper reporter Arthur Felson were joined by Bobbi Campbell, who flew with them back from Denver to New York, to plan a national group. In New York, an ad in local gay papers led to the formation of PWA–New York, a political organization for people with AIDS that foundered before long because of internal dissent, the deaths of many of its founders, and an inhospitable environment. From its ashes arose the PWA Coalition, a group still thriving today. Its monthly newsletter *PWA Coalition Newsline,* and a book it produced called *Surviving and Thriving with AIDS: Hints for the Newly Diagnosed,* became valuable sources of information for thousands of people with AIDS in New York, across the country, and throughout the world.

On the other coast, PWA–San Francisco also thrived. Bobby Reynolds, a gay man diagnosed with AIDS in June 1982, was on the first executive committee of PWA–San Francisco. Asked in an early interview what he thought about being public with his AIDS diagnosis in view of the stereotypes about people with AIDS, Reynolds said, "I felt that they were putting me on a file card and just sticking me away somewhere. So I made the decision to start speaking out, and I became known as Bobby Reynolds, the person with AIDS, and consequently they're going to know that I'm Bobby Reynolds, a gay man who has AIDS."

Reynolds likened the experience to "coming out" as homosexual. He said, "We've talked in group [therapy] about how coming out with AIDS is similar to coming out of the closet as a gay person: a lot of questioning, a lot of trying to find your identity, who am I as a gay man, who am I as a gay man with AIDS? It's like crawling— starting out in diapers and then crawling, then standing up, then taking your first step, and it's very similar, I think, to what people go through coming out."[2] The images of infancy spring easily to mind for anyone describing how someone learns something new. Unfortunately, it was about the decline and end of life that PWAs were forced to learn.

The importance of personal identity as someone diagnosed with AIDS was recognized in the earliest days of the epidemic. Shortly after the first reports of AIDS in the press in 1981, Larry Mass asked Donald Krintzman in a *New York Native* interview about being a "cancer patient." Before AIDS had a name, someone with Kaposi's sarcoma was simply called a cancer patient. How, asked Mass, did this new identity fit with his other identities—including gay, male, American, Jewish, and New Yorker. Krintzman, the former lover of GMHC cofounder Paul Rapoport (who himself died of AIDS) and the first person with AIDS ever interviewed in the press, answered, "I think my new identity as a cancer patient is less powerful than my new identity as a man who may be facing death." In fact, Krintzman was only three months away from his death in November 1981.[3]

Many lives would have ended sooner had it not been for two gay men in San Francisco, neither of them infected with HIV, who understood the importance of information and self-determination to the well-being of people with HIV infection and AIDS. Martin Delaney was suffering from chronic hepatitis when he moved to California before the start of the AIDS epidemic. A treatment research program at Stanford University opened his eyes to the way people with life-threatening illness are treated in the medical system. Delaney says, "I was one who lucked out. The drugs worked." He referred to the "dark side" of research to describe the side effects of the drugs, and the fact that treatment didn't work for everyone. For those not even involved in the study, the effectiveness of treatment was a moot point because for them there simply was no treatment. "It became clear," said Delaney, "that the same issue was involved with PWAs. Once scientists identified the cause, and knew that there are things out there that may be helpful to you, they said, 'You can't have them. We in our largesse in the government will decide.'" He added, "This is the Big Brother way they've dealt with other life-threatening illnesses."

In 1985 Delaney founded Project Inform, to study the benefits and drawbacks of PWAs' taking treatment issues into their own hands. The project, originally an academic study expected only to last six months, turned up other issues that were clearly important to address in defining the scope of self-empowerment in the area of medical treatment: How did people make decisions? How would they know the way to use medications? Said Delaney, "Doctors had no answers, the government had no answers except to say wait, we'll figure it out for you." Project Inform's message of "hope and empowerment through information" was appealing to people with AIDS whose combination of fear and fearlessness drove them sometimes to take desperate measures in their efforts to survive. In providing information through its hotline and newsletter, *PI Perspective*, Project Inform helped to create what would become a unique relationship between many people with AIDS and their health care providers— "changing the doctor-patient relationship from 'priest-supplicant' to 'co-conspirator,'" as Delaney put it.[4]

I was struck by the sheer size of John James, a tall man whose Levi's measure forty-two by thirty-eight, when he answered the front door of his house in the Castro district. The house is well known as the site, at one time or another, of a number of gay and AIDS organizations, ranging from the National Task Force on AIDS Prevention to the Gay and Lesbian Medical Association. I had often heard that James held a concern for the gay community in proportion to his stature. In 1986, James began writing a weekly column for a local gay newspaper on experimental AIDS treatments, which evolved into *AIDS Treatment News,* a bimonthly newsletter he publishes out of his home. In the mid-eighties, said James, "Treatment information was unrespectable because the view then was that everybody with AIDS dies and service organizations felt they weren't supposed to be involved between doctor and patient."[5] James, however, understood that information was essential even in the absence of effective treatment.

Commonly during the AIDS epidemic patients—particularly gay men, because AIDS treatment information was frequently discussed in the gay press and among friends—have been better informed about emerging treatments than their physicians, especially if they are in a part of the country with a low incidence of AIDS. If learning about AIDS seemed optional for some doctors, for the gay men they treated it was a matter of life and death. Mervyn Silverman says that not only was AIDS a different kind of disease in medical terms, but gay AIDS patients were different from the typical patients who pass through a doctor's office or hospital. "The average gay man knows more about HIV/AIDS than the average physician," Silverman told me. "This can be daunting for physicians to deal with. It speaks to the need for a partnership between the doctor and patient." Silverman said that gay PWAs, besides being well-informed and actively involved in their own care, also benefited from their connections to the gay community. "This was the first time in history that a community of individuals, linked by various media and socially, were afflicted, so the response was a collective response," he said. Because gay physicians were both members of the community and typically the first to treat AIDS in their gay patients, Silverman noted, "The doctor looked at himself as a potential patient, so was more willing to work with the patient."[6]

In some cases, the doctor himself actually became a patient. Atlanta physician Stosh Ostrow has a thriving HIV practice—and is himself living with HIV. His own experience has led Ostrow to prefer working with patients who participate in their own health care decisions. Until he began to treat people with HIV and AIDS, though, Ostrow said these "activist" patients were rare. "I quit medicine on a couple of occasions," he said, "because I couldn't make people well. It took me a long time to figure out that my job is to present people with opportunities and allow them to make choices." Ostrow noted that, for gay men with HIV, the beginning point of taking an active role in their treatment—as it is in prevention—has been self-acceptance. As he put it, "How can you be comfortable dealing with your disease when you're not even comfortable about who you are?"[7]

Dennis Altman points out that one uniquely important benefit of people with AIDS taking an active role in their own care is that it provides medical science with firsthand information about the disease from those who actually have it. This adds a level of information about the disease usually unavailable to science and medicine. Gay men have been particularly successful at contributing to the understanding of AIDS because of their willingness to put themselves forward and speak forthrightly of their experience. "I have spent time with some remarkable men with AIDS," writes Altman, "and have listened to their presentations at conferences, and I am struck by their capacity to understand the social and political implications of their illness and to communicate this to others."[8]

Even as gay people with AIDS helped educate doctors and scientists about AIDS, they continued to share information with one another through PWA coalitions, in the gay press, and in town meetings. When the Food and Drug Administration (FDA) in March 1987 approved AZT—azidothymidine—"the world of clinical research was turned upside down," as the National Academy of Sciences put it.[9] The first drug ever approved by the government to treat HIV brought an exciting burst of sunshine into the gloaming world of people with AIDS desperate for any kind of relief from the mounting physical ravages of the virus. But the excitement was immediately tempered by the $10,000 annual price tag that Burroughs Wellcome, the manufacturer of AZT, said was necessary to recoup its research costs. Six years into the epidemic, the first seemingly effective drug ever approved to treat HIV was going to be out of reach of most of the people who needed it.

As they had before, gay people with HIV and AIDS, together with their supporters, took action. ACT UP (AIDS Coalition to Unleash Power) formed in New York to insist on access to experimental treatments. In San Francisco, thousands of people gathered in the Castro area to kick off a thirty-mile, two-day march to

Burroughs Wellcome's offices in a bid to draw attention to the drug's high price. From the protests emerged an organized effort to circumvent the government's lethargic drug development process by procuring drugs approved in countries outside the U.S. and making them available to people with AIDS who were willing to take them. Under an FDA regulation that allows individuals with life-threatening diseases to import for personal use drugs approved elsewhere, "buyers' clubs" were formed to buy such drugs in bulk for distribution among people with AIDS throughout the country.

Michael Callen and Tom Hannan, another man with AIDS, announced the launch of a buyers' club, the PWA Health Group, in New York in April 1987. The two had formed a partnership to import a food substance manufactured in Israel from egg whites, called AL-721, believed to have some effect against HIV, based on test tube studies. Callen said, "If a substance cannot hurt and may help, we will make every effort to see that those PWAs who desire to obtain such a substance may do so."[10] Desperate times called for desperate measures. For Callen and other people with AIDS, the issue was a matter of self-determination: If they were willing to try an experimental treatment, why should they be denied the opportunity to do so by a paternalistic government's drug regulation system? Speaking on behalf of people with AIDS and everyone else who was puzzled by the slow pace of treatment research, Callen said, "Why do PWAs themselves have to take time and energy from their own individual struggles for survival to do the job that others are supposed to be doing?" Callen said he hoped not to be in the "business" of importing drugs for long.[11]

AL-721 turned out to be essentially useless, like so many other substances and drugs lauded and then dismissed as the hoped-for cure. In 1988, a Japanese drug called Dextran Sulfate was the rage. In 1989, the PWA Health Group imported two drugs from England that would indeed prove effective, as well as receive the FDA's imprimatur as treatments for AIDS-related infections. Fluconazole was brought in after appearing to be useful in treating cryptococcal meningitis, an inflammation of the lining of the brain affecting 10 to 15 percent of AIDS patients. Aerosol pentamidine, used to prevent *pneumocystis* pneumonia, was already available in the U.S. but was very expensive. The drug typically cost $125 to $175 per dose in the States, but the PWA Health Group imported it and made it available for only $40. Naturally the American manufacturer didn't appreciate the profits it lost because of people with AIDS who refused to be ripped off and found a way to avoid paying the inflated domestic price of the drug.

As sales of AL-721 reached the $1 million mark in its first year, the PWA Health Group knew that it needed someone to organize and run its underground medication distribution operation. Derek Hodel was volunteering as a crisis intervention worker at GMHC in the late eighties when he realized that his volunteer work was more interesting and important to him than his day job. After seeking a job in what he called the "AIDS business," the PWA Health Group hired Hodel to be its first paid executive director. Hodel, who led the group from 1988 to 1992, says the PWA Health Group always saw its mission as going beyond simply importing drugs for people with AIDS. "They tried real hard to be thoughtful and to take actions that would have a larger policy implication, rather than simply providing drugs," he told me.

Sally Cooper, Hodel's successor as director of the PWA Health Group, explained that the group had always pursued a "twin mission" of giving people with HIV the information they need to make their own choices about which treatments to pursue, and "to show the system what it could be doing." She noted that the group—"a very good community-based FDA," as she put it—grew out of its founders' will to live and willingness to organize. "The underground is brilliant," said Cooper. "It's an incredible thing—and it's what happens when a community wants to survive."[12]

Nevertheless, said Hodel, the buyers' clubs didn't represent a viable long-term solution to the desire of people with life-threatening illness for access to emerging or experimental treatments. "My intention," he said, "was always to promote a larger, more systemic response to get the system to adjust, rather than to create another piece of the health care delivery system. That was not our intention." One reason the clubs could not be viewed as the best solution was that not all people with HIV or AIDS had access to them. As Hodel put it, "The buyers' clubs fulfilled a need for people who were relatively plugged in, had access to this kind of information, and had the wherewithal to negotiate that kind of transaction. But it didn't really take care of a lot of other people who still deserve to be helped."[13]

A group of people with AIDS who met regularly at the Metropolitan Community Church, on Eureka Street in San Francisco, to share support and information about possible treatments, decided they weren't going to wait to get drugs from the FDA. Like the PWA Health Group in New York, the group decided to bring unapproved drugs into the country and make them available to people with AIDS through a buyers' club that they formed in April 1987 and named the Healing Alternatives Foundation. A couple of them began to smuggle a drug called ribavirin from Mexico. Then it was AL-721 and dextran sulfate. "They would bring these drugs back to the church," explained Matt Sharp, the foundation's director at the time of our interview, "and after their treatment exchange meeting they would go and purchase some of the drugs that were being smuggled into the country."

Demand was huge, and the foundation soon became a combination health-food store and pharmacy, selling at reasonable prices vitamins, nutritional supplements, and "foreign products" (unapproved drugs). Underscoring its role as simply a conduit for possibly useful therapeutics, a brochure for the organization notes that "H.A.F. makes no medical claims for the products it distributes." As Sharp explained, "The most important issue for us is safety, because we want to make sure that we have clinical trial data that show that whatever somebody brings to us is safe. After that, in terms of efficacy, we feel like it's up to the individual patient to make the decision. As long as it's safe, they should be able to try anything they want."

Sharp himself is typical of the kind of self-motivated client who pays the nominal one dollar membership fee to use the foundation's services. Nearly nine thousand people had become members to the point when I interviewed Sharp at the foundation's modest offices on Market Street. He described the road that had taken him from his home in the Midwest to San Francisco, and his own sense of empowerment. Sharp was a thirty-five-year-old professional ballet dancer in Oklahoma City when he was diagnosed with AIDS. Although he loved dancing and wanted to continue, he kept thinking he should move to San Francisco, where he would have excellent care and access to the latest information. The AIDS support group he was in didn't help; everyone in it had mostly resigned themselves to inevitable death. Looking and feeling healthy at the time we met, Sharp justifiably cited himself as an example of "what motivating yourself will do to keep you alive."[14]

Of the buyers' clubs throughout the country, only three hold tax-exempt status by the IRS: the PWA Health Group, Healing Alternatives Foundation, and the AIDS Treatment Initiative in Atlanta. The Atlanta buyers' club was founded in 1991 by Tom Blount, an architect who became a full-time AIDS activist after his business partner was diagnosed and died in 1986, and his own lover tested positive. "I think the first thing I did was call Project Inform's eight hundred number," Blount recalls. "I called AID Atlanta, and it was all sort of 'let's hold hands and sing Kumbuya on the way past the graveyard.'" Blount was impatient with this palliative approach and determined to save his partner's life. "I didn't want to find a way to feel good about this," he said. "I wanted to find a way to cure it."

Blount's lover, Jim, died only a month before our interview, after exhausting every possibility that the resourceful activist could muster through his nationwide network of contacts in the scientific community and treatment underground. Jim had an HIV-related brain tumor. An Internet search turned up only one clinical trial, at the University of Southern California, an old chemotherapy that had been discarded thirty years earlier because of its side effects. The doctor who studied the drug had only about a 22 to 30 percent success rate in destroying central nervous system lymphoma, which is what Jim had.

Despite the low success rate and possible side effects, Blount wouldn't give up. "All the doctors had thrown up their hands," he said. "But I forced it through." Blount arranged to have the drug flown in from L.A. and given to Jim. Days of waiting and watching followed. An M.R.I. ten days later revealed that the drug had had no effect. Blount said, "That was the day I gave up [hope for Jim's survival]. After ten years of this epidemic, we never gave up. I only had to spend two and a half days of hopelessness, and I consider that a real blessing. Most people give up the moment they're declared positive."

As Blount's and his partner's experience demonstrated, there were no instruction manuals to guide the way in dealing with AIDS. Faith, and a willingness sometimes to take potentially serious risks, is all there was for many people with AIDS. As Blount described it, "It's like swinging through a jungle in the middle of the night, from vine to vine. You have to let go at the high point and reach out and grab whatever you can out there. I have swung through that jungle in the night for ten years, and there's always been something." Despite his lover's death and a serious setback to his own faith in an eventual cure, Blount added, "There is a way to get through this, I know there is."[15]

Michael Callen, like all his fellow PWA activists and their uninfected supporters, pursued the same belief. But their faith and involvement carried a steep price in terms of their own emotional well-being. In his book *Surviving AIDS*, Callen observed that one of the consequences of being involved in the PWA self-empowerment movement was having to endure the deaths of new friends. The energy and drive required was terrific for someone like Callen, who was living with HIV infection, busy following leads on promising treatments to try to save himself, and at the same time trying to inspire hope and pass along information to other people with AIDS.

One way that Callen, Bobbi Campbell, and other gay men with AIDS and their supporters worked to empower their fellow PWAs was in the creation of the National Association of People with AIDS (NAPWA), which they founded after the 1983 Denver AIDS forum. Located in Washington, D.C., NAPWA continues to serve as "the voice of the people," as its literature describes the organization. The Denver Principles of PWA self-empowerment are its "guiding light." Advocating on behalf of people with AIDS in the nation's capital, providing speakers who share their personal stories at schools and businesses throughout the country, operating a mail-order prescription drug service called MedExpress, and serving as a cosponsor of the annual National Skills Building Conference for AIDS service organizations, "NAPWA's mission is broad but its vision is simple—a world without AIDS," as the group's *Community Report* puts it.

Like its founders, NAPWA is committed to disseminating accurate information to and about people with AIDS with the simple belief that information is power, and that having information gives one the ability to live as well and as long as possible with HIV. In

1995, the group launched a national campaign to encourage people to be voluntarily tested for HIV, declaring June 27 to be "National HIV Testing Day." NAPWA believes the information about one's HIV antibody status is an essential first step in preventing oneself from becoming infected if HIV-negative, and both preventing others from becoming infected and receiving appropriate medical attention if HIV-positive.[16]

While its fiscal condition has fluctuated over the years—in late 1996, the organization had to cut back on staff and programs because of a significant shortfall in projected income[17]—NAPWA has played an important role in keeping attention focused on the human face of people living with HIV. In 1992, NAPWA released a report that offered the most comprehensive look to date at the needs and problems of people living with HIV and AIDS. Drawing upon survey responses from more than eighteen hundred people with HIV, the report, *HIV in America,* revealed that in addition to the challenge of simply trying to stay well, one in five people with HIV had been a victim of violence at home or in the community. More than half the respondents said they had difficulty in obtaining and paying for health care. Out of every ten people with HIV infection, nearly three were living on less than $500 a month, and another three lived on $500 to $1,000 a month. As if it wasn't challenging enough to obtain and pay for health care, the report noted that fear and discrimination against people with HIV by health care providers continued to stand in the way of receiving appropriate care.[18]

A. Cornelius Baker, NAPWA's executive director, is a black gay man with a mirthful laugh. He has been active both in the federal government—he worked on AIDS issues in the Bush administration—and in the local Washington, D.C., community, where he helped to organize a group called Best Friends, to provide emergency funds to black and Hispanic men with AIDS. Baker had been living with HIV for a dozen years when I interviewed him for this book. His remarks illustrate both his own character and NAPWA's advocacy role. On a day in early spring, Baker said, "Today is such a beautiful day, and I think about the daffodils. It's another sign that after the winter there still will be some life. I think we have to look for our signs. For me one of the signs now is whenever any friend tells me that they're negative, or whenever I meet somebody who has been positive for fifteen years and they're still healthy. Or when I meet an eighteen-year-old gay man, and I think that in the midst of all this horror here's a person who says, 'I will be what I am.' Those are all signs of hope. It gets you through."[19]

Despite the lift provided by taking charge of their lives, living with HIV and losing friends and loved ones to AIDS was sometimes too much, even for PWA activists. When Bobbi Campbell died in 1984, Dan Turner, his early partner in the fight against AIDS, thought to himself, "Where will we get another Bobbi? Bobbi was not only fighting for himself; he was fighting for all of us. And when he went into battle, he was carrying the standard for all of us. And then suddenly he was gone." Turner added, "I cried for fifteen minutes solid when I heard Bobbi had died. I remembered him wearing his 'Survive' button."[20]

*

On July 3, 1985, a Boston furniture salesman became the first person with AIDS to take AZT, a drug that had been shelved as a useless cancer treatment since the 1960s.[21] The date is significant because it was precisely four years to the day after the first mention of the epidemic in the "newspaper of record," the *New York Times*, when many gay men first learned of the disease that would kill so many of them and forever change their world. Having passed the bare minimum first phase of the federally mandated three-phase drug development process, AZT was deemed "safe" after being tested in only nineteen AIDS patients.

Next came the phase-two trial, to determine the drug's efficacy and correct dosage. A 1986 study of 282 patients with AIDS and a milder, preliminary form of the illness then referred to as AIDS-Related Complex (ARC), found that those given AZT lived longer and had fewer of the opportunistic infections associated with AIDS. Forty-five subjects being given placebo developed opportunistic infections, compared with twenty-four who were on AZT. By the end of the study, nineteen of the 137 patients who were given placebo, and only one of the 145 taking AZT, had died. The causes of death of those on placebo read like a laundry list of the various infections that run amok in the body in the presence of an immune system compromised by HIV: *Pneumocystis carinii* pneumonia (PCP) killed eight; disseminated *Mycobacterium avium-complex* four; cryptococcosis two; cerebral toxoplasmosis two; disseminated cytomegalovirus infection one; B-cell lymphoma one; and another individual died from severe debilitation with wasting. The one person on AZT who died was the casualty of disseminated cryptococcosis.

At the beginning of the study, participants already were well along in the course of HIV infection, evidenced by their baseline CD4 counts. The normal count of these white blood cells (commonly called T-cells, they are an important part of the immune system and the primary target of HIV) is around one thousand per cubic millimeter of blood. For the AIDS patients who entered the study, the damage to their immune systems was evident in their dangerously depressed CD4 counts: an average of only 65.6 for those on AZT, and 77 in those on placebo. Even those who had AIDS-Related Complex had an average of less than two hundred CD4 cells, which today is the cutoff point below which an HIV-positive individual is diagnosed as having full-blown AIDS. The researchers, led by University of Miami scientist Margaret Fischl, noted that the slowed pace at which CD4 cells were destroyed by HIV in those who were taking AZT warranted further investigation of the drug's possible benefits for individuals with HIV but without symptoms.[22]

The monitoring board overseeing the AZT development process for the Food and Drug Administration (FDA) recognized that AZT was having what at the time seemed a dramatic effect in the early trials. In September 1986, the "blind" was taken off the study, and patients who had received placebo were offered AZT. Burroughs Wellcome, the pharmaceutical company that held the patent on AZT, provided the drug, free of charge, to some forty-five hundred people with AIDS between September 1986 and March 1987—about a third of all those living with AIDS in this country at the time.

Phase three, in which a drug's safety and effectiveness is tested in a larger group of patients, was waived for AZT. Instead, Burroughs Wellcome rushed to submit all the new drug application paperwork required by the FDA to consider a drug for approval. Ellen Cooper, who at the time was director of the FDA's Antiviral Drug Division, overseeing the development of AIDS drugs, recalls, "The company worked around the clock to get the data into shape to submit to the FDA. Then basically we worked almost around the clock to approve it."[23]

On March 19, 1987, the FDA approved AZT, despite reservations over the limited knowledge about the drug, its hasty six-month phase-two trial, and the lack of a phase-three trial. Desperation for any kind of treatment meant that corners were cut throughout the process. Their consequences would become apparent in the coming years as patients suffered sometimes serious side effects from the high dosages of AZT prescribed early on. More importantly, the drug eventually would prove to have limited effectiveness when used alone as a "mono-therapy." In the meantime, questions about AZT's speeded-up approval, and the right of Burroughs Wellcome to have an exclusive claim on a drug that had been created by taxpayer-funded government scientists, would keep the political waters roiling for a long time to come.

For the time being, however, the importance—as much symbolic as medical—of having some kind of treatment to offer patients, and the pressure to make it available as quickly as possible, was tremendous. San Francisco internist William F. Owen, Jr., who had used AZT on an experimental basis with a number of his AIDS patients, said, "For the first five years of the epidemic, there was so little we could offer to patients once they were diagnosed. Now the medical profession has *something* to offer. It may not sound like much, but the chance for some quality time is really important to patients who, just a few months ago, had nothing."[24]

Just over a week before the FDA approved AZT, Larry Kramer addressed a group of about 250 men and women at the Gay and Lesbian Community Center in New York on March 10, 1987. With thirty-two thousand AIDS cases in the country by that point—nearly a third of them in New York alone—Kramer reminded the group of his famous 1983 article "1,112 and Counting." Rephrasing the article that first alerted many gay people to the political ramifications of AIDS, Kramer warned, "If my speech tonight doesn't scare the shit out of you, we're in real trouble. If what you're hearing doesn't rouse you to anger, fury, rage, and action, gay men will have no future here on earth. How long does it take before you get angry and fight back?"

Kramer noted that FDA approval of a new drug could easily take ten years. "Ten years!" he said. "Two-thirds of us could be dead in less than five years." Kramer criticized the FDA's speeded-up trials of AZT and plans for the drug's imminent approval. One of his biggest targets was the FDA itself and what he called the "exceptionally foolish" double-blind studies ordinarily used to test drugs. (The studies are called "double-blind" because neither the patient nor the doctor knows whether the patient is getting the actual drug being tested or simply a placebo.) Kramer noted that people facing a life-threatening illness like AIDS would lie if they had to in order to get hold of a promising treatment. Cutting to the chase in his inimitable way, Kramer raised a challenge to the FDA: "We're willing to be guinea pigs, all of us," he thundered. "Give us the fucking drugs!"[25]

Formed in response to Kramer's rousing speech, ACT UP wasted no time in planning its first action for the twenty-fourth—five days after the approval of AZT. At the demonstration on Wall Street, the group distributed thousands of copies of an op-ed article by Larry Kramer that had run in the *New York Times* the previous day. "There is no question on the part of anyone fighting AIDS that the FDA constitutes the single most incomprehensible bottleneck in American bureaucratic history," wrote Kramer. "Double-blind studies were not created with terminal illnesses in mind," he noted, calling for the FDA to make experimental AIDS drugs available on a "compassionate usage" basis.[26] In response to Kramer's article, an effigy of FDA Commissioner Frank Young was hung in front of Trinity Church.

ACT UP explained its anger in a fact sheet that said, "For twelve long months AZT was proclaimed as promising, but in such short supply that it had to be rationed to a very few mortally ill patients. Once Burroughs Wellcome was licensed to distribute AZT, supply for thirty thousand was immediately on hand!" AZT became the most expensive drug ever marketed to that point when Burroughs Wellcome seemed arbitrarily to slap a $10,000 price tag on a year's supply of the drug, putting it well beyond the reach of most of the people who needed it. ACT UP noted the fact that many people with AIDS, if not already poor when they were diagnosed, were financially devastated as a result of not being able to work, had lost their health insurance if they had it, and were rejected by health insurers if they didn't. "Every major insurance company routinely denies benefits to

THE MAKING OF SOLDIERS

people with AIDS or at risk for AIDS," said the group. "That leaves only taxpayer-funded Medicaid, which will not pay for any form of experimental therapy."[27]

Now that AZT had been approved, AIDS activists finally had something concrete to rally around. Besides ACT UP in New York, a group calling itself Citizens for Medical Justice demonstrated against Burroughs Wellcome in San Francisco. After briefly changing its name to AIDS Action Pledge, CMJ became the San Francisco chapter of ACT UP. In cities throughout the country, and in Europe, ACT UP chapters sprang up, leaderless and only informally affiliated with one another. For its first six months, ACT UP's main goal was to get "drugs into bodies."[28] They were determined to shake loose any experimental therapies that might have been caught in the clogged bureaucratic pipeline at the FDA or the National Institutes of Health.

As the result of pressure from ACT UP, Burroughs Wellcome by the end of 1987 reduced the price of AZT by 20 percent to $8,000. Even so, *Barron's* predicted that the pharmaceutical giant would earn $200 million on AZT in its first year alone. Within four years after AZT's approval, Burroughs already had earned $1 billion on the drug that had been developed at the expense of the American people.[29] The company's extraordinary profits on AZT were the catalyst that finally sparked the interest of other drug manufacturers that had, until then, seen AIDS as a waste of their time and money.

Among ordinary citizens infected with or at risk for HIV, the availability of a drug that had even some promise for treating the virus was the catalyst for a political movement focused largely on pushing for the speedy approval and availability of new drugs to treat HIV and its attendant infections. As Peter Arno and Karen Feiden observe in *Against the Odds*, "The approval of AZT seemed to unleash a potent force into the world. Patient empowerment—the refusal to be passive victims, the insistence on fighting the system that would pronounce their doom, the willingness to take matters in their own hands—became a reality."[30]

Since its creation in 1927, the Food and Drug Administration has overseen the licensing, research, and regulation of foods, drugs, cosmetics, and medical devices in the United States. The 1938 Food, Drug, and Cosmetic Act made it illegal to market a drug in the U.S.

until it is proven safe. In 1962, Congress extended the FDA's mandate through the Kefauver amendments to the Food, Drug, and Cosmetic Act, requiring not only safety but also proof that a drug's claims of efficacy are legitimate. Not long after AZT's approval, FDA Commissioner Frank Young in June 1987 announced the agency's new regulations allowing the use of investigational new drugs (IND) to treat AIDS even as they were being studied in clinical trials. The treatment IND, as it was known, allowed patients to receive drugs that were safe and possibly effective while the companies testing them completed controlled trials and compiled, analyzed, and prepared study data for presentation to the FDA. Despite the expectations of a flood of new drugs that activists presumed were stuck in the pipeline at NIH and FDA, the truth was, there simply weren't any. In fact, AZT would remain the only FDA-approved treatment for HIV infection until 1991.

At the July 1988 national gay and lesbian health conference, in Boston, FDA Commissioner Young announced that the agency would permit individuals to import small quantities of unapproved drugs for personal use in trying to treat AIDS. The "new" policy merely codified the FDA's longstanding compassionate-use policy, essentially giving a stamp of approval to what the buyers' clubs already had been doing for a year at that point. Said Young, "In fighting AIDS, FDA is committed to two important, but sometimes conflicting, principles—compassion and good science." As the federal government had already demonstrated with respect to prevention, neither compassion nor good science counted when it came to politics. For the moment, though, gay people were pleased that their efforts seemed to have been acknowledged. Three rows of ACT UP protesters holding signs saying "FDA, You're Killing Me," and an audience inclined to be hostile toward the commissioner, were taken by surprise, and responded enthusiastically to Young's announcement with a standing ovation.

But ACT UP wanted more. The group's Treatment and Data Committee prepared an *FDA Action Handbook* and conducted teach-ins for ACT UP's general membership, educating activists about the FDA and its drug approval process. When ACT UP demonstrators from across the country converged on FDA's Rockville, Maryland, headquarters on October 11, 1988, they knew what they wanted and articulated it forcefully to the news media. Among their demands, ACT UP insisted that the FDA shorten its drug approval process to "ensure immediate free access to drugs proven safe and theoretically effective," eliminate double-blind placebo trials and instead measure new drugs against other approved or experimental drugs, and "include people from all affected populations at all stages of HIV infection in clinical trials." ACT UP contended that in the case of a new disease like AIDS, the testing of new drugs itself was a form of health care—and that everyone should have the right to receive health care.[31]

Eight days after the demonstration, the FDA announced new regulations to speed up the drug approval process, formalizing the expeditious process that had been used the previous year to move AZT quickly through the pipeline to the market. Besides the changes at the FDA, the 1988 demonstration was "one of the most cataclysmic and definitely milestone activist events of the eighties," says Robert Bray, who assisted in promoting the event to the media in his role as director of public relations for the Human Rights Campaign Fund, the Washington-based gay lobbying organization. Looking back, Bray said, "I would say the FDA action represented not only an escalation of activist tactics, but a newfound professionalism, media savvy, and strategic organizing of AIDS activism."[32]

It also represented an important shift in the tactics used by activists, as they realized that venting their rage outside of empty government buildings could only go so far in changing the policies and procedures followed by the federal agencies housed inside them. FDA's agreement to streamline the drug approval process had at least as much to do with meetings between agency officials and key members of ACT UP as it did with the verbal drubbing by demonstrators who had learned how to manipulate the media to advance their cause. David Barr, a member of ACT UP's Treatment and Data Committee, said, "Not only had we been able to show our firepower out on the street, but when we sat down at the table we had a list of issues that we understood." Barr said that while ACT UP's demonstration was "theater," the small, select group of informed activists who met with the FDA had to distill their issues to a short list of priorities. "We learned how to do a meeting," he said.[33] As it turned out, this particular skill would serve the activists far more effectively than the talent for drama they continued to display over the next couple of years.

As activists worked both inside and outside the federal government to push for more and better AIDS drugs, two innovative research programs looked at experimental treatments in untraditional settings in local communities, rather than in university hospital settings where medical research typically is conducted. In San Francisco, Don Abrams helped to launch the County–Community Consortium (CCC) in March 1985. A group of physicians from the Bay area who originally came together to talk about their AIDS patients and experimental drug protocols, CCC members soon decided to design a clinical drug trial that they could conduct from their own offices. After AZT became available, the group launched a study of aerosol, or inhaled, pentamidine, a drug that had showed promise in preventing *pneumocystis carinii* pneumonia—the leading killer of people with AIDS. A hundred patients were enrolled at twelve sites throughout the Bay area, with sixty-nine physicians participating in the study. Abrams says the federal government refused to provide funding for the CCC study because "it was too novel and too community-based."[34]

Meanwhile, in New York, the PWA Coalition organized their own treatment research program, called the Community Research Initiative, and described by Larry Kramer as "an historic attempt by the gay community to test drugs on ourselves."[35] Modeled after San Francisco's CCC, the goal of the initiative was to test drugs in a community setting—CRI was located in rooms adjoining those of the PWA Health Group, on West Twenty-Sixth Street in Manhattan—rather than in an impersonal, intimidating medical research center. The goal of CRI's founders—PWA activists Michael Callen and Tom Hannan, their physician Joseph Sonnabend, and Mathilde Krim, the director of the American Foundation for AIDS Research—was, as Callen described it, to conduct "rigorous scientific research on promising AIDS therapies in a community-based setting faster and more cheaply than traditional systems do." In keeping with the Denver Principles, Callen said, "CRI utilizes study designs that are sensitive to the needs of PWAs, because PWAs and physicians who care for us are involved at every level of the decisionmaking process."[36]

A group of people with AIDS met in May 1987 with Dr. Anthony Fauci, director of the National Institute of Allergy and Infectious Disease (NIAID), to plead that the government issue guidelines advising physicians to use inhaled pentamidine to prevent *pneumocystis* in their AIDS patients. Fauci refused. Michael Callen announced that people with AIDS would test inhaled pentamidine themselves. Ninety New York City physicians and two hundred people with AIDS agreed to participate in the study.

Two years later, on May 1, 1989, Lyphomed, the drug company that held the patent on pentamidine, presented data from the CCC and CRI studies to the FDA. Physician-researchers from the CCC in San Francisco spoke about the effectiveness of inhaled pentamidine, and speakers from New York's CRI offered additional information about the drug's safety. In a final, personal plea, Michael Callen told the FDA committee, "I have witnessed firsthand the tremendous, unnecessary suffering caused by PCP—people with AIDS gasping for breath, twitching on respirators, unable to speak." He noted that, despite the desperate need for prophylaxis against *pneumocystis* and the promise that inhaled pentamidine had showed when used by physicians, "No one in the AIDS establishment seemed to have any interest in the clinical observations of the physicians on the front lines of this epidemic." As was the case with the buyers' clubs, Callen said, "The AIDS community has done an end run around federal incompetence and indifference."[37]

Based upon the information provided by the CCC and CRI, the FDA committee voted unanimously to approve aerosol pentamidine to prevent *pneumocystis* pneumonia—the first time a drug had ever been approved based on research conducted at the community level. Although the research wasn't as "pristine" as traditional academic medical research used to decide for or against a new drug, Ellen Cooper, the former FDA official, said, "I guess the lesson is, first, that important information can come from rather primitive trials as long as certain key elements are followed," including randomization, two "arms" of the study that are different enough to detect whether one was superior over the other, and reasonable "endpoints," in this case the development of PCP.[38]

As much as the scientific knowledge generated by the community-based studies, Cooper said, "just doing it was important." Important because it showed that there are alternatives to the traditional way of conducting clinical research—in the cases of the CCC and CRI, involving both the doctors who actually cared for AIDS patients and the patients themselves in the design of the research studies. By putting research in the hands of the doctors on the front lines providing care, and the people with AIDS receiving it, community-based trials emphasized that the need to gather scientific information can be balanced with not merely caring for, but also caring about, patients as human beings, friends, and neighbors. The active involvement of people with AIDS in community-based trials served—like the support groups, coalitions, and buyers' clubs they had formed—to strengthen their own will to survive. As Peter Arno and Karen Feiden put it, "Because it empowered patients and fostered strong ties with their physicians, community-based research offered, above all else, something whose value could not be measured: a sense of hope."[39]

The Presidential Commission on the HIV Epidemic mentioned the CRI in its June 1988 report, urging the federal government to fund similar community-based AIDS research. An October 1988 congressional report quoted CRI director Tom Hannan as saying, "Open communication and trust are more common in relationships between the community physician and the patient than in those between university-based investigators and clinical trial participants whom they may see once every three months or less frequently unless the patient is hospitalized. The AIDS patient is more likely to believe his or her personal health is a top priority with the community physician than with the investigator whose first goal is to study the effects of the drug."[40]

Addressing the matter of whether care and research are mutually exclusive categories, the House of Representatives Committee on Government Operations noted in its report, *AIDS Drugs: Where Are They?* that in conducting research on cancer, the federal government had no problem resolving this conflict. "HIV infection," said the report, "may have brought us to the time when it is necessary to reevaluate the dichotomy between research and treatment for all life-threatening conditions." It went on to quote from an earlier report, produced by NIAID in January 1988, which said, "The primary intent of [NIAID's clinical trials program] is not the delivery of medical care to AIDS patients, although providing excellent medical care is a component of every good clinical trial."[41]

The committee wasn't satisfied with that assessment. "In the context of AIDS and other life-threatening conditions," it insisted, "clinical trials cannot be considered solely scientific experiments. Access to clinical trials becomes access to therapy, access to quality health care, and for many, access to hope." Of the twenty-five thousand Americans known to be living with AIDS at the time—with as many as 1.2 million more estimated to be HIV-infected—the committee noted that only about forty-six hundred, or 0.3 percent, of the estimated total had participated in clinical trials.[42] Put another way, this meant that 99.7 percent of Americans believed to be infected with HIV did not have access to drugs that could potentially save their lives.

Following the recommendation of the presidential commission, Congress in the fall of 1988 approved a $6 million pilot program to conduct clinical trials in local hospitals, health centers, doctors' offices and clinics, and drug treatment facilities around the country, to be managed by NIAID. The Terry Beirn Community Programs for Clinical Research on AIDS (CPCRA) were intended to complement NIAID's AIDS Clinical Trials Group (ACTG), which began in 1987 to conduct trials in academic medical centers across the country. In its first year the CPCRA supported eighteen treatment research programs based in fourteen cities where large numbers of people with AIDS lived and received medical care. Local physicians and their patients were enlisted in clinical trials of new drug therapies. The program was designed especially to reach out to blacks, Hispanics, women, and intravenous drug users—overrepresented in the AIDS population, but grossly underrepresented in clinical research.

Advocates interpreted the new support for community-based research as an acknowledgment of what they had been criticizing as a flawed clinical trials process. By reducing the cost of research on prospective AIDS drugs, and providing access to promising treatments directly through the physicians who were caring for AIDS patients, the advocates felt community-level, grass-roots, research would speed up the historically glacial pace of the three-phase drug development process required by the FDA. As Martin Delaney said,

"The clinical trials model we use is designed for the convenience of the FDA and drug companies. It has nothing to do with making patients better. It has only to do with licensing a product."[43]

Physicians were concerned about the drugs and other substances their AIDS patients were taking, many of them available through the drug underground and buyers' clubs, and saw community-level research as an opportunity to evaluate these agents.[44] Despite the benefits of the research, it was probably inevitable that, at some point, patients and advocates would be brought up short by the guesswork and lack of hard information used in trying untested treatments. Compound Q, the derivative of a Chinese cucumber root, did precisely that.

After promising animal studies, the FDA approved phase-one clinical trials, to be headed up by Paul Volberding at San Francisco General Hospital. Word about the animal studies spread quickly. Martin Delaney, together with San Francisco pediatrician Larry Waites and allergist Al Levin, decided to launch their own four-city trial, sponsored by Project Inform. Jim Corti, who had been nicknamed "Dextran Man" for his role in smuggling dextran sulfate into the country, now traveled to China to obtain Compound Q for the study. Delaney recalls the reasoning behind the underground trial, launched in May 1989. "Our fear was that if the drug was as helpful as we hoped, it would be forever before we got the answer on it," he said. "If it was as dangerous as we feared, large numbers of people could be hurt from self-experimentation."[45]

Unfortunately, a participant in the Project Inform study, Robert Parr, died on June 24, 1989. A national spotlight now lit up the shadowy world of the AIDS drug underground. Delaney claimed that Project Inform was simply monitoring patients who were being treated with Compound Q, rather than conducting a study per se. However it was defined, the Compound Q study cut corners that threatened the credibility of community-based research. In addition to using a form of the drug that the FDA would not consider pure enough, the Project Inform study didn't bother to obtain the approval of the local review boards that are convened to protect the interests of participants in scientific research. These institutional review boards include doctors, scientists, clergy, and others who determine whether a study has sufficient promise to let participants assume whatever risks may be involved, and ensure that they are informed of any significant aspects of the research. Still, Delaney argued that the physicians involved deserved credit for at least monitoring the use of the drug, which he said patients would have used anyway, and with potentially even more dire consequences.

The FDA asked Project Inform to stop the Compound Q trials, and asked Delaney to meet with Ellen Cooper and other FDA officials in Washington. In the meantime, two more participants in the trials died, one a suicide and the other a young New York actor named Scott Sheaffer, who died after surviving three bouts of PCP and numerous opportunistic infections. Michael Callen criticized Project Inform for not having the ethical stamp of the institutional review board. Mark Harrington, a member of ACT UP/New York's Treatment and Data Committee, said it was incumbent upon activists who conducted clinical research to meet "the highest standards of scientific integrity and medical care."[46] Although he expected to be reprimanded, and possibly even charged criminally in the death of Robert Parr, Delaney instead was surprised and relieved to get the FDA's blessing. On March 8, 1990, the FDA approved Project Inform's plan to move forward with Compound Q, requiring only that it use a synthetic version of the drug and test it on people who had already used it.

Looking back on the troubled and troubling history of this one drug, destined to disappear into the miasma with the many other drugs that ultimately proved ineffective against HIV, Ellen Cooper, who initially had been impressed by Project Inform's data when she met with Delaney at the FDA in 1989, said, "Compound Q is an example of too many risks being taken too quickly."[47] Despite the flawed Compound Q study, and his role in sponsoring the renegade drug trial, Delaney's experience of working with the FDA led to a shift in his advocacy. Rather than being an "outsider," Delaney came to be viewed as an "insider" whose views and connections to the vocal gay AIDS community were actively sought by the federal institutes conducting research on AIDS treatments. This suited Delaney fine. As he explained, "We concluded we'd have a better impact on finding the cure for AIDS not by running trials, but by advising on which trials [would] get done."[48]

During the hiatus forced by the FDA on Project Inform's

Compound Q study, and shortly before Delaney's meeting with the agency, the federal government made an announcement that sent shock waves through the scientific and advocacy communities. Dr. Louis Sullivan, the Secretary of Health and Human Services, announced on August 17, 1989, that a NIAID study had found AZT to be effective in delaying the onset of AIDS in people who were infected but had no symptoms. "Today we are witnessing a turning point in the battle to change AIDS from a fatal disease to a treatable one," said Sullivan.[49]

A front-page article in the *New York Times* the following day quoted Dr. Samuel Broder, director of the National Cancer Institute and one of the first to use AZT against AIDS, as saying, "This is a true breakthrough, and I don't use those words often." Excitement was tempered among AIDS advocates, however, by the fact that AZT was still extremely expensive. Thomas Sheridan, speaking on behalf of the Washington, D.C.–based AIDS Action Council, told the *Times*, "The announcement is historically significant because it is the first time that the government is actually offering a treatment for those who are HIV-positive. But now the question is who will pay for these people to get the drug."[50]

ACT UP asked the same question. The answer it arrived at was quite different from what might have come to the minds of scientists or even other advocates: Make Burroughs Wellcome pay for the drug. On September 14, 1989, former bond-trader-turned-AIDS-activist Peter Staley and six other men, dressed in business suits and wearing falsified ID badges, made their way past the guards into the New York Stock Exchange. ACT UP had returned to Wall Street.

As it had done in its first demonstration there two and a half years earlier, the group was once again protesting the cost of AZT. As the opening bell rang at nine-thirty a.m., five of the men chained themselves to a bannister and unfurled a banner from a balcony overlooking the trading floor—"Sell Wellcome," it said. They drowned out the traders with foghorns, and tossed fake hundred dollar bills into the crowd of traders below. On the bills was imprinted the message, "Fuck your profiteering. We die while you play business." Meanwhile, the other two men snapped photographs, walked outside, and handed them to waiting ACT UP members, who spirited them to the Associated Press.

Of course the actual traders didn't take the situation lightly. "Kill the faggots!" they yelled. Clearly they didn't understand that without access to effective treatment, there would be no need for macho gay bashing; a microscopic organism was already doing a damned good job on its own in killing homosexuals. The five protestors were eventually cut loose from the bannister and, with the two photographers, arrested. An hour later, though, fifteen hundred ACT UP demonstrators appeared at the scene. There were more foghorns, much yelling, and a leaflet saying "Sell Wellcome, Free AZT" was distributed to startled and fascinated onlookers. ACT UP's "bottom line," said the leaflet, was its demand for free AZT. "With a million and a half Americans infected with HIV and millions more infected worldwide," it said, "Anything Else Would Be Genocide."

Four days later, Burroughs Wellcome announced another 20 percent reduction in the price of AZT. Even at the reduced price of $1.20 a capsule, though, AZT still would cost more than $6,000 a year. ACT UP decided to continue its boycott of Burroughs Wellcome's other over-the-counter drugs, affixing "AIDS Profiteer" labels on packages of Sudafed, Actifed, Neosporin, and other common Burroughs Wellcome products.[51]

*

After behind-the-scenes meetings with Larry Kramer during the Fifth International Conference on AIDS, in Montreal in June 1989, NIAID director Tony Fauci announced in San Francisco that month that the institute was going to implement what he called a "parallel track" program for AIDS drug development. One track of the program was the closely monitored clinical trials used to test drugs for efficacy, while the other track would enable physicians to provide drugs that had passed the phase-one test of safety to patients who were unable or unwilling to participate in regular clinical trials because they didn't meet the entry criteria for the standard trials, the trials were full, or they lived too far away from a trial site. Kramer lambasted Fauci in his 1989 book *Reports from the holocaust*, but wrote in a conciliatory afterword, "In crusading for the notion of 'parallel track'—a plan for making experimental drugs available while they are still in Phase Two efficacy protocols under the FDA, in so doing bringing them to us a minimum of two years faster—[Fauci] has indeed become the 'hero' George Bush once named him."[52]

As a comfortably heterosexual man, Fauci was a far cry from his predecessor at NIAID, Dr. Richard Krause, a closeted homosexual man. After a January 1984 lunch at Krause's official residence on the bucolic NIH campus in Bethesda, Maryland, Larry Kramer realized the director was, in Kramer's words, "a closeted gay man so terrified of being discovered to be gay that he didn't want AIDS in his fraternity."[53] Fauci made up for Krause's resistance to involving the institute in AIDS research, going so far as to meet with gay activists and actually involve them in the development of clinical trials. Besides his deputy director, Jim Hill, Fauci had two other openly gay scientists in key positions within NIAID. He hired Jack Killen, formerly a National Cancer Institute researcher who had served as the first paid medical director at Washington, D.C.'s Whitman-Walker Clinic, to help organize the AIDS Clinical Trials Group in 1987. Fauci also hired "Bopper" Deyton in 1986 to help coordinate AIDS research at the institute. Deyton, who was acting director of NIAID's $1 billion-plus extramural research program when I met him, said that Fauci "saw in me, Jim Hill, Jack Killen and others, a professional interest, but also a personal interest that he wanted."[54]

Killen, director of NIAID's AIDS Division, said that as a gay man himself, he was concerned about a disease that was striking down people he knew. As a scientist, however, it was a new experience altogether to have members of the patient community actually involved in the decision-making process. "It's been an interesting two-way learning process by activists and scientists," said Killen. He is convinced that it has been a humanizing process as well. "You go to an AIDS meeting," he said, "and you see scientists in ties and people with turned-around baseball caps, and you see people who are obviously sick. It brings a very human dimension to this epidemic, which I think anybody going to a scientific meeting about AIDS experiences."[55]

Robert M. Wachter, the program director of the 1990 international AIDS conference in San Francisco, describes the increasingly cooperative relationship between AIDS activists and scientists as a "fragile coalition." But the coalition grew stronger over time in much the same way that successful relationships of all sorts develop: by spending time together, working jointly to get through the rough patches, and always being willing to return to the table because of a shared belief in the ultimate value of the relationship. Of course another important way that business or social relationships are strengthened is through the breaking of bread together. A series of "working dinners" at Jim Hill's Capitol Hill home allowed scientists and activists to meet informally and solidify their relationship as they developed simple human comfort with one another.

Hill, a NIAID scientist working on whooping cough and other vaccine research before becoming Fauci's deputy director in 1986, met Gary MacDonald, the first director of the AIDS Action Council and first full-time AIDS advocate in Washington, for dinner in early 1985. Hill later introduced MacDonald to Fauci. In the following years, Hill served as an advance man for Fauci, meeting with AIDS activists, then arranging meetings for them with his boss. "They always knew that if they wanted to talk to Tony Fauci about something, they could get to him through me," said Hill.

One of Hill's dinners brought together Fauci and members of ACT UP shortly before a May 21, 1990, ACT UP demonstration at the National Institutes of Health. "That demonstration was fascinating," said Hill. "We had Peter Staley and Mark Harrington here for dinner the weekend before. They had come down to Washington to meet with Tony. They left a package in my house, a big yellow envelope full of stuff. The next morning I FedEx-ed it to Mark Harrington without looking at it. It was the plans for the demonstration. Then they came and had the demonstration."[56] On the twenty-first, about one thousand demonstrators tossed smoke bombs and chanted "Ten years, one billion dollars, one drug, big deal" and "One AIDS death every twelve minutes." The protest lasted four hours and resulted in eighty-two arrests.

Looking back on those tense years, and the tentativeness on all sides, Tony Fauci says the relationship between scientists and activists has "matured." He attributes its maturation to a fundamentally similar and shared agenda. "I think one of the reasons I've gotten along so well with the gay activists," he told me, "is that we've always understood each other. As friendly as we've become—we've actually become very friendly over the years; you can't help that when you're working against or with somebody ten years or longer and you start spending so much time together that you actually become friends—we kind of have a tacit agreement that we will feel comfortable agreeing to disagree on things that we just can't come to agreement on. Yet we agree on a lot more than you'd think we'd agree on."[57]

Clearly much had changed since the days when Fauci was harshly condemned by Larry Kramer and ACT UP. How did it feel to have been the target of such wrath? Fauci said he didn't take it personally because he realized it wasn't himself as an individual but Dr. Fauci, the Director of NIAID, who was being condemned. "I noticed early on that they were criticizing not me, Tony Fauci, but they were criticizing what they perceived as the establishment—particularly people like Larry. Then I extended myself to them, and tried to listen to the issues that they were criticizing, instead of being very defensive that they were burning *me* in effigy, calling *me* a murderer the way Larry did on the front page of the *San Francisco Chronicle,* and things like that."[58]

So Fauci began to meet regularly with activists like Kramer, Martin Delaney, and members of ACT UP/New York. He said, "That's when we started to develop the bonds and friendship that now, when I get criticized publicly, I know it's an issue they're criticizing, not me. That type of evolution in the relationship between activists and myself has led to what I consider an extraordinarily good relationship between Larry and myself. Interestingly, Larry publicly called me a murderer, but I think the world of Larry; we're actually quite good friends."

The "fragile coalition" had evolved to the point that the lines blurred in everyone's mind as to who was friend and who foe. Said Fauci, "Once they got our attention and they began to understand the issues, and we understood their issues more, they made a decision that it would be best, and they could work better, by actually being part of the process. That's why they're on the advisory committees and ad hoc groups."

By July 1990, Fauci had announced that activists would have representation on all of NIAID's committees and in the AIDS Clinical Treatment Group, where he established the Community Constituency Group (CCG) to provide them with formal involvement in the ACTG.[59] Were the activists co-opted by effectively becoming part of the system they had criticized so vehemently from the outside? No, said Fauci. "They certainly haven't turned into the metaphorical 'Uncle Toms' at all," he explained. "However, there are other groups of activists who perceive them as having given in to the system, and they prefer to remain more strident on the outside. But now there's much less of that because, I think, even the outside activists realize that there is something to be gained by becoming part of the process so long as you don't give up your principles."[60]

But principles weren't the only thing the activists had hung on to in their efforts to move the scientific research establishment. Rage—as much from feeling let down in their middle-class expectations of what America owed them as from their grief and sense of impotence against the viral enemy—was something the activists had nurtured at least as closely as the principles they brought to the table. But, as in all adult relationships, rage and temper tantrums ultimately accomplish little more than alienation. In Larry Kramer's 1992 play, *The Destiny of Me,* the playwright's alter ego Ned Weeks—introduced in *The Normal Heart*—seemed to speak for the activists who were now consulted by government scientists, when he said, "When we were on the outside, fighting to get in, it was easier to call everyone names. But they were smart. They invited us inside. And we saw they looked human. And that makes hate harder."[61]

After a December 1990 conference on women and HIV sponsored by NIAID, ACT UP's Women's Action Committee proposed a six-month suspension of all face-to-face meetings with government officials. The women were angry at the cozy relationship between some of the men on the Treatment and Data Committee and government officials such as Fauci. But after all the meetings, dinners, and promised slots on the committees and advisory boards, the men from ACT UP's Treatment and Data Committee weren't about to give up their newfound access now. As Mark Harrington put it, "As soon as we got the seat at the table, which we had fought for, and which had been a part of our rhetoric for years, there was a faction in ACT UP that didn't want us to claim it."[62]

In addition to complications from gender and race, the growing tension between the activists who had become insiders and their fellow ACT UP members was exacerbated by what sociologist Steven Epstein calls "the politics of expertise." As he explains in *Impure Sci-*

ence, "It was not simply that some people were working on the inside while others were outside—just as important, those who were on the inside were increasingly mastering specialized forms of knowledge with which their fellow activists on the outside did not come into contact."[63] Before his involvement with ACT UP, Mark Harrington probably had one of the more extensive backgrounds in science to be found among the activists who fashioned themselves into lay scientists—and that was nothing more than childhood reading of his father's copies of *Scientific American.*

If the goal of the PWA self-empowerment movement was to help people with AIDS live longer by making informed choices, treatment activists represented a kind of hyper-informed version of the PWA activist, devouring information, and now working inside the federal system to influence choices and policy-making that would affect tens of thousands of Americans. As *AIDS Treatment News* editor John James put it, "Treatment activism takes an immense amount of commitment because of the work involved in becoming informed enough to make a real contribution when you sit down with M.D.s and Ph.D.s."[64]

Activists like Harrington and Peter Staley became proficient enough in the arcana of science that they could indeed sit down with doctors and scientists and both speak and listen with intelligence. Although the proposed moratorium on meetings with government officials failed, Harrington, Staley, and a small group of others from the Treatment and Data Committee realized the time had come to part from ACT UP. Frustration with the group's growing fractiousness, often chaotic attempts to make decisions by consensus, uncertain funding, and, more than anything, a desire to work within the system, propelled the men to break away from ACT UP and form the Treatment Action Group (TAG) in 1992. According to a leaflet for the group, TAG's purpose was to "analyze and watchdog our nation's public and private AIDS research efforts and advocate for greater efficiencies and resources."

The "TAG boys," as they are described by critics and supporters alike, were businesslike—and they certainly meant business. As TAG spokesman Spencer Cox put it, "We tend to want to function within the system. Our feeling is you should cooperate with people who are actually doing the research. You also get tired of standing outside of empty buildings and yelling." Cox, who said he "dropped out of ACT UP because [he] was tired of all that infighting," is one of a second generation of AIDS activists, those who are young enough not to have known a gay community without AIDS—and not to have done anything else professionally before becoming an AIDS activist. As the twenty-eight-year-old told me, "I had no background professionally before I did this. I came to AIDS straight from college, where my field of study was Victorian literature."[65] Now his conversation was saturated with esoteric terms from medical science and words like "groovy," the cutting edge and the retrograde. When he talks about "dating himself" because he can recall the approval of AZT in 1987, the newness of the scientific patina is evident.

TAG's 1992 report, *AIDS Research at the NIH: A Critical Review,* suggested reforms that were later incorporated into the NIH Revitalization Act of 1993. Among other things, the act created an Office of AIDS Research to oversee all of the federally funded AIDS research conducted on the campus of the National Institutes of Health and in universities, hospitals, community clinics, and private doctors' offices throughout the country. TAG participated in a number of prominent federal policy review committees, including the executive committee of NIAID's AIDS Clinical Trials Group, the Office of AIDS Research's AIDS Research Program Evaluation Working Group (the Levine Committee), and the National Task Force on AIDS Drug Development. But among treatment activists across the country, the group is best known—and, for many, notorious—for its insistence in 1994 that the FDA not approve the first of the protease inhibitor drugs because of the relatively short trial and limited information about its long-term effectiveness. Look at what happened with AZT, argued TAG.

In 1993, a large European trial found that AZT benefits asymptomatic HIV-positive individuals for about a year, after which it neither staved off the progression to AIDS nor prolonged life. In the so-called Concorde study, more than seventeen hundred HIV-positive people—the largest and longest study of AZT, which in 1993 was still the most popular drug to treat HIV infection—were randomly assigned to get either AZT or a placebo until they developed symptoms, at which time they were given AZT. As in earlier trials, the Concorde study showed a survival advantage for those on AZT up to one year. But by the third year of the study, most of the advantage had disappeared. Concorde spurred a reassessment of what had become the common practice after 1989 of prescribing AZT when an HIV-positive person's CD4 cells dropped below five hundred cells per microliter of blood, regardless of symptoms. It also made researchers question the usefulness of small, quick trials.[66]

TAG extrapolated the experience with AZT to the drug development process in general. "Now we had all these questions about how to use [AZT]," said Moisés Agosto, a former member of ACT UP/ New York, a member of TAG's board, and director of research and treatment advocacy for the National Minority AIDS Council. "Everybody was so confused. We had advocated so much for that drug—instead of building knowledge of pathogenesis and basic research."[67]

Saquinavir was the first of a new family of drugs called protease inhibitors—literally designed to inhibit an enzyme needed by HIV to infect new cells. Used in combination with AZT, ddC (Dideoxycytidine, like AZT, is a drug that disrupts the virus's reproduction), or both, saquinavir had showed promise in a six-month clinical trial in 1994. The two hundred people with AIDS on the new drug had increases in their CD4 counts, and decreases in viral load, gauged by a more recently developed test that actually measures the amount of virus present in the blood. The higher the viral load, the greater the chances of developing AIDS-related symptoms and infections. Based on its data, Hoffmann–La Roche prepared to ask the FDA to grant it accelerated approval of saquinavir under the FDA's two-year-old policy that allowed the agency to license drugs with minimal evidence of their effectiveness based upon the blood markers.

TAG in August 1994 urged the FDA to hold off on approving Hoffmann–La Roche's application for accelerated approval of saquinavir. Instead, TAG called for an eighteen-thousand-person long-term trial to ensure the collection of in-depth data—precisely the kind of clinical trial that ACT UP and other activists had protested only a few years before. TAG broke away not only from virtually all other treatment activists in the country, but from the FDA itself, which had granted accelerated approval in the first place because of the persistent pushing of AIDS activists. More than fifty organizations united to urge the FDA to save the accelerated drug process they had worked so hard to get. Pharmaceutical companies that had champed at the bit under the FDA's former regulatory policies welcomed the activists' success in doing what they had been unable to do themselves. In fact, the unlikely alliance of politically conservative multinational corporations and the extreme leftists of the AIDS activist movement had been profoundly successful in reforming the FDA. Now the "TAG boys" wanted to go back to the future.

But even in 1994, TAG was "behind the eight ball," says Ellen Cooper, now in the NIH Office of AIDS Research, overseeing the development of new drugs through NIH-sponsored clinical trials. "They came out recognizing the value and need for trials," she said. "But the field is moving ahead. That was an appropriate position four or five years before. But with viral load testing in particular, and with combination therapy, a new approach is needed to evaluate those drugs."[68] By monitoring the viral load and CD4 counts—generically referred to as "surrogate markers" because the increase in the former and decrease in the latter signify the progression of HIV infection—it was possible to know fairly quickly whether a given drug had any effect against HIV.

Other treatment activists were furious with TAG. "TAG breaks my heart," said Larry Kramer. "It's as if they'd never been in ACT UP at all, as if all their experiences in grass-roots activism taught them nothing."[69] For once, Kramer's words were tame compared to the opinions of TAG expressed by others. Bill Bahlman, a charter member of ACT UP/New York who worked with the TAG founders on the Treatment and Data Committee, said that in opposing the accelerated access to new drugs that activists had pushed for since ACT UP's founding, TAG had betrayed the activist agenda. He noted, "If any individual outside the community—whether a pharmaceutical company, the FDA, NIH, or Congress—was pushing for the things that TAG has been pushing for, we'd be picketing their apartments at one o'clock in the morning."[70] Even John James, widely respected as a moderate voice among treatment activists, said, "We have TAG saying they want the large trials that are going to take thousands of people and years for every drug studied. Now we need small, rapid studies to find out what the best drugs are to put into the larger trials. That's not just between me and TAG, but the whole community is going in that direction."[71]

Even if the science had moved beyond the need for what are

called large, simple trials—in this case, comparing saquinavir to a placebo—TAG's rationale was "altruism." Writing in *POZ* magazine, TAG founder Peter Staley said, "Perhaps the time has come to defer immediate hypothetical benefit—often couched in terms of right-of-access—in favor of near-term and long-term benefits for all of us. This is known as altruism. By definition it means that individuals give up some immediate benefit for the longer-term benefit of the group." Staley continued, in words that would ring hollow a few months later. "It may be harsh to frame this debate in terms of selfish individualism versus altruism or symptomatic versus asymptomatic, but demanding access for the individual without insuring a process to benefit the entire group becomes just that: A small circle of people in the know may benefit while the majority is left with nothing. We should strive to do better."[72]

Hoffmann–La Roche rejected the idea for a large trial, though it didn't file a New Drug Application for saquinavir until August 1995. In a November hearing of the FDA's Antiviral Drugs Advisory Committee, the drug company was asked about its incomplete research. But enough evidence had been gathered to suggest that saquinavir had at least a modest, short-term benefit. The committee recommended approval, and the FDA granted it three weeks later—a record ninety-seven days after the company applied.

TAG was there with everyone else demanding immediate access to the drug.[73] Altruism be damned, survival was the main thing, as it had been for empowered people with AIDS throughout the epidemic. But the issues raised in the case of saquinavir, and TAG's call for individuals to nobly consider the greater good above their own interests—presumably including their health, possibly even their lives—went well beyond the development of promising new drugs. TAG had become what Peter Staley referred to as "a small circle of people in the know." Not coincidentally, they were overwhelmingly white, middle-class, and had private health insurance. They also have connections with scientists at the highest levels of American biomedical research. Their notions of what is right, wrong, and necessary didn't always jibe with the realities of others with HIV who don't meet regularly with government officials and corporate CEOs.

Although he is a board member of TAG, Moisés Agosto's job

with the National Minority AIDS Council keeps him grounded in the reality of the lives of people of color, who comprise ever-increasing numbers of those with HIV in this country. Agosto noted that treatment advocacy has never been a major priority for people of color, for a variety of reasons including their traditional mistrust of the medical establishment, social and health burdens in addition to AIDS, and the need for political skills to insist upon a place at a table surrounded by white, male faces. As much as anything else, they hadn't made treatment activism a priority because they figured they were unlikely to have access to new treatments anyway. "When you have good insurance," said Agosto, "when you have a good doctor, when you have education, when you have access because you're a white man or you have money, your priorities change. You don't have to deal with all those social issues we have to take care of in communities of color. You can go right straight to the cure and treatment."[74]

For poor people of color who don't have good insurance, education, or political access, there are other priorities. As for everyone else, survival ranks high on the list. Like the white gay men who demanded access to experimental drugs in the late eighties, poor people of color, after years of underrepresentation in clinical trials, despite the disproportionate number of AIDS cases among them, had come to see participation in clinical trials as the only way to receive medical care. But in late 1994, NIAID announced it was axing three of its four community-based trials in New York. Naturally the motive given was scientific: these particular trials simply did not meet the right research criteria. Within three years, the number of people enrolled in trials in New York—with more than seventy thousand AIDS cases at the time—was expected to drop from 2,130 to only 534.

NIAID's Jack Killen said at the time, "Do we have an obligation to provide everyone access to clinical trials? No, we don't. The purpose of health care is to provide health care. The purpose of clinical trials is to provide research to provide health care." He added, "Fundamentally, it's a problem of the health care system. If they could go and get treatment that is currently available we wouldn't be having this discussion."[75] But "this discussion" had been going on since at least 1987, when AIDS activists first called attention not only to the protracted drug development process but to the flaws in the health care system itself as well. Perhaps the single biggest flaw was (and still is) the fact that only those with private health insurance, linked to employment, get the best treatment. Those without it are left to fend for themselves, or to do something like hook up with a clinical trial where they can get medical care and possibly even effective treatment for HIV infection.

The three New York programs, which were in fact phased out, accounted for 25 percent of all African-Americans, as well as 59.5 percent of Hispanics, 38 percent of the women, and 45 percent of the intravenous drug users enrolled in NIAID's program nationally. Unlike the middle-class, gay, white men with health insurance plans that gave them access to physicians who were affiliated with research studies based in university hospitals, these people had no other options. Nevertheless, Gregg Gonsalves, another member of TAG, told the *New York Times* that the demands of outraged New York researchers and politicians to preserve the programs could be construed as "political pork." As if intentionally flouting the vision of ACT UP and the arguments of AIDS activists across the country and throughout the epidemic, Gonsalves said, "We're getting into politics. This is research. Research does not equal health care. Are we going to treat research as pork? It's really hard."[76]

It's even harder to understand where and why the cherished principles of AIDS advocacy had changed so drastically for treatment activists like Gonsalves and TAG. Actually, the "where" seemed to have been the meeting rooms in Washington in which TAG worked on the "inside." The "why" seemed to have to do with their desire to continue to be invited into those rooms. Not only did they sound like the "junior scientists" others accused them of thinking themselves, but they seemed to have adopted the pre-AIDS mindset of the actual scientists whom activists had denounced for looking at human beings as nothing more than "subjects" and for regarding clinical trials of promising treatments as nothing more than scientific experiments.

It was the activists' own argument that AIDS research and care are inextricably linked which led to the expedited release of new drugs, lower drug prices, and community-based drug trials. It was their arguments that led to a shift in thinking about clinical trials as sources of care rather than only dispassionate scientific experiments. As Ellen Cooper explained, before AIDS activists argued for access to clinical trials as a "right," such trials were seen historically as risk situations for patients. "That was the model until AIDS," she said. "Then it became much more a right to enter trials, and the government ought to support trials so anybody who wants to get in one can—which is really a remarkable change."[77]

For these things alone AIDS activists could claim credit for some of the most tremendous changes in the history of American medicine. As Robert Wachter noted in an editorial in the *New England Journal of Medicine*, "Because AIDS activists have demonstrated the degree of influence that a well-organized, highly motivated advocacy group can have, we can be certain that the empowerment of patients will be a major part of the American social landscape of the nineties."[78]

But with prominent AIDS activists now a part of the system they had once condemned, parroting words like "altruism" in the hope that others—certainly not themselves—would make sacrifices for the sake of medical science, the medical landscape for poor people of color with HIV seemed as bleak as ever. It's easy to ask others to be "altruistic" when you can get immediate access to a promising new drug because of your connections. Privilege has its rewards. But what of those who had never known privilege, whose best hope for good medical care was the clinical trials they participated in—the same way it had been for white gay men in the eighties? Gay activists had once complained bitterly that the scientific establishment didn't care about gay lives, and they refused to accept the idea that some lives might have to be sacrificed now to secure better health for later generations. Had gay lives suddenly taken on added value when a few of those leading them became a part of the establishment?

It was hard to believe the brilliant legacy of AIDS activism and PWA empowerment could devolve to a small circle of people in the know who repudiated the movement's charter beliefs, called upon others to sacrifice their personal interests for the greater good—and then were first in line to get the best treatment for themselves as soon as it became available. Of course they continued to call what they did self-empowerment. Most others called it selfishness.

No matter how highly TAG members valued their own lives,

gay lobbyists in Washington regularly downplayed the impact of AIDS on the lives of gay men in this country to win political support and funding for treatment and services. Like TAG members, the "coat-and-tie" politicos thrived on working inside the federal system. Doing so, they would accomplish impressive political feats with tremendous benefits for people with AIDS. But in the process they struck bargains with the devil of a homophobic political system, and were denounced by "street" activists who, after making their own significant contributions began to spin out of control in fits of rage they increasingly directed at gay leaders. Mud wrestling was never as dirty as what went on between the street activists and Washington lobbyists.

6

We'd spent so many years huddling in the ghetto that it never occurred to us to turn to the federal government.

EDMUND WHITE, *THE FAREWELL SYMPHONY*

AIDS has often been described as history's most "political" disease. Because it mainly afflicted gay men at first, the combination of the morally and politically charged issues of homosexuality and death— as well as everything associated with them—ensured that the politics of AIDS would shake the nation's political system to its core. The refusal of gay people to accept the stigma society attached to AIDS— hell, they'd been stigmatized for years anyway—and their willingness to stand up to the federal and medical establishments to demand what they felt was rightfully theirs as Americans, further infused the AIDS "movement" with angry drama. How gay people learned, and didn't learn in some cases, to focus their anger strategically is the story of a despised minority group learning to play the American game of politics. Too many times it meant accepting second-class status as the price of playing.

"Unless we fight for our lives, we shall die," wrote Larry Kramer in his 1983 article "1,112 and Counting."[1] Kramer described what little was known about AIDS at that point, excoriated public officials for ignoring the growing epidemic, and lambasted gay men and the gay press for their refusal to take the threat of AIDS seriously. The only praise Kramer had was for the National Gay Task Force—"our only hope for national leadership, with its new and splendid leader, Virginia Apuzzo." And he set the stage for the kind of direct-action

AIDS activism that hadn't to that point happened anywhere. Before "1,112 and Counting," gay people were doing what they could to care for the sick and to mourn their dead with quiet dignity. After the article's publication, they continued to do those necessary things, but they grew increasingly unwilling to be quiet about the deaths of gay men and the preternatural silence about the epidemic from elected officials.

Kramer's article was accompanied by a call for three thousand volunteers to join in "demonstrations of civil disobedience" that Kramer said might include sit-ins, traffic tie-ups, and arrests. The appeal for volunteers to protest was unsuccessful. Kramer says that only about fifty people showed up to "meet for instruction with a straight black man who had worked with Martin Luther King, Jr." The group called themselves the AIDS Network Public Events Committee. In a letter to New York Mayor Ed Koch that he wrote on behalf of the AIDS Network, Kramer said the gay community's frustration and anger at the city's inaction on AIDS "will manifest itself in a manner heretofore not associated with this community and the gay population at large." AIDS, he said—accurately, though a bit prematurely—"has, ironically, united our community in a way not heretofore thought possible."[2]

Kramer's article and letter to the mayor were the last straws for GMHC's board of directors, who were angry at his outspokenness and insistence that the organization should play a more active political role. In New York, Kramer was denounced by some gay leaders as "sex-negative" and accused of using AIDS "to deliver his post-*Faggots* 'I told you so.'"[3] But while GMHC fumed and other gay men in New York continued to downplay the growing epidemic, "1,112 and Counting" was reprinted in gay newspapers throughout the country. Kramer was just starting to have a political impact—which was ironic in view of the fact that just a month earlier he had said in the GMHC newsletter, "There is one thing we must not allow AIDS to become, and that is a *political* [Kramer's emphasis] issue among ourselves. It's not. It's a health issue for us."[4]

Before the AIDS epidemic, Larry Kramer wasn't a politically active gay man. In fact, he steered clear of gay political activism because, in his view, "All that activism was focused around sex, around the freedom to fuck wherever, whenever, however, and whomever."[5]

His circles of friends consisted of upper-middle-class white gay men in Manhattan who spent summer weekends at Fire Island Pines and winter weekend nights in the city's hottest dance bars, like The Saint. But Kramer's world was rocked when those who peopled it began to get sick and die. He immediately began to use his reputation, media connections, and the gifts he had displayed as a polemicist in *Faggots* to draw attention to AIDS. His anger at the lack of interest with which the city and federal governments—and the gay community—were handling the epidemic while his friends were dying sparked what before had only been a latent activism in himself. As he puts it, "I'd been an angry kid since I was born. So it was all a marriage made in heaven."

A year before the appearance of "1,112 and Counting," the Centers for Disease Control reported in March 1982 that 285 cases of what was being called Gay Related Immune Deficiency (GRID) had been diagnosed in seventeen states. Half the cases were in New York and a quarter were in California.[6] In San Francisco that month, the gay Stonewall Democratic Club sponsored the city's first forum on the new disease, calling it "Gay Cancer." Bobbi Campbell, the sixteenth person in San Francisco to have been diagnosed with Kaposi's sarcoma and the self-proclaimed "K.S. Poster Boy," came to show the group what the unusual skin cancer looked like. Twelve people showed up.

The other gay political groups were preoccupied with trying to line up delegates to the Democratic National Convention, which would be held in San Francisco in 1984. After the forum the Stonewall club also moved on to the more pressing business of organizing a gay rights march to be held during the Democratic convention. As the gay political groups prepared for the convention, San Franciscans were taken aback by a "Startling Finding on Gay Disease," reported by Randy Shilts in the *San Francisco Chronicle:* One out of every 350 gay men in the city was believed to be suffering from AIDS.[7]

A hundred thousand people showed up for the National March for Lesbian and Gay Rights on July 14, 1984, in a characteristically San Franciscan version of Bastille Day. On the eve of the march, the Sisters of Perpetual Indulgence staged a mock exorcism of a woman dressed as arch-conservative Phyllis Schlafly and ripped off the pants of a Reverend Jerry Falwell look-alike to expose fishnet stockings and a black corset.[8] Both Schlafly and Falwell were in San Francisco at the time, rallying their own antigay forces.

The momentum generated by the July march spiraled into support for an independent gay AIDS activist group in San Francisco. Thirty-one-year-old Paul Boneberg, then president of the Stonewall Democratic Club, was tapped by other gay community leaders to head the new group. Mobilization Against AIDS came into existence in the fall of 1984 with the express goal of organizing street demonstrations, a goal it accomplished by staging monthly protests. In addition to its street demos, Mobilization, beginning in 1985, took on the task of organizing the annual AIDS candlelight vigil that the San Francisco PWA Coalition had started two years earlier. Another San Francisco group, Citizens for Medical Justice, began in early 1985 to do nonviolent civil disobedience. The group constructed their "AIDS Vigil," an encampment of a half-dozen tents that the *New York Times* said "stood as a silent, if unsightly reproach to indifference" on the grounds of the old Federal Building in the civic center until hundred-mile-an-hour winds flattened them in December 1995.[9]

Shortly after the candlelight vigil in May 1985, Mobilization sponsored the first PWA lobbying day in Washington, D.C. Michael Callen was there, issuing a challenge to President Reagan, who still had not spoken publicly about AIDS, "Say the word 'AIDS,' Mr. President!" The lobbyists also attacked friends in Congress, such as California Representative (now Senator) Barbara Boxer, demanding that Congress hold hearings on AIDS in San Francisco. Boneberg explained, "There was a definite influence in the strategy by the old Vietnam war organizers, who said the Vietnam war was never ended when you attacked Republicans. The Vietnam war was ended when you attacked the moderate Democrats, and therefore what we have to do is, in effect, attack our friends to move forward."[10]

Meanwhile, in New York, a group of gay activists with roots in the gay liberation movement of the early seventies formed the Swift and Terrible Retribution Committee. After William F. Buckley published an article in March 1986—in which he claimed "it is both a fact and the popular perception that AIDS is the special curse of the homosexual" (despite epidemiological figures at the time showing that worldwide AIDS was afflicting far more heterosexuals), and called for the tattooing of gay men with AIDS on the rear end and drug users on the arm—the reaction by gay people was indeed swift. The Retribution Committee swung into action, protesting—in concentration camp uniforms—at the Manhattan headquarters of Buckley's *National Review.* That summer, the group struck again, this time picketing a visit to New York by Supreme Court Justice Warren Berger, not long after the Supreme Court handed down its ruling in the *Bowers v. Hardwick* sodomy case. The hometown of Broadway wouldn't let San Francisco outdo it in the street theater department, and a group calling themselves the "New Supremes" serenaded the twenty-five hundred protestors with their version of "Stop that kind of love, before you break the law."

About twelve people from the Swift and Terrible Retribution Committee began to meet at the apartment of Bill Bahlman, in the West Village, planning the kind of "zaps" that gay activists had used in the years immediately following the 1969 Stonewall riot. Calling itself the Lavender Hill Mob, the breakaway group began in late 1986 to direct its attention at targets like the Catholic Church and the *New York Times.* The mob surfaced nationally at a March 1987 conference sponsored by the CDC, in Atlanta, to discuss mandatory HIV antibody testing. Bahlman recalls venting his own anger at the gay community leaders at the meeting, letting loose during a press conference they held after the participants in the meeting voted against mandatory testing.

Bahlman said the activists were "congratulating themselves" on the adoption by conferees of a position opposing madatory testing. Bahlman shouted at them, "Where is your anger? PWAs are dying! Our community is being decimated, and here you are patting yourselves on the back for what was a foregone conclusion—no one was for mandatory testing at this conference. And here you are speaking in front of the press as if we had some major victory—and we're all dying."[11]

The Mob's next national appearance was at the Third International AIDS Conference, in Washington, D.C., the first week of June 1987. The protestors marched outside the Washington Hilton, where President Reagan had been shot in 1981, chanting, "We're dying of red tape"—a reference to the interminable federal drug approval process. One of the banners the protestors held up said, "Hey

Mr. President. Just Say Yes to More: AIDS Funding, Education, Research, Drugs, Safe Sex, Anonymous Testing." Another slogan that would become internationally famous also made its national debut that day: "Silence = Death."

The boos that had greeted President Reagan's first-ever speech on AIDS the night before were echoed that Monday, June 1, when Vice President George Bush endorsed the president's call for mandatory testing in a speech to the assembled scientists. Returning to his seat afterward and thinking he was off-mike, Bush asked Assistant Secretary for Health Robert Windom, "Who was that, some gay group?"[12]

Bahlman recalls the boos that had provoked Bush's gaffe: "Of course it was Henry [Yaeger], Martin [Robinson], and myself." The anger that Bush elicited in the morning spilled over at noon in a planned civil disobedience demonstration at the White House. About 350 people gathered in Lafayette Square, across from the White House, to protest a lack of funding for AIDS research and the snail's pace of federal AIDS education programs. "Reagan, Reagan, too little, too late," they chanted. Led by former Legal Services Corporation head Dan Bradley, who had AIDS at the time, a group of sixty-three protesters stepped over a concrete barrier onto Pennsylvania Avenue and blocked traffic by sitting on the street. Wearing riot helmets and bright yellow rubber gloves, D.C. police escorted the protesters—among them, Dan Bradley, Larry Kramer, Larry Mass, and Ginny Apuzzo—to waiting police buses where they were photographed and handcuffed.[13]

Vivian Shapiro, then the national co-chair of the Human Rights Campaign Fund (HRCF), a gay lobbying organization in Washington formed in 1983, said of her arrest, "Truly, being arrested was the only action I knew to begin to release my frustration at the insanity of this [Reagan] administration. It was a primal scream."[14] The photographs of prominent gay leaders being arrested ran in newspapers across the country, and the nation was given its first taste of a new kind of AIDS activism.

It was called ACT UP.

"The fact that everybody responded to ACT UP, I think was more just a question of time, and moment, and frustration," says Larry Kramer. "It was the right time for it to happen."[15] In Kramer's speech at the New York Gay and Lesbian Community Center on the night of Tuesday, March 10, 1987, he laid into the gay community in the way that only Larry Kramer could: "I sometimes think we have a death wish," he railed. "I think we must want to die. I have never been able to understand why for six long years we have sat back and let ourselves literally be knocked off man by man—without fighting back. I have heard of denial, but this is more than denial; it *is* a death wish." The crux of the speech, though, was Kramer's simple question: "Do we want to start a new organization devoted solely to political action?"[16]

Two days later, about three hundred people again showed up at the center. They answered Kramer's question with the formation of ACT UP, the AIDS Coalition to Unleash Power, a leaderless protest group, "democratic to the point of near anarchy."[17] Bill Bahlman and other veterans of the Lavender Hill Mob, just back from the CDC conference in Atlanta, provided training to the seventy-five people who formed the initial core of ACT UP. Marty Robinson taught ACT UP how to negotiate with the police. Henry Yaeger taught people how to wheat-paste notices about upcoming actions on streetlights. Jean Elizabeth Glass taught them how to train marshals for demonstrations. Bahlman himself provided instruction on writing flyers and dealing with the medical research establishment.[18]

These early members of ACT UP may have needed training in the finer points of civil disobedience, but they were more than eager students. For them this was hardly an academic exercise. Bahlman explained, "This wasn't something where they said, 'Someone should do something about AIDS, and I guess I should do something.' These were people who had lost their lovers, who had lovers who were sick, who had AIDS themselves."[19]

ACT UP's first demonstration—a protest on Wall Street against the exorbitant price of just-approved AZT—introduced what became the group's distinctive brand of street theater. Older activists were gratified to see a return of the colorful demos and zaps they had pioneered in the early seventies. But the rage! The rage was more than anger at the suffocation of the closet. These gay people were furious that they weren't getting the treatment they expected as tax-paying Americans. They were furious about the neglect they were experiencing from the government because of a sexual orientation and now a disease that rendered them expendable—just like the nation's poor, who suffered the same fate.

As with other AIDS organizations that were started by middle- and upper-middle-class white gay men, the angry energy that drove ACT UP came at least in part from a sense of betrayed entitlement, a feeling that they weren't getting their due. Allan Robinson, a black gay man active in ACT UP, said, "One of the things I picked up, especially among the upper middle class, is that they were goddamned angry. They were angry because they thought they had everything—trips to Brazil, and Fire Island, hanging in the clubs, boyfriends, drugs, money, and living perhaps on Eighty-First Street and Central Park West. They were angry because they were being treated like everybody else."[20]

Two months before President Reagan would finally utter the word "AIDS"—six years into the epidemic—the group asked, "Who is in charge?" The demonstration and arrests made national news. And when FDA Commissioner Frank Young announced several weeks later that the FDA was speeding up its drug approval process, CBS anchor Dan Rather credited ACT UP's pressure.[21]

The energy and early successes of ACT UP sparked the formation of ACT UP chapters in cities throughout the United States and in several other countries as well. In San Francisco, for example, activist Hank Wilson recalls, "We formed ACT UP here because we liked the name, we got off on the energy of the people in New York, and we loved their graphics."[22] And in Atlanta, Jeff Graham, director of the city's AIDS Survival Project, joined the local ACT UP chapter because he saw it as the only group with "the enthusiasm, commitment, and energy" he wanted.[23]

ACT UP members were predominantly gay, and the group's sensibility often drew deeply from gay camp humor. In 1989, for instance, it launched a campaign against New York Health Commissioner Stephen Joseph called "Surrender Dorothy!"—a title taken from *The Wizard of Oz*, the 1939 film that launched the career of Judy Garland, an icon of many gay men. In the years before the Stonewall uprising, gay men often referred to themselves as "friends of Dorothy," and familiarity with the expression conveyed to another man that one was gay. Strangely, ACT UP downplayed its gay identity, insisting it be known only as an AIDS activist organization. One of ACT UP/New York's more ubiquitous members, Michael Petrelis, claimed in a letter to the editor in the *Wall Street Journal* that "ACT UP isn't 'gay'" because the group welcomed heterosexuals and anyone else interested in stopping AIDS.[24]

ACT UP's real moment in the sun—actually the spotlight of media coverage—was its October 11, 1988, protest against the FDA. A year to the day after the second March on Washington for Lesbian and Gay Rights, and just after the second showing of the AIDS Memorial Quilt in Washington, D.C., "Seize Control of the FDA" was the most widely publicized of ACT UP's early demonstrations.[25] The demonstration was organized by ACT NOW—a network of ACT UP chapters throughout the country that had formed during the 1987 march, primarily to protest the FDA's hidebound procedures for the testing and approval of new drugs.

Michelangelo Signorile, who oversaw the media coverage of the demonstration as head of ACT UP/New York's media committee, recalls, "What we had done was organized a well-rehearsed circus. What we were doing was exploiting each other in order to get our message across." As a former gossip columnist, Signorile said, "I dealt in sleaze and dirt and I spoke the language of the masses."[26] All of Signorile's skills were put to use on behalf of the FDA action, as ACT UP's media committee began months in advance to promote the event to the media throughout the country, distributing more than five hundred press kits that included what he described as a "really hokey, tear-jerking cover letter."

ACT UP was assisted in promoting the demonstration—touting it as "the largest act of civil disobedience since the storming of the Pentagon over twenty years ago"—by Urvashi Vaid, then the media coordinator for the National Gay and Lesbian Task Force (NGLTF), in Washington, D.C. Signorile said, "She seemed to know everyone at the networks and newspapers, and almost every reporter seemed to know 'Urv.'"[27] A veteran gay organizer and press spokesperson, Vaid put together a press conference to be held during the demonstration, and provided reporters from across the country with activist "spokespeople" from their own towns and cities.

Activists in T-shirts that said "We Die, They Do Nothing!" plastered the front of the Parklawn Building, the suburban Washington

FDA headquarters, with ACT UP graphics and banners that said things like "Time isn't the only thing the FDA is killing" and "The Government has blood on its hands. One AIDS death every half hour." Others provided a nonstop theatrical spectacle for television cameras that ate it up. One group did "die-ins," lying on the ground in front of cardboard tombstones with "epitaphs" such as "R.I.P. Murdered by the FDA." Another group wrapped themselves in red tape. For Signorile, the spectacle was exactly what ACT UP had intended. As he put it, "This was going to be a spectacular demo and a wonderful show for the media. ACT UP *always* delivered." But "It wasn't all show biz," he added. "We were angry."[28]

The ten-hour demonstration more or less shut down the FDA and resulted in 176 arrests. ACT UP was intoxicated with a sense of its own power. America certainly found out about ACT UP as the group lunged onto the front pages of the nation's newspapers and into the living rooms of millions of Americans in lead stories on the TV evening news. Signorile says, "Suddenly every street activist was a 'press whore,' and all of us were speaking in sound bites. In-your-face activism took shape nationally, and being out of the closet and in the media became the ideal for a new generation."[29]

On October 24, nearly two weeks after the ACT UP demonstration at the FDA, Commissioner Young called for researchers to help speed the process for developing and approving AIDS drugs. On the twenty-eighth, President Reagan signed a bill making October—of course the month was just ending—AIDS awareness month. And on November 8, George Bush was elected the forty-first president of the United States, calling for a "kinder, gentler nation." As Bush and many others in the federal government—as well as among the gay community's own political groups in Washington—would soon learn, kind and gentle would not be on anyone's list of adjectives for describing the attacks that ACT UP made in the coming years.

*

"It had all the right trappings," recalls Tim Westmoreland. "Real people, scientists, policy-makers, people from the CDC and NIH— Marcus Conant was there."[30] But the first congressional hearing on what was then called Gay Related Immune Deficiency (GRID) on

April 13, 1982, could be described as the silence heard around the world if you were talking about the media coverage it did not attract. Westmoreland, then chief counsel to the House Subcommittee on Health and the Environment, organized the one-day hearing at the Gay and Lesbian Community Services Center, in the heart of sub-committee chair Representative Henry Waxman's district in Los Angeles. Waxman functioned as a one-man subcommittee at the hearing, other members apparently preoccupied back in Washington with more important business than what in a year would be deemed the "nation's number one health priority."

To open the hearing, Westmoreland wrote a statement for his boss that underscored the congressman's disdain for the Reagan administration's creeping response to the growing epidemic, and what he thought were the reasons for it. "This horrible disease afflicts members of one of the nation's most stigmatized and discriminated against minorities," said Waxman. "The victims are not typical Main Street Americans. They are gays, mainly from New York, Los Angeles, and San Francisco. There is no doubt in my mind that, if the same disease had appeared among Americans of Norwegian descent, or among tennis players, rather than gay males, the responses of both the government and the medical community would have been different."[31]

The symbolism of holding the first congressional hearing on AIDS at the gay community center would not be lost on anyone, least of all members of Congress, in the coming years. In fact, Congress's response to AIDS would become intimately connected with how much power—which in Washington means the ability to influence public opinion, contribute money to political campaigns, and, above all, to deliver votes—members thought the gay community possessed and could wield. In those early days, though, neither Congress nor anyone else in Washington was paying much attention to the epidemic because there weren't yet gay people insisting that they pay attention and do something as minimal as increasing the government's funding for research into the mysterious new disease.

Before the AIDS epidemic, gay people had no experience in Washington dealing with federal budgets and appropriations, and certainly not with the Department of Health and Human Services (HHS). The only gay political presence in Washington was Steve

Endean's Gay Rights National Lobby and the National Gay Task Force's efforts to push the federal gay and lesbian civil rights bill, a revision of the 1964 Civil Rights Act, introduced by the late Bella Abzug in 1975.[32] Ginny Apuzzo, who became the executive director of the National Gay Task Force (NGTF; the word lesbian would be added to the name later) in 1982, says, "What you have to understand was that the gay and lesbian community in 1980–81 had only one experience with lobbying—that was how to get the gay rights bill through. Every session you'd go in and add two or three sponsors, get people to write from home. That's where this community's expertise was, and it had to turn around on a dime."[33] Apuzzo attributes the gay leaders' political education to Westmoreland and some of the staff of the late Representative Ted Weiss, one of whom was Patsy Fleming, President Clinton's second AIDS "czar."

In the early years of the epidemic, Westmoreland spent a great deal of time on the telephone with gay community leaders who were running the country's fledgling AIDS organizations. They were learning about politics in the same way they had to learn about caring for dying young men: by doing it of necessity. Westmoreland suggested ways they might get involved in the political system. "Many," he said, "were totally unaware of how government worked." Westmoreland provided political "tutorials" for GMHC cofounder and *Advocate* writer Nathan Fein. He also worked with another of GMHC's cofounders. He said, "I spent lots and lots of time on the phone—*lots* of time—with Larry Kramer, helping him understand the Public Health Service and the budget process."

At first, says Westmoreland, gay organizations didn't want to take on a major public health issue like AIDS. They had their hands full—that is, the very few hands there were in the professional gay civil rights movement at that point—trying to deal with discrimination issues and getting a few more supporters for the federal gay rights bill. But there was a collective epiphany. Said Westmoreland, "They came around quickly to the realization that this was threatening to undermine progress they might make in any other area."[34]

Jeff Levi, who became NGTF's Washington director in 1983, says that not only did gay people have to learn about Washington politics, but they had to make a major shift in their thinking about the role of the federal government as well. "The traditional gay and lesbian agenda," explained Levi, "is 'Stay out of our lives. It's a privacy issue. Let us live. Let us be who we are.' The antidiscrimination protection we were seeking is a more involved way of saying the same things." When AIDS appeared, gay leaders suddenly realized how essential the government's involvement—particularly its financial resources—would be to deal with a crisis of such magnitude. Said Levi, "Now we're saying we need affirmative programs that will save our lives, not get out of our lives, and that we need a much closer relationship with the government."[35] You can be sure Apuzzo is being as diplomatic as her many years in politics have taught her to be when she says, "Getting people to change their perspective was like trying to turn a ship around."

For many gay people, especially those whose financial wherewithal provided a cushion against antigay discrimination in areas like employment and housing, AIDS brought the shocking realization that they were at risk and that their government didn't seem to give a damn. Kramer's article "1,112 and Counting" was a revelation for politically apathetic gay people, and those who—like Kramer himself before the epidemic—thought gay community politics were either irrelevant or beneath them. Slowly but surely, the grass roots began to sprout around the country as gay people mobilized themselves into action. And in Washington, the gay community's few spokespeople at the time learned their own lessons—under duress and under the circumstances—very well.

By the time Apuzzo testified at a congressional hearing on August 1, 1983, the former Catholic nun would bring all her sources of strength to bear on the federal government. In an interview nearly twelve years to the day after that hearing, Apuzzo said, simply, "I demanded $100 million for AIDS." Total federal spending for AIDS at the time was only $14.5 million.[36] But Apuzzo went further than just to ask for more funding. She ticked off the "failures" of the federal government's response to AIDS—about which she made it clear that her constituents were very angry. They included the failure to expedite funding for AIDS research, the failure to educate the public to stem hysteria about AIDS, the failure to address specific questions about the safety of the blood supply, the failure to include affected groups in decision-making, and the failure to recognize a right to confidentiality and privacy.[37]

Besides sharpening their skills in lobbying Congress, gay politicos in Washington cultivated relationships with people inside the executive branches, particularly at HHS. Apuzzo recalls that when she first met Ed Brandt, number two in Reagan's HHS, "he looked at me like I'd lost my mind." But Apuzzo wouldn't leave the conservative Oklahoma Republican doctor alone. "I kept working on him," she said, "giving him data, giving him facts." Brandt eventually came to support Apuzzo's efforts, even if he had to do so on the sly to avoid being caught by other hawk-eyed Republicans. Apuzzo remembers that after Brandt sent what was supposed to be a confidential memo to HHS Secretary Margaret Heckler, in 1984, asking for $55 million more than the administration's $51 million request for AIDS, "it ended up in our mailbox in a plain brown envelope." Tim Westmoreland leaked a copy of the same memo, which he'd also received in a brown envelope, to the *Washington Blade*, where a story about it ran on page 1.[38]

Not only did Brandt furtively send copies of his memos to key players on the Hill and in the gay organizations that had come to embrace AIDS as a political issue, but he seemed to have learned to appreciate the humanity and decency that people like Ginny Apuzzo, Jeff Levi, and Tim Westmoreland brought to their political work. After his leaked memo had become what Randy Shilts called "the watershed event in the AIDS budget battle of 1984,"[39] Brandt announced his resignation from HHS. Before he left, though, he spent his last day with Apuzzo, and later sent her a handwritten letter saying he wished he'd spent more time with her.

Gay politics was coming of age in the nation's capital. But before anything significant could be accomplished, it would take some odd twists and turns and even camouflage itself for protection against hostile politicians.

After eight years in the Middle East with the Foreign Service, Gary MacDonald was glad to be back in the States, and ready for a job in which he could feel more comfortable about being gay. Jeff Levi told MacDonald about a job opening with a new group called the Federation of AIDS Related Organizations (FARO). FARO was formed by thirty-eight community-based AIDS organizations at the June 1983 Second National AIDS Forum, in Denver, to provide members with a means to network with one another. The group also wanted a presence in Washington, and in August 1983 hired a health lobbyist to singly man their "lobby project," which they called the FARO AIDS Action Council. MacDonald was interviewed at Whitman-Walker Clinic, then a tiny operation in Washington's Adams-Morgan neighborhood. GMHC's board president, Paul Popham, came down from New York to scope out MacDonald on FARO's behalf. He gave the nod, and MacDonald was hired to be the first executive director of what today is simply called AIDS Action Council.

MacDonald's job was to lobby Congress and the administration to increase funding for AIDS research and education. It was "extremely lonely," he told me, looking back at those early years when he was literally the only person in Washington working full time on AIDS political issues. Working out of the second bedroom of his Capitol Hill apartment, MacDonald and the fledgling AIDS Action Council faced daunting odds against the success of their mission. As MacDonald put it, "There was no AIDS industry, no public consciousness, no fundraising, no prevention—in short nothing." Within a year and a half after MacDonald started his new job in 1984, the virus that causes AIDS was discovered, an antibody test became available, and Rock Hudson died. "The barometer shot way up," he said, and the telephone at AIDS Action Council—like that early hotline in San Francisco that Cleve Jones recalled—now "rang incessantly."

A lot of MacDonald's time in those early years was spent educating people in the government about homosexuals. Because of his willingness to be open about being gay, MacDonald was invited to join the government's early advisory panels on counseling and testing, prevention education, and, as he says, "really in some sense on the gay community." He explained, "There was enormous ignorance in the early days: 'Who are these people? How many of you are there? Where do you live?' I'd get calls from people at CDC asking, 'What percentage of the population is gay male?' They were doing all this projecting and numbers and statistical models trying to figure out just how bad this really was."[40]

Despite the perception of policy-makers and everyone else in Washington that AIDS Action Council was a gay organization that represented a group of gay-run AIDS organizations, MacDonald said, "The council had deliberately decided not to position itself as a gay organization. That was a board decision, which I supported." While AIDS Action represented organizations that derived from the gay community, the council itself never saw itself as a gay organization—just like ACT UP. Said MacDonald, "I think it helped to establish the fact that this disease does not just strike gay men, it's not just a gay disease—which was at that point, and still is, a common perspective."[41] A board of directors who took a laissez-faire approach to the fledgling AIDS Action Council—mostly because, as MacDonald puts it, "The board didn't know diddly about Washington"—allowed the executive director to mold the organization and its image as he deemed fitting and necessary to the business of doing politics in Washington.

There were gay AIDS organizations—including D.C.'s own Whitman-Walker Clinic and Chicago's Howard Brown Memorial Health Center—that resisted joining AIDS Action Council. "They never believed it was an important priority," said MacDonald, ever the diplomat as he resisted adding that of course the groups likewise didn't refuse any federal money that came their way because of AIDS Action Council's lobbying efforts. Because membership dues for AIDS Action Council were proportional to the size of the annual budgets of member agencies, the larger, wealthier agencies kicked in considerably more money to the council's war chest than their smaller counterparts. When Paula Van Ness was director of AIDS Project Los Angeles, the group contributed $60-70,000 a year. The San Francisco AIDS Foundation was good for another $70,000 a year.[42] And GMHC, the "world's oldest and largest" AIDS organization, as it touted itself, was pumping $275,000 a year into AIDS Action Council.[43]

Other AIDS lobbyists—virtually all of them gay—began to appear on the Washington scene in the late eighties. Besides contributing to AIDS Action Council, large agencies like GMHC, APLA, the San Francisco AIDS Foundation, and Seattle's Northwest AIDS Foundation created policy departments and hired lobbyists to look out for their particular interests. Paula Van Ness hired APLA's first policy director in 1985. In 1987, Tim Sweeney had recently left his job as director of Lambda Legal Defense and Education Fund, when GMHC director Richard Dunne took him to lunch. GMHC needed to "get more political," said Dunne—of course Larry Kramer had been saying exactly that for years—and he wanted Sweeney to come aboard and form a policy department.

As AIDS organizations were formed by and for people of color in the late eighties and early nineties, AIDS Action Council was buffeted by charges of being elitist, racist, and beholden to the white gay men who originally had formed it. Dan Bross, who was director of the council from September 1990 until November 1994, told me that he responded to such charges against the council by saying, "People with AIDS deserve better than charges of racism." He added, "The easy part of my job at AIDS Action Council was dealing with Capitol Hill and the administration. The difficult part was dealing with the diversity of the epidemic, of the AIDS community, because people's first reaction is to blame and to personalize and to divide, and that really is not healthy."[44]

AIDS Action Council's struggle to articulate its identity was the same as with every other AIDS organization originally formed by white gay men in the early eighties: Are we a gay organization? Are we an AIDS organization? What's the difference? And what does being one or the other mean, exactly? Finding the answers—there doesn't seem to be only one, and there definitely are not easy ones—to these questions continues in the late nineties to vex everyone involved. When I asked Bross how AIDS Action Council answered these questions during his tenure as the group's leader, he recalled his years at GMHC that revealed a nostalgia for an earlier, easier time when most people with AIDS were gay white men and AIDS groups had a clearer sense of their identity as gay community organizations.

Unlike in the early years, when most people with AIDS were gay men, Bross noted that as the people affected changed, "the circle has changed." Now there were some gay white men, some injection drug users, some women, and a lot of people of color. "The only thing they share is they're all living with HIV," said Bross. He added that the loss of a feeling of community—from the years when the epidemic was homogeneously homosexual—is "tearing some of these AIDS organizations apart." AIDS Action Council's job of speaking on behalf of the AIDS "community" became complicated by the inability of that community to agree on exactly who its members are, and who should speak on their behalf. Which of course made it nearly impossible to speak with one voice to the Feds whose bureaucratic minds naturally resist ambiguity in any form.

Fortunately, in the late eighties, before the intracommunity discord became the kind of civil war it did in the mid-nineties, the council spearheaded a political coalition that was effective, powerful, and accomplished tremendously important feats in Washington that benefit all people with AIDS in this country to this day. Unfortunately, the strategy it used to win support and funding for AIDS would wind up alienating many gay people who were already tired of feeling scolded, slighted, and generally viewed as second-class Americans. In a city whose residents are practically required to learn a new language consisting entirely of acronyms, the coalition was known as NORA, National Organizations Responding to AIDS.

*

AIDS Action Council's board members were very interested in Jean McGuire's two children when they interviewed her in early 1988 for the position of executive director. Although she was at that point identifying herself privately as bisexual, no one in the interview process asked directly about her sexual orientation. In a follow-up phone call from one board member, though, McGuire recalls that the individual "was trying to impress on me how important they felt it was not to have a gay image of AIDS Action Council. And a woman with two kids who was committed to this issue despite the fact that so many people affected by it are gay. . . ." McGuire told me, "I stopped the conversation and said, 'What about having two kids makes you think I'm straight?'"[45]

The day I interviewed McGuire in Cambridge, Massachusets, where she was pursuing doctoral studies, happened to be the tenth anniversary of Rock Hudson's public announcement that he had AIDS. The timing of McGuire's remarks about the desire of AIDS Action Council not to be seen as a gay organization couldn't have been more appropriate. It was in fact Hudson's July 25, 1985, announcement—and the public fear and attention it brought to AIDS because Hudson was perceived publicly as a heterosexual man—that provided gay AIDS activists with a strategy they hoped would finally increase the political and financial commitment from Washington that had been in short supply since the beginning of the epidemic. They reasoned that this would happen if they played down the fact that the vast majority of AIDS cases in the country at that point were among gay men, and instead emphasized that, as *Life* magazine put it, "Now No One is Safe From AIDS."

"De-gaying" the epidemic, and playing upon the fears of heterosexuals that they also were at high risk, became the main strategy of gay AIDS advocates, including AIDS Action Council. So when a woman whom they perceived as heterosexual simply because she had children (today McGuire lives with a female partner) wanted to be their executive director, they were elated at the prospect of being able to tell politicians, "See, it's really not a gay disease, as this 'straight' woman's involvement proves."

The de-gaying strategy was necessary, according to Vic Basile, director of HRCF from June 1983 until June 1989, who jokingly referred to himself as "something of a political whore" in our interview. For him, playing down the overwhelming number of gay men affected by AIDS, and playing up for politicians the relatively few American women and children with AIDS at the time, was merely a political move to win sympathy and support from antigay politicians. Brooking no disagreement, Basile said, "To the extent that gay people are offended by that, the hell with them. It's stupid not to use your most effective weapons here."

For Basile, the "moral imperative" of AIDS politics "is to find a cure for AIDS . . . not to see any more of my friends die." Basile, with that laudable goal in mind, saw the strategy for attaining it as simply "by whatever means necessary." Pragmatism, what is achievable, mattered above all else. As Basile put it, "If it takes Mary Fisher [white, wealthy, and heterosexual] to speak at the Republican National Convention [as she did in 1988], let's have Mary Fisher talk about it. She's a charismatic speaker, she's rich, she's mainstream—she's all the things that break down those stereotypes" about people with AIDS being only gay men and injection drug users. Basile said anyone who disagrees with this strategy is "egotistical, self-centered, and selfish" for not realizing that the ends (more funding and ultimately a cure for AIDS) justify the means (soft-pedaling the fact that the majority of people with AIDS in this country in the late eighties—and still today—were gay men). As Basile said, the National

Rifle Association—which he cited several times as an example of savvy politicking, albeit one at the opposite end of the political spectrum from himself and which is frequently criticized for "buying" politicians—"don't want you to see a redneck out there; they want you to see a family man. Nobody relates to the redneck, or, if they do, they [NRA] want to keep a distance from them."[46]

The board of AIDS Action Council was pleased enough to have Jean McGuire at the helm of the organization because she was perceived as a heterosexual woman. Fortunately for people with AIDS, who would benefit from the political accomplishments of McGuire and other lobbyists and activists, the council wound up getting in McGuire a gifted political strategist who understood the necessity of working within coalitions to advance the mutual interests of participating organizations. McGuire brought to the council an impressive Washington résumé that included stints working on issues related to the elderly, substance abuse, and, what would become most crucial to her work with AIDS, people with disabilities. She was used to bringing together a number of organizations that had a particular interest in an issue, getting them to agree to speak with a unified voice, and then going to Congress as a bloc that could wield considerable political clout. She also was used to surrounding herself with others who could play the game of Washington politics by the same rules, and as well, as she did.

McGuire's right-hand man at AIDS Action Council was Tom Sheridan, a former social worker turned lobbyist who went to the council from the Children's Defense Fund. Like McGuire, Sheridan understood the importance of coalition politics, the give-and-take that members must agree to in the interest of a greater good. Sheridan says, "Coalition politics is effective because it's the hardest to get people to do. The Hill really respects it because they figure that if you can get up here with a coalition that big and that diverse and have everyone agreeing on something, you must have hit on something."[47] Also like McGuire, Sheridan was "horribly closeted at the time," as Basile described him. "At the first mention of 'gay' he would go ballistic."[48]

McGuire and Sheridan were instrumental in organizing a coalition of organizations in Washington that in some way had a vested interest in AIDS, either because of the nature of their business (medical groups, for example) or the clients they represented (such as disability organizations). The coalition, called National Organizations Responding to AIDS (NORA), included the national gay groups. But for the first time since the beginning of the epidemic, those groups were no longer the principal spokespeople on AIDS. NORA depended on the "mainstreaming," or "de-gaying," strategy—something that couldn't be accomplished if the coalition was perceived as simply a gay ploy for attention and money. Sheridan explained, "We tried to make sure that 'the table' looked like the epidemic, and that no one was left out and no one was distanced. HRCF had a seat at the table, NGLTF had a seat at the table. But the nurses' association had a seat at the table as well. Disability rights groups had a seat at the table. The ACLU had a seat at the table."[49]

NORA had a membership of about sixty organizations at the time. Among those representing "mainstream" national organizations were Curt Decker, who, besides helping to organize the MACS study in Baltimore, lobbies on disability issues in Washington, and Pat Wright, a lesbian who is a lobbyist for the Disability Defense and Education Fund. There was Bill Bailey, a powerhouse lobbyist for the American Psychological Association who pushed Congress and the administration relentlessly on HIV prevention. And there were others as well whose willingness to be open about their sexual orientation within their organizations, to demonstrate the relevance of AIDS to their organization's interests, and to devote untold hours to AIDS policy work despite their employers' expectations that they also work on other policy issues, served not only to bolster support for NORA but in some cases to affect entire professional disciplines. When Bailey died from AIDS in 1994, for example, the American Psychological Association established a William A. Bailey Congressional Fellowship Fund "in recognition of his advocacy on behalf of AIDS-related psychological research, training, and services."[50]

Besides AIDS Action Council's McGuire and Sheridan, the inner circle of NORA during the years when it scored big wins on Capitol Hill, 1988 to 1990, included a young lawyer, frequently described in Washington's gay political circles as "brilliant," named Chai Feldblum. Just finished with a clerkship for Supreme Court Justice Harry Blackmun, Feldblum followed her longtime friend Tim Westmoreland's suggestion that she explore her interest in public law at AIDS

Action Council. Like McGuire, Feldblum was identifying herself as "bisexual" at the time. Hired for a salary that was equivalent to what her fellow Harvard Law School grads were being paid as bonuses for joining the nation's major law firms, Feldblum was soon in the thick of AIDS politics. In her second week at the council, Senator Jesse Helms introduced his "No Promo Homo" amendment. The AIDS lobby was caught offguard with no strategy to counter Helms's gay-baiting, and with no one else at that point to take their side. Feldblum said, with considerable understatement, "For me, that was a very poor start." Within three months she left AIDS Action Council, and went to the ACLU's AIDS Project. Shortly afterwards, Jean McGuire became the council's director.

The pieces were in place—at the power center of the coalition two sexually ambiguous women and a closeted gay man—to propel NORA into the winner's circle it hadn't yet occupied since the group was first convened in 1986. McGuire became the group's strategist, Sheridan its key lobbyist, and Feldblum, now at the ACLU, was the coalition's "legislative lawyer"—a term coined by Feldblum for the team member who, through research into a bill's legislative history (the accumulated committee reports, testimony, and records of discussion surrounding legislation being considered by the House or Senate), provides the group with the language it needs to frame its argument in a way that will win support on Capitol Hill. As Feldblum puts it, "'Winning' in the congressional process means winning *something*, and then if you're a good player you win the *most* that you can get given the constraints."[51]

NORA mobilized its forces to take away as its spoils the Ryan White Comprehensive AIDS Resources Emergency (CARE) Act and the Americans with Disabilities Act (ADA), both in 1990. Named after the Indiana teenager who died of AIDS just four months before the bill was passed, the CARE Act provided funding to the cities and states hardest hit by the AIDS epidemic to pay for services for people with HIV and AIDS. Crafted by Jean McGuire, Tom Sheridan, GMHC's Tim Sweeney, and Pat Christen, who at the time was the policy director for the San Francisco AIDS Foundation, the CARE Act's first two years alone provided more than $847 million to fund AIDS services nationwide. When Congress in spring 1996 finally reauthorized the CARE Act for another five years, it was being funded to the tune of $738.5 million in fiscal 1996 alone.[52] The government's proposed fiscal 1999 budget would fund the CARE Act at more than $1.3 billion.

The CARE Act certainly was a juicy plum for AIDS Action Council's member organizations, and has been a tremendous source of funding for much-needed services for people with AIDS. But the ADA, also passed in 1990, offers an even clearer example of how the council was able to achieve a significant legislative win for people with AIDS by maneuvering within the NORA coalition. The ADA expanded on earlier federal antidiscrimination laws protecting people with disabilities, in such areas as employment and public accommodations, by redefining discrimination to include not only outright discriminatory actions against a disabled person but also the absence of taking certain affirmative steps to *accommodate* disabled people. Under the law, for example, an employer is required to make "reasonable accommodations" for applicants and employees who are disabled but who are otherwise qualified to do a job.[53] People with AIDS are covered under the law because the Supreme Court in 1987 ruled in *School Board of Nassau County v. Gene H. Arline* that contagious diseases, including AIDS—though technically an infectious, not a contagious, disease—are considered a handicap or disability, and are therefore protected under federal disability law.[54] In its first AIDS-specific decision, the Supreme Court in 1998 ruled that asymptomatic HIV infection qualifies as a protected disability.[55]

Curt Decker and Pat Wright were seasoned team players in the Consortium of Citizens with Disabilities. Decker and Wright showed both the consortium and the NORA coalition how AIDS was relevant to the disability lobby, and why the AIDS lobby would gain from an alliance with the established disability groups. Decker recalls that he tried to interest disability organizations in AIDS well before the passage of the ADA. "I kept pushing the disability community to look at AIDS as a disability before there was NORA," he said. "I told them that if they couldn't embrace it, they should realize that a fair amount of their constituency—such as substance abusers and the mentally retarded—might become infected." If that didn't persuade them, Decker added that "given the stigma associated with this disease, it was going to backlash."[56]

As the ADA made its way through Congress, from its earliest

drafts in 1987 to its passage in 1990, there were a number of attempts by hostile members to split apart the disability and AIDS coalitions by driving a wedge between the mentally ill and people with AIDS. Fortunately, said Decker, "The disability community realized what was going on, and said we may not be thrilled about AIDS, but we realized this was trying to slice off unpopular communities—and twenty years ago that was us, with forced sterilizations."[57]

One attempt to "slice off" protections for people with HIV and AIDS from the ADA was the so-called Chapman food-handler amendment, which would have prevented HIV-positive food handlers from claiming protection against discrimination. When the amendment passed the House and Senate in the spring of 1990, the disability lobby and NORA joined forces in opposing it. The disability and AIDS coalition argued that AIDS is a disability and must be protected under the ADA. Chai Feldblum, recognized by *The American Lawyer* as one of the nation's leading experts on the ADA, says "What was key was that the disability community as a whole was fighting the amendment. When we went to meetings at the White House there would be fifteen people around the table—ten of them with disabilities, and only two of them whose disability was AIDS. People in wheelchairs, people with cerebral palsy, people who were blind—they were all saying this is a bad amendment."[58]

Despite the major political victories in the ADA and the CARE Act—the first and only disease-specific law in U.S. history[59]—Jean McGuire never wavered from her belief that AIDS Action Council's ultimate objective, indeed that of all AIDS organizations, was to mainstream the AIDS issue to the point that AIDS organizations per se would no longer be needed. "Our goal," she recalls saying at the time of the fight for the ADA, "has to be some level of integration of this obligation into the other health care structures."[60]

Mainstreaming, or de-gaying, AIDS was a shrewd strategy and worked to bring about major legislation with tremendous benefits for people with AIDS. In the process, though, what happened is that politicians ate up the idea that they could "do something for AIDS" by helping women and kids—as small a segment of the AIDS population as they may have been. Gay men with AIDS certainly benefited from the ADA and Ryan White CARE Act. But it was hardly coincidental that the CARE Act was named after a white teenager from middle America who contracted HIV in a "respectable"—nonsexual—way from blood products to treat his hemophilia. Despite the widespread attention his diagnosis and death brought to AIDS, it was politically inconceivable there would be a "Rock Hudson CARE Act." To win support on Capitol Hill, the unprecedented suffering of a seemingly selected group of Americans was downplayed by lobbyists virtually forced to play by the rules of a political system that doesn't value the lives of gay people.

Only in retrospect is there acknowledgment that playing by those rules may have been deleterious to the gay civil rights movement, whose main goal, after all, is to get the nation's political leaders to value the lives of gay Americans as much as those of nongay Americans. Urvashi Vaid says, "Today, there is broad acknowledgment among gay and AIDS leaders that the de-gaying of AIDS was a conscious political choice made by gay organizers in the mid-eighties." But, she adds, "With our frequent pleas to the government to spend funds for AIDS because straights can get ill too, we promoted the homophobic subtext that AIDS would not be as important if only gay or bisexual people were susceptible."[61]

Looking back on the effort to "de-gay" AIDS, former HRCF director Tim McFeeley puts a very fine point on his critique of the strategy that HRCF actually supported. It seemed the only viable option, he said, was to "make people afraid in the straight community." The lobbyists talked about women and children at risk, downplaying the fact that the overwhelming majority of AIDS cases in the country were among gay men and injection drug users (IDUs). Said McFeeley, "Gay people—leaders, organizers—were suffering from feeling that we need to portray ourselves as victims, and that nothing can come out of the government, so therefore we need to be slyly strategic by saying, 'This isn't about gay people; this is your sons and daughters, Mr. and Mrs. America.'"

But, as McFeeley adds, "There's no less hurt because it's affecting gay men and IDUs—and that's all we had to say."[62]

*

In the spring of 1995, AIDS advocates in Washington, now representing organizations that had become community institutions—

even referred to as "mainstream"—and part of a nationwide "industry" supported by the CARE Act, fought against each other and against any cuts that Republicans in Congress might try to make when the act came up for reauthorization. Meanwhile, a contingent of forty-five gay elected officials from across the country—including mayors and state legislators—was met by Secret Service guards wearing bright blue rubber gloves as they checked the officials' bags and briefcases before letting them into the White House, where they'd been invited for a June 13, 1995, meeting. Administration officials were appalled and apologized profusely. Vice President Al Gore made a point of shaking all the gay officials' hands at a reception afterward to show that at least he wasn't afraid of "catching" AIDS from them.

The week before this insulting action—which gay activists promptly dubbed "Glove-Gate"—the Clinton Justice Department had declined to file a friend-of-the-court brief challenging the constitutionality of Colorado's antigay Amendment Two, a measure intended to prohibit gay people from being protected by antidiscrimination laws, as it came before the Supreme Court. A year later the Supreme Court overturned the Colorado law as unconstitutional—with no input from the supposedly gay-friendly administration. Hoping once again to smooth over his bumpy relationship with the gay community, President Clinton used the occasion of the meeting with the gay officials to present his new liaison—the White House's first-ever—to the gay community: Marsha Scott, a nongay woman whose only qualification for the job seemed to be that she had gay friends and was, naturally, a longtime Friend of Bill's. Of course Clinton apologized for the glove incident, portraying it as nothing more than just another of the numerous lapses of judgment under his watch.[63]

Clinton offered unprecedented access to gay and lesbian leaders because they had given millions of dollars and strong political support to his 1992 campaign. He had won many gay hearts, and pulled in huge contributions from the community, when he recognized gay people's efforts and suffering in the AIDS epidemic. In a historic speech during the 1992 campaign, Clinton said to a group of gay and lesbian supporters in Los Angeles: "I just want to thank the gay and lesbian community for your courage and your commitment and your service in face of the terror of AIDS. When no one was offering

a helping hand, and when it was dark and lonely, you did not with-
draw, but instead you reached out to others. And this whole nation
has benefitted already in ways most people cannot even imagine from
the courage and commitment and sense of community which you
practice."[64]

Once in office and put to the test of hostile opinion from conservatives in Congress, however, Clinton did not keep his word to the
gay community. As Urvashi Vaid points out, "All the access in the
world has not strengthened our ability to pass pro-gay legislation
or to hold the president to his campaign promises."[65] "Glove-Gate"
brought home once again the fact that even an invitation to the
White House didn't mean gay people had been invited finally to
participate as equal citizens in the land of *e pluribus unum.* The influx
and visibility of so many gay men and lesbians in the gay political
movement in the late eighties because of AIDS had not led to genuine political clout at the national level. The political strategy to "de-
gay," or mainstream, AIDS had worked to gain support from frightened heterosexuals—but then it backfired by having the unintended
effect of separating AIDS advocacy from the gay rights movement.
The gay organizations effectively turned over the leadership role on
AIDS to de-gayed, so-called mainstream organizations, such as AIDS
Action Council.

The treatment of the gay officials at the White House made clear
that, no matter how vigorously gay lobbyists denied and downplayed
the connection of gay people and AIDS, the American public and
its leaders still viewed all gay people as potential vectors of HIV,
regardless of their antibody status and no matter how casual the
contact with them. Ben Schatz, who wrote AIDS policy papers for
Clinton's 1992 campaign, said that even the accessible, often gay-
supportive president saw "no differentiation" between the politics of
AIDS and the movement of gay people for equal rights.[66]

As happened with young gay men who believed that "gay" and
"AIDS" were synonymous, even the president didn't distinguish the
two. Why, then, did the gay groups believe their own "de-gaying"
rhetoric about women and children first and gay men last? Where
and how did AIDS advocacy split apart from the gay rights movement? And what were the implications of turning over the political
reins on AIDS to advocates and organizations that sometimes went

out of their way to distance themselves from the gay community? Clearly the advocates hadn't succeeded in de-gaying AIDS in the minds of the public. But what did it mean that they had de-gayed it in their *own* minds?

Some argued that gay people needed to look beyond AIDS, to resume the work of gay liberation that had begun in the seventies and was interrputed to a great extent by the community's desperate need to mount a response to the epidemic. In a seminal article in the *Nation,* Darrell Yates Rist, a gay writer who has since died from AIDS, challenged gay people to look beyond the AIDS epidemic in thinking about a community with many long-term needs and challenges that were largely set aside because of the immediate demands of all the sickness and death in the community. The gay civil rights movement shouldn't be subsumed by the AIDS epidemic, said Rist, because not all gay men, and certainly not many lesbians, would die of AIDS. He said that the divorce of AIDS from the gay movement was a "route to respect for homosexuals not open to unapologetic gay activists." But the support that gay people received from nongays too often came at the price of their gay identity. As Rist put it, "Even homophobes who'd never want to see a homosexual holding a lover's hand, especially in front of the children, can cry (and contribute) at the thought of so many gay men dying."[67]

In an *Out/Look* article that sounded similar themes to Rist's, Eric Rofes asked, "De-gaying AIDS might bring more funding, but isn't the cost too high?" Rofes cited a number of examples of AIDS organizations that were created by gay people, still largely staffed by, and providing services to, gay men with HIV and AIDS, but that downplayed their connection to the gay community. He noted, for example, that although the majority of participants in an AIDS Project Los Angeles walkathon were gay men and lesbians, there was no acknowledgment during the opening ceremony of this community, while speakers mentioned other affected populations. Flyers for Boston's AIDS Action Committee's "Pride Dance," during a lesbian and gay pride weekend, hadn't even mentioned the gay and lesbian community. Perhaps most remarkable of all, Gay Men's Health Crisis advertises itself only by its initials, with the letter "H" underlined to emphasize "health" and to deemphasize the word "gay."[68] I have been told by GMHC staff that the agency retains the word "gay" in its name simply to honor its six gay founders.

Urvashi Vaid says that AIDS service organizations are compromised by the receipt of government money. "They don't want to rock the boat," she told me. "They have to work with Republicans and Democrats to get their money. So they end up not taking forceful political positions."[69] This is why, she added, the HIV-related interests of gay people can be represented only by independent gay organizations, not "mainstream" AIDS groups on the public dole from the Ryan White CARE Act. But the gay rights organizations are only too happy to leave AIDS to the AIDS groups, even if they marginalize gay men in the same way as do the mainstream organizations they were meant to supersede.

In his *Out/Look* article, Rofes articulated what really was behind the de-gaying strategy of gay AIDS advocates, and what led the gay rights organizations to surrender their stake in the politics of the epidemic to the de-gayed AIDS industry: embarrassment about gay male sex. Diverting the spotlight that had been shined by the news media and others from what gay men do in bed, as well as what some do in less private places, helped AIDS advocates to win support and funding from the government. So gay advocates downplayed gay men's sexuality, pointing out that gay men really had become "good" homosexuals, evidenced by declining rates of new HIV infections.

By de-gaying AIDS, advocates won government funding for AIDS services—but gay men were made eunuchs in the process.

Some, mainly people with AIDS, argued that the gay community had abandoned AIDS because it was too distracting from other political priorities. In a probing cover story in the *New York Times Magazine* in late 1993, reporter Jeffrey Schmalz, who died from AIDS just before the article's publication, asked, "Whatever happened to AIDS?" The gay movement, he wrote, "has pushed AIDS to the sidelines." As proof he contrasted the overriding "themes" of the 1987 and 1993 gay and lesbian marches on Washington. In 1987, AIDS carried the day as people with AIDS led the march and the AIDS Memorial Quilt was displayed for the first time. The 1993 march, on the other hand, was dominated by the issue of gays in the military—which previously had been a low-level priority on the gay movement's agenda until it was catapulted to the forefront by President Clinton's 1992 campaign promise to end discrimination against gay people in the armed forces.

Schmalz quoted former NGLTF director Torie Osborn, who argued that the shift in gay political priorities was inevitable with the election of a Democratic president, renewed attacks from the right wing, and just plain burnout. Schmalz noted that many gay people, particularly those who are not HIV-infected, do not want the gay community to be defined by a disease. Osborn said, "There is a deep yearning to broaden the agenda beyond AIDS. It's one thing to be fighting for treatment, believing you're going to get a cure that will have everyone survive. But it's an incredibly depressing truth that AIDS has become part of the backdrop of gay life."[70]

But not all gay people, including men who are not HIV-infected, believed that AIDS should simply be relegated to being "part of the backdrop of gay life." As they continued to see their friends get infected with HIV and struggle to pay for treatments to keep them alive, they still viewed AIDS as a profoundly "gay" issue. But they questioned whether the gay community's political organizations were willing and able to keep AIDS on the front burner as they simultaneously worked to address other community priorities. They also questioned whether a compromised and de-gayed AIDS industry could effectively serve the gay men who still comprised the majority of new infections and AIDS cases in most areas of the country.

The street activist in him shows when Paul Boneberg says, "I would argue that we should go back to what was before AIDS activism—that is, community activism, constituencies who are at risk—and serve those constituencies relative to AIDS." AIDS organizations are doing what they need to do *as* organizations, by raising money and trying to garner political and community support for their work. But they are unable to be forceful voices for gay people with AIDS because they are compromised by taking public funds—however necessary those funds are to their operation. Boneberg told me, "The lesbian and gay community's leadership has to reassert responsibility, and that will mean disagreeing with AIDS groups, many of which are led by gay people. But so be it."[71]

Many among the community's leadership had come into the gay civil rights movement because of AIDS. In fact, says John D'Emilio,

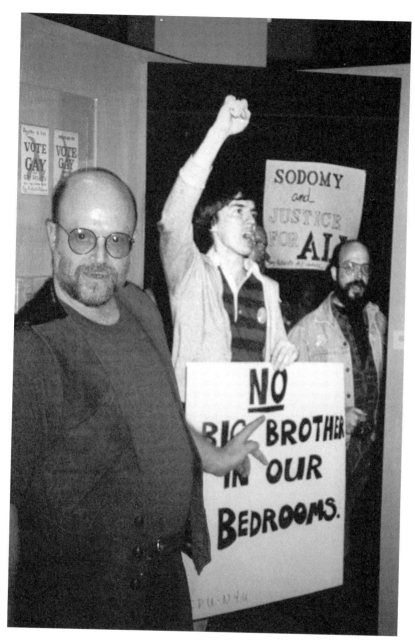

"We elected to be open," wrote Arnie Kantrowitz in a 1973 op-ed article in the *New York Times*, "and face the oppression that would come with it because that was more dignified than being frightened and hiding." Two decades and many AIDS-related losses later, Kantrowitz stood before a poster depicting him and others at a protest in New York, circa 1973. It was part of the New York Public Library's 1994 exhibit *Becoming Visible: The Legacy of Stonewall* marking the twenty-fifth anniversary of the Stonewall uprising that launched the modern gay civil rights movement.

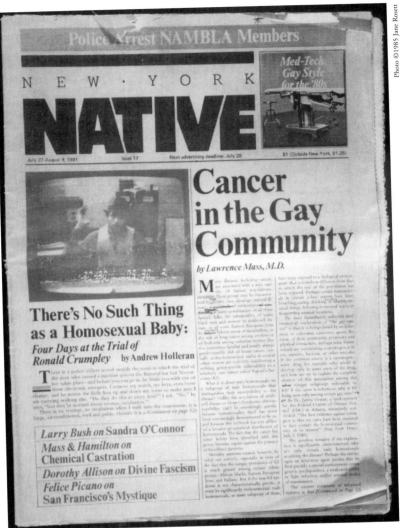

The pioneering AIDS reporting in the *New York Native* of New York physician and GMHC co-founder Lawrence D. Mass alerted gay people throughout the country to the mysterious and deadly epidemic just beginning to unfold. "Cancer in the Gay Community" was the first news feature on AIDS anywhere in the world. It is displayed, with other history-making journalistic memorabilia, at the Newseum, in Arlington, Virginia.

Right, On the night of May 2, 1983, a dozen people with AIDS led the first of what became an annual candlelight march in San Francisco and throughout the world. Their banner encapsulated the hopeful determination of gay people with AIDS and those who cared about them. It became the motto for PWAs who insisted on an active role in their own care, pushed the federal government to reform its protracted drug approval process, and armed themselves with as much information as they could find in their effort to live with HIV.

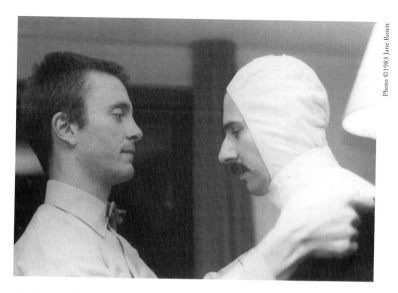

Photo ©1983 Jane Rosett

San Francisco "K.S. Poster Boy" Bobbi Campbell (left) was the first person with AIDS (PWA) ever to go public about his disease. A member of the campy Sisters of Perpetual Indulgence, Campbell fitted his habit—and passed the activist mantle—to New Yorker Phil Lanzeratta, during the Second National AIDS Forum in Denver in 1983. With their fellow PWAs, the two men eschewed the "victim" label and showed the world that neither AIDS nor the stigma society attached to it could break the spirits of people committed to their own and one another's survival.

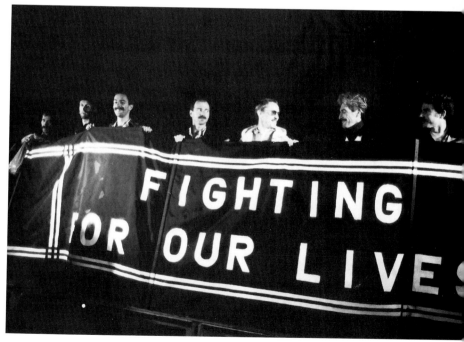

Rink / San Francisco

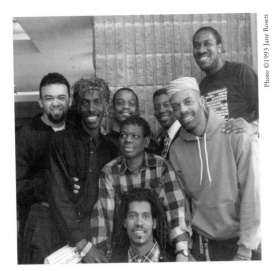

Black gay men pioneered efforts in the African-American community to address AIDS directly and without judgment. By tying personal survival to cultural and community values, prevention educators who serve blacks and other people of color found ways to bolster self-esteem and prevent the spread of HIV among those who have been treated as second-class citizens because of their skin color, socioeconomic status, or sexual orientation. Among those pioneering men were these activists at a 1993 meeting in Secaucus, New Jersey. Left to right, back row: (unidentified), Reggie Williams (founder of the National Task Force on AIDS Prevention), Charles Nelson, H. Alexander Robinson, and Donald Burch. Second row: André Fallen, Ernest Hite. Bottom: Troy Fernandez.

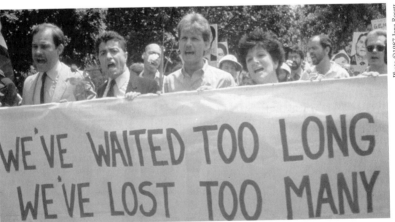

WE'VE WAITED TOO LONG
WE'VE LOST TOO MANY

More than three hundred protesters shouted, "Reagan, Reagan, too little, too late!" in front of the White House when they demonstrated on June 1, 1987. By the time President Ronald Reagan had finally spoken publicly about AIDS the night before the protest—six years into the epidemic—36,058 Americans had been diagnosed with the disease and 20,849 had died. D.C. police, wearing riot helmets and bright yellow rubber gloves arrested sixty-three of the protesters—including some of the nation's most prominent gay and lesbian leaders.

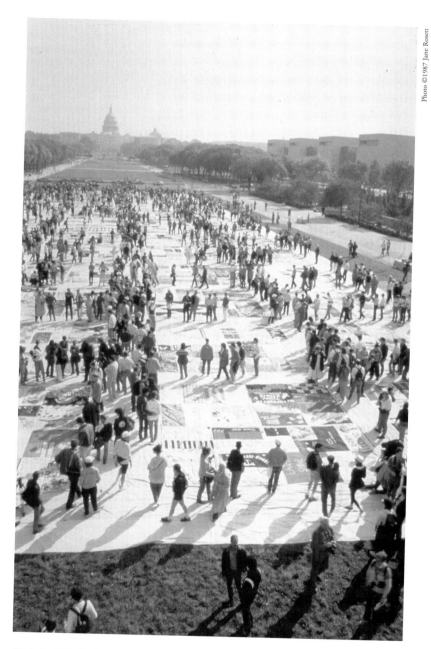

With the U.S. Capitol in the background, the AIDS Memorial Quilt was displayed for the first time during the second March on Washington for Lesbian and Gay Rights, on October 11, 1987. The quilt's 1,920 panels, covering the equivalent of two football fields, represented a fraction of the 24,698 Americans who had died from AIDS by then. When the quilt was displayed again in Washington, in 1996, 45,000 panels covered twenty-five acres on the Mall—and still represented only about one in eight of the total number of Americans who had died from AIDS at that point.

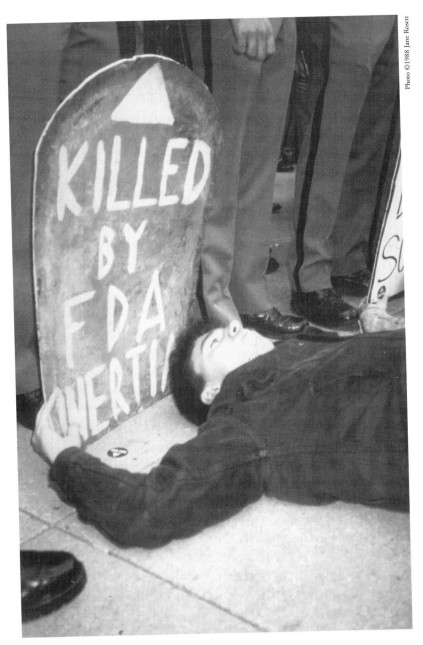

A year to the day after the second March on Washington for Lesbian and Gay Rights, ACT UP members from across the country rallied in Washington to "seize control of the FDA," as the October 11, 1988, demonstration was called. The news media swarmed over the made-for-television demonstration, with the dramatic images— "epitaphs" such as this one, "die-ins," and much fake blood—demonstrators consciously used to gain attention for AIDS. But "It wasn't all show biz," noted ACT UP media director Michelangelo Signorile. "We were angry."

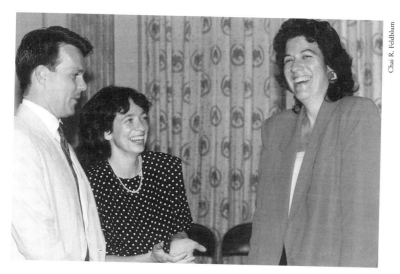

The power triumvirate behind the Washington AIDS lobby at a 1990 Capitol Hill reception celebrating passage of the Americans with Disabilities Act: Lobbyist Tom Sheridan (left), lawyer Chai Feldblum (center), and AIDS Action Council Director Jean McGuire (right). The three savvy coalition builders, in alliance with a range of national organizations, won major victories for people with AIDS and the AIDS organizations that serve them. The game of homophobic politics, however, required them to downplay the vast impact of AIDS on gay men, emphasizing the relatively few women and children affected by AIDS, to win support from skittish and conservative politicians.

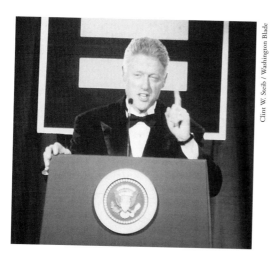

When President Bill Clinton became the first sitting president to address a gay rights organization, he was cheered loudly by the 1,500-member audience at the Human Rights Campaign's fundraising dinner on November 8, 1997. A heckler in the audience who shouted, "People with AIDS are dying!" was jeered by others in the tony crowd. To the heckler they yelled, "Sit down!" while they reassured their important speaker, "We love you Bill!" Times for AIDS and gay political organizations in Washington had changed since Larry Kramer heckled Ronald Reagan in 1987.

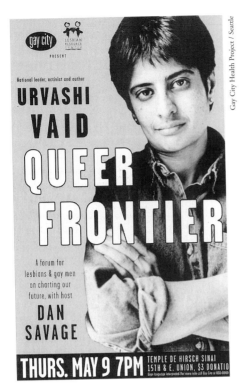

gay city PRESENT

LESBIAN RESOURCE

National leader, activist and author

URVASHI VAID

QUEER FRONTIER

A forum for
lesbians & gay men
on charting our
future, with host

DAN SAVAGE

THURS. MAY 9 7PM TEMPLE DE HIRSCH SINAI
15TH & E. UNION, $3 DONATIO
Sign language interpreted. For more info call Gay City at 860-6969

From its beginning as a Seattle–King County health-department task force exploring prevention options for gay men, "Gay City [Health Project] wasn't just about something bad that we wanted to prevent," says the group's director John Leonard, "but about something really good that we wanted to create." Gay City's programs and community forums don't "look like" HIV prevention programs. Yet, explains Leonard, they serve as vehicles for "building community, promoting communication, and nurturing a culture where gay men see their lives as worth living"—necessary ingredients in motivating gay men to continue protecting themselves against HIV.

Camp humor has been a cornerstone of gay people's ability to survive the physical and spiritual attacks of homophobes, neglect by their government, and the devastation wrought by a deadly microbe. Despite the "all clear" signal some have inferred from the early successes of new drug therapies, "the epidemic isn't over," as this poster from Boston's AIDS Action Committee points out. Until gay men all make healthful and responsible sexual choices, and until the federal government finally spends its hundreds of millions of HIV prevention dollars on relevant programs that target those who really need them, posters such as this one will be part of the landscape of gay life.

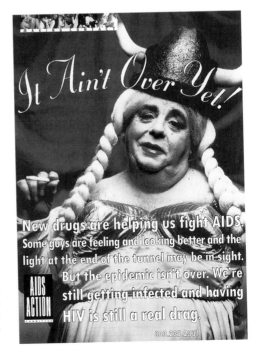

It Ain't Over Yet!

New drugs are helping us fight AIDS. Some guys are feeling and looking better and the light at the end of the tunnel may be in sight. But the epidemic isn't over. We're still getting infected and having HIV is still a real drag.

AIDS ACTION

800.235.2331

"AIDS built the gay movement. It shook loose the resources to transform a movement that was small and based almost entirely on volunteer labor into a movement of full-time people who were devoting themselves to this work and getting paid for it." He added, "Slowly in time that transition would have happened, but the epidemic compressed all of the change that might have taken a generation basically into a decade."[72]

The growth of both the AIDS groups and the professional gay political organizations "created a shift in the leadership of the gay movement, accentuating the trend toward leaders who can claim professional expertise instead of activist credentials," as Dennis Altman put it.[73] But, as he also points out, these "new bureaucrats" faced alienation from the gay and lesbian rank-and-file who became involved in AIDS work because the epidemic was affecting people they knew, or even possibly themselves. Credentials as a gay activist or even, at times, experience working in the "field" of AIDS were no longer necessary prerequisites for leadership positions in the AIDS organizations created by and for gay people.

A 1996 advertisement for AIDS Action Council executive director captured this quite clearly. Although the ad was placed in the *Washington Blade*—presumably the job would be open to a lesbian or gay man reading the gay community newspaper—the only mention of the word "AIDS" itself was in the title of the organization. Neither AIDS activist experience nor gay political leadership experience was required. Besides the experience necessary for managing a not-for-profit organization of a similar size, required skills included financial and budget management, fund-raising, and excellent communications abilities. "The executive director," said the ad, "should be a team builder, coach and a highly skilled consensus manager."[74]

The de-gaying of AIDS was now complete in the minds of AIDS advocates as the nation's leading AIDS advocacy group, created in 1984 to represent the AIDS organizations that had been founded and run by gay people, looked for an executive director who was simply a well-spoken fundraiser and "coach." Now gay rights organizations felt they could return to the business of gay and lesbian liberation—despite an ongoing epidemic that continued to kill tens of thousands of gay men—because AIDS was being "taken care of" by the AIDS industry. Few stopped to think that any industry, even one created by gay people, is above all interested in its bottom line. In the case of AIDS organizations, that meant preserving their funding at all costs, even when they felt it required them to dissociate themselves from the community that gave them life in the first place.

Of course this set up a curious paradox for these organizations: How could they continue to be *in* the gay community but not *of* it? More to the point, how would they keep gay people giving money and serving as volunteers in unprecedented numbers in organizations they helped to create but that now at times wouldn't even acknowledge them?

*

While the gay movers and shakers were doing their thing in Washington, of course, ACT UP and other activists "outside the Beltway" also were doing theirs. Sometimes there was synergy between the direct-action activists and the professional pols in Washington. At other times there was disagreement, even rancor, over strategy. And every once in a while, a split personality would emerge in Washington who had a sense of when politics should give way to protest, who could appreciate the exigencies of federal politicking while still believing there are limits to politeness and times when what is expedient and achievable must come second to what is necessary and right.

Urvashi Vaid had thrived on the excitement and challenge of direct-action activism since her early gay community-organizing days in Boston. Her assistance with publicizing ACT UP's 1988 FDA demonstration to the press was only natural given her love of street politics and the extensive media contacts she had cultivated throughout her years as NGLTF's media director. But in Washington, Vaid sometimes ran up against the hard-headed pragmatism of polished gay politicos who didn't have much use for direct action. As she puts it in *Virtual Equality,* "Although some veterans of the post-Stonewall generation embraced ACT UP as a return to the radical politics they felt the gay movement had wrongly abandoned, most gay political veterans looked down on direct action in general."[75]

Vaid recalls that at the meeting between gay and AIDS lobbyists and FDA bureaucrats immediately after the FDA demonstration, the lobbyists put forth the same message as ACT UP, yet they consciously positioned themselves as the "more reasonable" alternative. For their part, Vaid says ACT UP members "were contemptuous of and hostile to the mainstream gay and lesbian rights movement." Small wonder, then, that often there was such ill will between the coat-and-tie lobbyists and the in-your-face protestors.

Jeff Levi, who was NGLTF's executive director at the time of the FDA demonstration, is critical of the limited awareness of gay history prevalent among many in ACT UP, those, he said, who "think there was no organizing, no politics before ACT UP." Nevertheless, Levi credits ACT UP's media-grabbing protests with providing a useful backdrop against which gay political operatives could move and shake the Washington power establishment. "While we recognized that we did the coat-and-tie routine more often than not," he said, "the street activists played a critical role in helping us get that access. They moved the range of reasonableness more to the left than it might otherwise have been."[76]

To Larry Kramer and many other advocates of direct action, the gay Washington lobbyists were little more than sycophants of the system. In a strongly worded letter to HRCF, Kramer wrote, "I resent your organization. I resent just about every gay and AIDS organization in Washington. For you see, I don't know what you *do*. I don't know what *any* of you *do,* down there." To underscore his lack of understanding of what the gay lobbyists were doing in Washington, Kramer distilled his complaints to a typically enraged, self-interested, and highly personal closing jab: "What are you doing to save my fucking life?"[77]

Kramer was not the only one in ACT UP who didn't understand what the gay AIDS lobbyists do in Washington. Chai Feldblum described the tensions between pragmatic lobbyists, who played to win as much as they could in Congress, and those who were not familiar with this Washington style of politics. She said, "That caused conflict between the 'inside the Beltway' folks and the 'outside the Beltway' folks who said, 'Why are you putting forward this amendment that seems to be giving something up? We want to fight to the max.' Well, if you fight to the max and, as we say, go down in flaming glory on the Senate floor, you've got a lot of flaming glory and a lot of ashes. But you don't have any program that helps people with AIDS."[78]

Most of the gay and lesbian Washington lobbyists I interviewed for this book, like Levi, were quick to say that ACT UP helped them do their work. The activists pushed the limits of lawmakers' patience to the point that the legislative language offered by the lobbyists—often a legalese version of the activists' own demands—looked reasonable. Some lobbyists went so far as to credit ACT UP's trailblazing for much of their success in getting the government finally to help people with AIDS. On the receiving end of both the lobbying and demonstrations, President Clinton's first two AIDS "czars" also credit ACT UP with moving the government to make necessary changes.

Kristine Gebbie said, "I think the anger displayed through ACT UP protests was very useful. The intriguing thing it did was make 'the suits' look suddenly very wonderful and reasonable and paved the way for some conversations that might have been more difficult."[79] Gebbie's successor, Patsy Fleming, said, "There were times when there was an adversarial relationship between them and us. But I think in general and on balance, it was a very close relationship and it developed and it flourished over the years."[80]

Not all the coat-and-tie lobbyists, however, are willing to give unqualified praise to ACT UP. Most of them feel that ACT UP didn't understand or value the lobbyists' role the way the lobbyists valued ACT UP's. Tim McFeeley said, "By 1989, ACT UP had done the necessary shock troop work, which is shocking people, making people understand this was being ignored and was very serious. Then as solutions started to get crafted, it turned a lot of people off and it made it very difficult to work with politicians. There was never any particular collaboration; we just sort of tolerated one another." He added, "Do I think we would have gone further without [ACT UP]? Probably not. I just wish that some of that energy had gone into more permanent activism, the activism of political organizing, as opposed to a one-hour catharsis."[81]

Urvashi Vaid learned that direct action was okay to do while she was an NGLTF staffer but that it took on added significance when she became executive director. A few months after she organized a December 1, 1989, civil disobedience in front of the White House by the executive directors of a number of gay and AIDS organizations—sixty-five of them were arrested—Vaid, by then NGLTF's director, was invited to a meeting sponsored by the National Leadership Coalition on AIDS. The organization's membership, corporate CEO types, were to be treated to President George Bush's first and only speech on AIDS—which included mention of his support for the ADA, then pending in Congress, despite the opposition of many Republicans who wanted to protect businesses from the costs of making their workplaces accessible to people with disabilities.

Vaid helped organize a demonstration outside the Crystal Gateway Marriott Hotel, in Arlington, Virginia, where President Bush was to speak on that Thursday, March 29, 1990. She also tried to get other gay and AIDS organization leaders to join her in demonstrating inside. She said, "I thought it was just a matter of phoning people who had gotten arrested—they'd already protested Bush, what the hell did they have to lose?!" In the end, no one else would join her—not Tim McFeeley, not Jean McGuire, not even San Francisco rabble-rouser Cleve Jones, who was going to meet with Bush at the White House the next day. They offered their encouragement but, one by one, all of them begged off actually joining her with demurrals like "I'll have to get my board's approval," and "There are going to be funders in the room."

Vaid followed along in a printed copy of Bush's speech she'd gotten from her media friends. "It was a very straightforward speech about non-discrimination," she recalls. "He didn't mention gay men; it was all babies and women." Toward the end of the speech Vaid, in her "little black dress and 'Barbara Bush' pearls," stood up and said, "Mr. President, you're not doing enough. We don't need your leadership once a year; we need it every day." The crowd was stunned. They applauded Bush when he responded to his diminutive heckler and told the audience, "I understand the concern that these people feel. If we do nothing else, I hope we can make them understand that not only you care, but we care, too."

"These people" indeed. At that, Vaid stood again and shouted as she held up the sign she had made the night before and smuggled into the room. One side of it said, "Talk is Cheap, AIDS Funding is Not," and on the other, "Don't Forget Gay People with AIDS."

The Secret Service escorted Vaid and another heckler, from ACT UP, out of the building, threatening to arrest them if they returned. After Bush finished, Jean McGuire and Tim McFeeley held a press conference. Vaid recalls, "They took this empty chair and put it in the middle of the press conference and said, 'Urvashi Vaid would have sat here if she hadn't been kicked out of the speech. And we agree with what she said!'" McGuire noted at the press conference that Bush's speech was the first time he'd formally expressed compassion for PWAs. She added, however, "It was long on compassion but short on commitment."[82] Vaid says she was glad that her protest at least seemed to inspire the news media to scrutinize Bush's remarks more closely than they likely would have done otherwise.

But then she had to answer to some of NGLTF's board members who "flipped" at what she had done without their approval. For them, her visibility as director of the organization gave legitimacy to activism that they were ambivalent about, now that they were at least getting a taste of political access. They thought it was unseemly for the director of the National Gay and Lesbian Task Force to stand to protest a speech by the president which, in her judgment, included statements that, if translated into policy, would be harmful to gay people with AIDS.

Years later, Vic Basile still steams over Vaid's 1990 protest. He speaks of Vaid as "a purist, an ideologue" who "basically doesn't get politics." He elaborated, "She thought it was a good idea to challenge Bush in front of this corporate community. I thought it was a disaster because we had a captive audience of corporate executives who were inclined to be supportive on AIDS. And they became a captive audience to a very embarrassing demonstration. I can't tell you how serious that was."[83]

Afterward, as she rode the Metro to NGLTF's U Street offices, Vaid felt vulnerable. She had put herself and the reputation of her organization on the line by literally standing up for what she believed—to none other than the president of the United States. Her fellow gay and lesbian leaders had not stood with her. Being the savvy pols they were, of course, they were able to capitalize even on this rather embarrassing breach of protocol.

But Vaid didn't have too much time to reflect on all of this once she got back to the office. "The minute I walked into the office the phone was ringing," she recalls. "It was Larry Kramer."[84] Naturally he was calling to congratulate Vaid for her courage and brazenness, much like his own when he heckled Bush's predecessor in the White House when he finally spoke publicly about AIDS after six years of abject silence about the epidemic. Vaid had embarrassed gay lobbyists who were willing to do whatever they had to do—even downplaying the suffering of their own people—to be allowed a place at the table. Many other gay people, however, were proud to know that not all their leaders in Washington were willing to grovel under the table for political crumbs.

Of course Larry Kramer had never groveled under anyone's table, and he wasn't about to start now. In March 1990, the same month as Vaid's one-woman protest, Kramer shocked even some of his own "shock troops" in ACT UP. In his monthly "Kramer vs. . . ." column in ACT UP/New York's *OutWeek* magazine, he called upon "every human being who wants to end the AIDS epidemic" to be in San Francisco from June 20 to 24, at the Sixth International Conference on AIDS, "screaming, yelling, furiously angry, protesting, at this stupid conference." Lest anyone miss his point because of its subtlety, Kramer continued, "WE MUST RIOT! I AM CALLING FOR A FUCKING RIOT!"[85] Kramer elaborated in an interview with the *Wall Street Journal* in May. "It hurts me to say I think the time for violence has now arrived," he said. "I don't personally think I'm the guy with the guts to do it, but I'd like to see an AIDS terrorist army, like the Irgun which led to the state of Israel."[86]

Barely three months earlier, ACT UP/New York had staged its "Stop the Church" protest against what the group considered the Catholic Church's "assault on lesbians and gays," "bias," "ignorant denial," "endangering women's lives," "no safe sex education," "no condoms," and "no clean needles." On December 10, 1989, ACT UP members invaded St. Patrick's Cathedral to incarnate their anger within the church itself. Douglas Crimp and Adam Rolston participated in the protest. This is how they described it: "During high mass inside the church, angry protestors forced [Cardinal] O'Connor to abandon his sermon. Affinity groups lay down in the aisles, threw condoms in the air, chained themselves to pews, or shouted invectives at the cardinal. One former altar boy deliberately dropped a consecrated Communion wafer on the floor. (The media had a field day with that one: by the day after the event, it had become legions of 'homosexual activists' desecrating the host.) Forty-three activists were arrested and dragged out of the cathedral; another sixty-eight were arrested in the streets."[87]

ACT UP members seemed surprised that so many people, including many gay activists, were shocked and disgusted by their use of intimidation tactics so like those of Operation Rescue, the anti-abortion group they deplored. But even gay activists were beginning to tire of ACT UP's shenanigans, concurring with Randy Shilts in his *San Francisco Chronicle* column after the demonstration at St. Pat's and several similar protests by AIDS activists in other cities, "If I didn't know better, I'd swear that the AIDS protestors who have been disrupting services and vandalizing Catholic churches . . . were being paid by some diabolical reactionary group dedicated to discrediting the gay community."[88]

And now Larry Kramer, the nation's most prominent AIDS activist, was calling for a riot in San Francisco during the world's premier scientific conference on AIDS. As it happened, the conference would be going on at the same time as the Lesbian and Gay Freedom Day Parade, which typically drew upwards of three hundred thousand people to San Francisco. Conference organizers feared there would be massive disruptions by people who took Kramer at his word. Ron Stall, a medical anthropologist at the University of California–San Francisco's Center for AIDS Prevention Studies, said in a letter to the conference's local organizing committee, "The size of this year's parade will swell as a result of the understandable wish to use the conference as a stage for a show of force by a community under attack. This has created what seems to me to be a scary situation: There will be a lot of affected (and infected) people locked out of a conference that is about their survival and the survival of the people that they love. The closest analogy in American political history that I can think of is to the situation of Chicago in 1968."[89]

San Francisco activists also were on edge about Kramer's incendiary words, which they feared this time might spark actual fires and other destruction. Paul Boneberg, then director of Mobilization Against AIDS, believed strongly that leaders must take responsibility for protecting anyone who joins a political protest that they organize, and he was shocked that Kramer would launch a firebomb to land on San Francisco without necessarily planning to be there himself.

Boneberg sent a letter to Kramer on June 20, saying, "For God's sake, Larry, accept the responsibility of your position as the most famous AIDS activist in America and retract your call for violence around AIDS. You are putting our community in an even more dangerous position than it is already."[90] Looking back, Boneberg said, "For Larry to call on what in fact was my constituency, lesbian and gay people in San Francisco, to put themselves in harm's way without a willingness to put himself there as well was wrong. Nobody said so because he was Larry Kramer, but I said so."[91]

As it turned out, there was no riot in San Francisco. Kramer had gone too far even for ACT UP's street activists. ACT UP spokesman Alan Beck said, "Our policy is nonviolent, peaceful demonstrations. We may stage sit-ins to stop proceedings, but we'll have nothing to do with [rioting]."[92] While there was no full-scale riot, there were many arrests as ACT UP staged day after day of protests to grab the attention of the news media who had gathered like vultures waiting for post-riot carnage. About 350 members of the ACT UP women's contingent were arrested after staging a "die-in" that blocked traffic on Market Street for two hours. About a thousand protestors took over the downtown branch of Nordstrom's, claiming the department store discriminated against people with AIDS. For all its denial of being a "gay" group, ACT UP's roots were clearly showing as demonstrators beat drums, blew whistles, and chanted: "We're here! We're queer! And we're *not* going shopping!"[93]

ACT UP's biggest media grab during the conference was its disruption of a speech by Louis Sullivan, secretary of Health and Human Services. Typically the head of state in whichever country is hosting the international AIDS conference addresses the meeting. But President George Bush declined to speak at the conference, choosing instead to attend a campaign fundraiser in North Carolina for Jesse Helms and sending Sullivan in his stead. A number of AIDS organizations, including GMHC, were boycotting the conference because of the continued U.S. policy of denying visas to people with HIV infection. Activists were enraged at Bush's insulting slight as well as the ongoing senselessness of excluding people with HIV from obtaining visas to enter the country.

As soon as Sullivan's name was announced, recalls Robert Wachter, the conference's program director, "the Moscone Center was transformed into Times Square at midnight on New Year's Eve,"[94] as screaming, yelling, foot-stomping, whistle blowing, and anything else that could be done was done to drown out the secretary's speech. Sullivan defiantly and bravely continued to the end of his speech—but AIDS dropped to the bottom of his list of priorities from that point on.

While the temblor of activist anger jolted San Francisco, Kramer himself remained at a safe distance—a continent away; he hadn't even gone to San Francisco after all the Sturm und Drang he'd stirred up. Of course there were rumors that Kramer would be arrested and detained for the entire time of the AIDS conference if he showed up. The question was whether Kramer had called for a riot merely to be provocative. Was he once again speaking hyperbolically? Five years later, Kramer reflected, "No, I didn't mean that they should burn up everything, but I certainly think they should have been disruptive, and they were. Louis Sullivan was completely booed when he made his speech." He maintains that there should be "some kind of guerilla warfare," though he adds that he "unfortunately" isn't the one to do it. Harkening to his speech that led to ACT UP's formation, Kramer said, "Considering how many people have died from AIDS, we've been a remarkably docile lot."[95]

The distance ACT UP had put between itself and its founder reflected growing tensions within ACT UP itself as members disagreed about the group's priorities and whether or not direct action itself hadn't run its course and was no longer as effective as it had been. Only a couple of weeks after the events and nonevents in San Francisco, lesbian writer Donna Minkowitz said in the *Village Voice* that ACT UP was at a "crossroads." In a profile of the group, she revealed that ACT UP was in fact struggling to restrain its internal divisions.[96]

The internal split in ACT UP was essentially over whether the group should continue to focus exclusively on pushing for AIDS treatments and a cure, particularly by working cooperatively inside the system with government scientists, or pursue a broader agenda of social change on issues such as racism, sexism, and homophobia. On September 13, 1990, ACT UP/San Francisco split into two chapters because of the tension between these two positions. Now there was ACT UP/Golden Gate, devoted to treatment, and ACT

UP/San Francisco, which remained committed to broader social change beyond merely focusing on pushing medical science to find a cure for AIDS. ACT UP/New York, the Mother Church, also was splitting apart over similar issues, and in 1992 prominent members of the group's central Treatment and Data Committee split off to form the Treatment Action Group (TAG).

Something besides merely disagreeing over the group's focus also pushed ACT UP towards its seemingly inevitable demise. In an editorial in the *Advocate* a year after the San Francisco conference, Peter Staley, a member of ACT UP/New York who became a founder of TAG, speculated as to whether ACT UP had begun to falter. He felt that the group's power was beginning to corrupt it.[97] But what Staley didn't seem to realize, or at least admit, was that ACT UP's *perception* of its power was what had really led it astray. Certainly the group's high media profile—assisted considerably by the rationally made policy arguments of the Washington lobbyists—had moved federal policy-makers and scientists to change their minds about some things and, in some cases, make extremely important changes in the government's way of doing business, particularly in the area of drug development and approval.

But the view from Capitol Hill of ACT UP's "power" wasn't quite as clear as Staley and others in the protest group imagined it. From his vantage point in the House, Tim Westmoreland said, "ACT UP's role was to keep media attention on the issue. I think they actually had very little effect, pro or con, on the politics of it." He added, "ACT UP was a sort of flashbulb going off on a topic. I joked several times that ACT UP's major contribution was really good graphics—and that really matters. In the eighties and nineties, it's *all* about marketing your political issue before Congress."

Good graphics and a news-grabbing flashbulb notwithstanding, Westmoreland added, "I don't think it particularly helped or hurt Congress." Like the activists at the first PWA Lobbying Day in 1985, ACT UP typically hounded friendly lawmakers. "Most of ACT UP is situated in congressional districts that are already prone to be supportive on AIDS issues to begin with," said Westmoreland. "People didn't go around taking over rural Georgia offices, or picketing [former California Republican Representative] Bill Dannemeyer's office in Orange County. It was usually to get the attention of people who were already sympathetic. That doesn't make a big difference in Washington politics."[98]

The 1992 election of Bill Clinton, with his promise of a place at the table for gay people and a "Manhattan Project" on AIDS, robbed ACT UP of a target as big and blatant as Ronald Reagan and George Bush had been. Openly gay men and lesbians were appointed in considerable and visible numbers to positions in the Clinton administration. AIDS activists by now were fully integrated into the federal AIDS research establishment. Ginny Apuzzo became the highest-ranking open lesbian in the Clinton White House in the president's second term. Many others took jobs in AIDS service organizations, now collecting salaries to work on behalf of AIDS and sometimes even being required to dress in business attire—both of which had been anathema to ACT UP's radical counterculture sensibility.

ACT UP chapters throughout the country dried up for lack of interest. In early 1995, ACT UP/Kansas City was offered free, "to a good home." In Atlanta, Jeff Graham said ACT UP had faded from visibility because so many of its members had died. He explained, "There was a sense in the late eighties and early nineties that by force of sheer willpower we could keep people alive, and we could change the world. It's hard to continue to say with great force that, yes, we can cure AIDS, yes, we can stop people dying, when people continue to die."[99] And in Houston, ACT UP member Eugene Harrington echoed Tim McFeeley's critique, saying that if ACT UP had spent its energy drafting and pushing legislation rather than merely demonstrating, "we would have far more to show for that period of ACT UP activism."[100]

As ACT UP's demonstrations in the early nineties became more like guerilla assaults and less like the angry but campy street theater they were famous for, the group seemed to be spinning out of control. Some believed that the seeds of the group's destruction were sown at the 1989 demonstration at St. Patrick's Cathedral. Urvashi Vaid says, "The decline of ACT UP and direct action began, in my view, the instant concern about media coverage of actions displaced the political calculus of right or wrong." ACT UP/New York member and GMHC staffer David Barr said of the St. Patrick's demonstration, "The goal became more about personal expression and less about change."[101]

But the devolution of ACT UP into a group of individuals acting out their personal agendas shouldn't have been surprising, since the group was formed intentionally as a "pure democracy," with no apparent leaders. Its leaderlessness resulted in unchecked internal warfare as individuals formed committees and "affinity groups" to push their particular agendas. In such an atmosphere it was inevitable that one-upmanship would become the order of the day. Add to that the angry conviction that one is fighting for a "moral" cause, and it becomes apparent—to oneself, at least—that those who disagree are not only wrong, but immoral, even reprehensible, as well.

This was the attitude that many in ACT UP took toward gay leaders in Washington, the coat-and-tie set who may have been willing to shout in the streets and even be arrested in an act of civil disobedience when they felt it absolutely necessary, but who otherwise felt far more comfortable debating the finer points of legislation across a conference table. By 1992, ACT UP was taking direct action against the gay and AIDS lobby in Washington. ACT UP/Seattle member Steve Michael had moved to Washington, D.C., where he regularly harassed—even physically assaulted—gay leaders. In an action that has continued to reverberate negatively among gay leaders in Washington, ACT UP members in February 1992 actually handcuffed themselves to gay and AIDS lobbyists during a small meeting in Washington with CDC officials.

ACT UP asked Urvashi Vaid, who is a lawyer, to serve as their legal observer for the protest, which she agreed to do. Vaid recalls that the handcuffed lobbyists—including her immediate predecessor at NGLTF, Jeff Levi—said to her, "This is unacceptable. We won't even talk to you until you unloose us. This is preposterous." Vaid agreed with them. She announced, "This is not right. I'm not going to participate in this anymore. I think it's wrong that people are being held against their will. It violates everything I believe in, and this is nuts." So she walked out of the room. To this day, however, Vaid's participation in this demonstration—despite her withdrawal when she felt the protest had crossed a moral line she wasn't willing to cross—has left an uncomfortable mark on her relationships with some gay and lesbian leaders, including Levi.

For Vaid, that protest "is a perfect symbol of how at cross-purposes we became." ACT UP, she said, saw the "gay establishment" as giving up too much in its desire for mainstream access and respectability. She agrees that this sometimes was the case. "But the self-righteousness and smugness by some gay activists against the gay establishment was wrong," she says. "Hysterical statements—like calling people 'traitors' and 'Uncle Toms'—really cheapened the power of ACT UP's critique. ACT UP had really important things to say about gay leadership and its elitism, and it had important things to say about compromise and cooptation. But it wasn't going to be heard if it was going to be saying outlandish things." It was one thing to say gay leaders should be accountable, accessible, and democratic. But, said Vaid, "It's another thing to say we shouldn't have leadership, or to bully the leadership."[102]

Larry Kramer agrees that ultimately ACT UP's fatal flaw was its lack of, and hostility towards, leadership. By the time he and others realized things were out of control, Kramer said, "There was too much of an entrenched 'democracy' in place. This is a major problem of this [gay] community that we're going to someday have to face: its inability to organize, to accept leadership, to respond to that kind of altogetherness."[103]

When it was good, ACT UP was very good, helping to accomplish tremendous results. Said Kramer, "Singlehandedly we changed the image of gay people from limp-wristed fairies to guerilla warriors." But then it became not so good. "It fell apart," according to Kramer, "because it got out of hand, and there was no mechanism in any of the paperwork that allowed for getting rid of the crazies—and it became the haven for an awful lot of crazies—and they managed to vote down a lot of stuff that should have been done." Kramer said that those who wouldn't go along with the new agendas cobbled together from members' personal priorities "went off and started other organizations, went to work for GMHC, or disappeared."[104]

Or, as in the case of ACT UP's Steve Michael, they became complete strangers to anything like rationality. Seeking to draw attention to AIDS, he said, Michael—now a one-man ACT UP/Washington, D.C.—declared himself a candidate for president in 1996. David Smith, a spokesman for the Human Rights Campaign (the organization dropped the word "Fund" in an effort to downplay its connection to big money and the mocking name of the "Human Rights Champagne Fund" as it was sometimes called by gay people), told

Boston's gay newspaper *Bay Windows,* "I think that his running for president is so ridiculous and so bizarre that it really can't be dignified with any sort of rational comment."[105] Michael died from AIDS in 1998.

ACT UP/Golden Gate continued to be a respected source of information about treatment. ACT UP/San Francisco, on the other hand, insisted on perpetuating the protest group's worst features, choosing to throw public and petulant tantrums rather than work for constructive change. In 1996, a member of the group rushed the stage at a candidate forum in San Francisco, sponsored by the San Francisco AIDS Foundation, and threw twenty-five pounds of used cat litter at the forum moderator—none other than Pat Christen. The AIDS Foundation director said she would press charges against ACT UP. "It's very important that we draw a very clear distinction between healthy debate and acts of violence," she said.[106]

Other than a lone ACT UP member occasionally giving a provocative quote to a newspaper, or a flare-up of histrionics, the group by the mid-nineties was for all intents and purposes moribund, a toothless tiger. And what of ACT UP's founder? What of the man described by his friends as privately soft-spoken and gentle, but who yelled and wrote loudly and angrily when he saw his friends dying while the rest of the world—including the gay community early on—didn't seem to care?

Kramer directed my attention to a thick manuscript sitting on a table amidst piles of packing boxes in his apartment on Washington Square—the site of the first-ever fundraiser for AIDS research, and where plans took shape for the world's first AIDS service organization, GMHC. Kramer said the book he was working on would be his tell-all novel about the AIDS epidemic, and that it would be finished the day he dies. At age sixty he was living with HIV infection. And he was living with a man he loved after so many years of wanting love. Not only did he seem to have found his bliss, but his partner, David Webster, is the man Kramer dated in the seventies and demonized as "Dinky," the character in *Faggots* who rejects the monogamous love offered by the novel's Kramer-like hero.

If the *New York Times* is to be believed, Kramer had indeed been domesticated. In a profile of him in January 1995 that included a photograph of Kramer cuddling with Webster, the *Times* itself seemed to wonder what to do after all the years of invective and op-ed columns "when a roaring lion learns to purr," as the article's title put it.[107] Was it so? Kramer laughed as he recalled the angry letter he'd fired off the week before, criticizing the director of the Office of AIDS Research at the National Institutes of Health. "I faxed it to everybody—doctors, reporters, scientists, government officials," he said. "I thought it was a very strong letter. I in essence called him an idiot and asked him to resign." But he quoted Victor Zonana [HHS Secretary Donna Shalala's press secretary] as saying, "Larry, it's a very tame letter. You really have learned to purr." Said Kramer, "I think you're all used to me, in which case I'm not so effective anymore."[108]

Some people may have gotten used to Kramer, but neither they nor the "crazies" who took over ACT UP are the reason why the protest group faltered. Their arguments had come to be redundant after the government responded to their and the lobbyists' demands, now spending billions of dollars on AIDS research and services. A president who professed to "feel their [and everyone else's] pain" took away a primary target. Most importantly, in the place of activists there were now thousands of AIDS organizations throughout the country—the AIDS "industry" made possible by the Ryan White CARE Act. Where once there had been lone voices, like Kramer's, there now were publicity departments "spinning" the politics of AIDS in ways that protected their own interests and bottom lines. How the AIDS industry grew is a fascinating story of how the vision of a small number of dedicated people can make a tremendous differ-ence in this world—particularly when they are backed by large sums of money. It's also the story of how too many visionaries were tripped up by their own myopia.

INDUSTRIAL STRENGTH

Toil on heroes! toil well! handle the weapons well!

WALT WHITMAN, *AUTUMN RIVULETS*

Before there was an AIDS "industry," there were concerned individuals who banded together to care for their friends and neighbors. As AIDS spread, it became clear that a national "nerve center" was needed to link service providers with their counterparts in other areas of the country. Just as it was for people with AIDS, the sharing of "how-to" information among these organizations was vital to America's response to the epidemic. Of course no one knew then that as the nationwide network grew stronger when the federal government finally funded it, it would also grow, like a kind of Frankenstein's monster, into a massive creature that would turn on its creators. Those gay pioneers didn't know AIDS would last as long as it has done, or that the charitable services they once provided as volunteers would, with the CARE act's millions, provide careers for thousands of AIDS "professionals."

During AIDS Action Council's first national meeting on AIDS politics, hosted by Paula Van Ness in Los Angeles the first weekend of October 1985, the executive directors of the country's largest AIDS service organizations (ASOs) decided they needed to form another national organization devoted exclusively to providing information and technical assistance to the ASOs sprouting up throughout the country. Van Ness, then director of AIDS Project Los Angeles (APLA) recalls, "Whenever someone started an AIDS organization they would hop on a plane or in a car and drive to one of the big AIDS organizations. They would either call or just show up at your door and say, 'I want to know everything you do.'"[1] The older groups felt obliged to accommodate their visitors, but they were also trying to do their own jobs in the local community.

Although their initial idea was to incorporate the new organization under the umbrella of AIDS Action Council, Gary MacDonald, then director of the council, said that ultimately they "didn't want a group that was associated with a political entity; they wanted basically a service group for their organizations."[2] So three of the directors—Van Ness, Tim Wolfred from the San Francisco AIDS Foundation, and Richard Dunne from GMHC—invited the directors of the nation's other three largest ASOs—Larry Kessler from Boston's AIDS Action Committee, Jim Graham from Washington, D.C.'s Whitman-Walker Clinic, and Bea Kalleigh from Seattle's Northwest AIDS Foundation—to join them in founding and funding the new organization, which would be known as the National AIDS Network (NAN).

NAN's rise and fall provides a dramatic illustration of how well-intentioned but inexperienced people tried to cope with an exploding epidemic and a nationwide network of community-based organizations struggling to do their best to replicate "mainstream" health and social services for people with AIDS who couldn't get those services in mainstream organizations. NAN's story also illustrates how gay social networks became lifelines connecting communities around the country and in the process created an important component of the Ryan White CARE Act when the federal government finally did something on a scale commensurate with its resources and the needs of Americans living and working with AIDS.

Paul Kawata was working for the city of Seattle in October 1985 when Richard Dunne called him and asked, "Do you want to go to Washington?" Looking back, Kawata said, "Being really stupid and really naive, I said 'sure.'" Kawata flew to Los Angeles to meet with Dunne, Van Ness, and Wolfred. They all got along just fine. On Christmas Eve 1985, Van Ness called Kawata and asked how soon he could move from Washington state to Washington, D.C. So in January 1986, Kawata headed east to set up NAN's first office—above AIDS Action Council's office on Capitol Hill. NAN's founders pooled $5,000 to begin the new organization. The newly dubbed executive director Kawata literally moved into NAN's office because he had no other place to stay at that point. And while the idea for NAN seemed clear to its founders, Kawata said it was much less clear to him what, exactly, he and NAN were to do. As he put it, NAN started out as "one guy, $5,000, and a dream."[3]

Kawata could have been describing the experience of virtually everyone who ever started an AIDS organization. Without the benefit of years of experience—or even, necessarily, the awareness of existing organizations that could provide a blueprint of what to expect as their own fledgling agencies expanded—the growing AIDS organizations tended to lurch unsteadily forward as volunteers and what few staff there may have been tried as best they could to meet the growing demand for AIDS-related services. Although there were people involved who had professional experience in health care and social service organizations, many AIDS organizations, particularly in small towns, were run by people who tended to have more zeal than managerial experience. As John Paul Barnich said of his service on the board of AIDS Foundation Houston in the early eighties, "None of us had any experience at all at running a foundation. We were just a bunch of people who cared. We took care of people, we lost people, and we did the best we could."[4]

NAN was dedicated to helping the new AIDS organizations, such as AIDS Foundation Houston, to do even better by teaching them to manage the *business* of providing AIDS services. Jim Graham, who became the treasurer of NAN's board, told me that NAN's goals were threefold: advocacy, providing technical assistance, and facilitating information exchange among ASOs.[5] These functions are what NAN cofounder Tim Wolfred describes as "the self-help organizational development activities."[6]

In October 1987, NAN cosponsored a meeting of 150 representatives from government and private sector organizations to map out a plan to address "AIDS into the Nineties," as the meeting and report produced from it were titled. NAN was joined by the American Medical Association, the Association of State and Territorial Health Officers, and the CDC in producing this first-ever major collaboration among the various "players" involved in the nation's overall response to the epidemic. Representatives of the federal government, ASOs, gay rights groups, the insurance industry, the Catholic Health Association, public health organizations, minority organizations, Burroughs Wellcome Co., and many others met together to discuss and argue about why America had faltered in its response to AIDS—and where, exactly, it ought to be going.

The group concluded that community-based ASOs were the backbone of the nation's response but that those organizations needed to look to "a broader future when the AIDS response is concentrated within traditional mainstream institutions." Coalitions, partnerships, and community alliances were viewed as essential to a fully mobilized national effort. Among the conference's key outcomes was the recommendation that the new AIDS organizations develop strategic plans, more sophisticated fundraising efforts, collaborative partnerships with other mainstream groups—and, in effect, that they plan for an AIDS epidemic that would stretch into the foreseeable future.[7]

Peter Lee, who was hired as a consultant by NAN to produce the meeting and subsequently became NAN's program director, says the conference "in some ways was the blueprint for the Ryan White CARE Act in terms of community control and the need to interrelate services and education."[8] Just as the report was one of the earliest strategic assessments of the nation's AIDS response, the meeting itself was a prototype of the community planning councils mandated by the CARE Act to delineate services and distribute funding among local organizations.

In January 1988, I joined NAN's small staff as its publicist and staff writer. The agency's down-at-the-heels offices were connected to those of the Human Rights Campaign Fund in an old office building on Fourteenth Street NW, only a few blocks from the White House. The building was the home of a number of low-budget, left-leaning organizations. The staff at that point consisted entirely of gay men and lesbians, and NAN offered me and a number of others the first taste we'd ever had of what it's like to be comfortably gay in a work environment.

My job entailed writing and editing NAN's newsletters, giving occasional interviews to the press, writing speeches for Paul Kawata, and, of course, doing whatever else might have needed to be done around the office. NAN's biweekly newsletter *Network News* offered information about successful AIDS services in communities around the country, "how-to" stories that were told to us firsthand by the people who were pioneering AIDS services in America's big cities and small towns. We published articles on such topics as funding opportunities, AIDS informational hotlines, prevention campaigns, and the importance of having input from people with AIDS in the design of AIDS services, as mandated by the 1983 "Denver Principles." Above all, we wanted the information we provided to be practical and useful to the running of AIDS organizations.

Soon after my arrival at NAN, the organization embarked on a major binge of growth. The biggest boon to the two-year-old agency was its selection by the Ford Foundation in the spring of 1988 to house and administer the National Community-AIDS Partnership (NCAP, today the National AIDS Fund), a unique matching-grants fund intended to support and expand community-based AIDS education and services. Directed by Paula Van Ness, NCAP was launched with an initial $2 million grant from Ford, with another $2 million expected to come from other national foundations and corporations, and an additional $4 million to be matched with funds raised in local communities. NCAP funds, however, would not be distributed by NAN; rather, they were to be distributed by community foundations in the sites chosen by Ford.[9]

In keeping with its own name, NAN sought to network community-based AIDS groups with their counterparts throughout the country—making formal the informal networks that had been in place since the gay community first began to coalesce nationally in the seventies, and which had proved so vitally important in the earliest years of the AIDS epidemic. Many groups found all the technical assistance they hoped for in the *NAN Directory of AIDS Education and Service Organizations.* For a mere five dollars cost to a member organization, the directory provided listings of local AIDS organizations, state AIDS coordinators, local public health agencies, key federal agencies, and national private-sector organizations addressing AIDS. Like the "coming out" experiences of the gay people who formed them, the new AIDS organizations were bolstered merely in knowing there were others like themselves working to provide AIDS services. The NAN directory was paid for with part of a $125,000 contribution from New York-based Group W Television, which at the time was sponsoring a nationally syndicated series of documentaries, public service announcements, and feature-story segments called "AIDS Lifeline."

NAN was selected by the CDC in the summer of 1988 to oversee a consortium of AIDS organizations that were charged with the task of developing model prevention programs targeting minority women. In keeping with its role as a provider of technical assistance, NAN's part in the consortium was to develop informational materials based on the experiences garnered from three participating cities to assist ASOs in understanding and developing interventions specifically for women of color. In fact, NAN was one of the first national organizations to recognize the growing AIDS epidemic in communities of color and to try to address the needs of community-based organizations that were formed in the late eighties as the epidemic expanded among minorities.

Flush with a feeling of prosperity from its growing visibility and expanding coffers, NAN moved uptown into new offices across the street from CBS News in July 1988, after the staff returned from the annual gay and lesbian health conference, in Boston. Situated in the aptly named (in view of NAN's own expansion) Empire Building, NAN was reunited with AIDS Action Council, though only by virtue of their sharing contiguous offices. Jean McGuire, then the council's director, recalls, "I was very pissed off about the extent to which I was obligated to cohabitate, co-locate, and collaborate with the National AIDS Network."[10] When there was discussion in 1989 of merging NAN and AIDS Action Council, McGuire protested, believing that NAN's image as a "gay" organization would be a hindrance to AIDS Action Council's just-emerging political clout in Washington.

To stoke and support the entrepreneurial spirit that pervaded NAN, more than seven hundred staff, board members, and volunteers from community-based AIDS organizations gathered in the Hotel Inter-Continental in New Orleans, October 20–23, 1988, for NAN's first management "Skills Building" conference. Sandi Feinblum, GMHC's first deputy director, organized the conference for NAN. Participants were offered presentations and workshops that dealt with the nitty-gritty of running professional organizations—including financial management, case management, fundraising and development, human resource management, public relations, and information systems. Robert A. Beck, the chairman emeritus of the Prudential Insurance Company—and father of Stephen Beck, who was then director of the National Association of People with AIDS, which shared office space with NAN at the time—spoke in his plenary speech about the need for AIDS advocates to recognize that "the market is crowded with worthy causes competing for limited funds."[11]

Encouraged by the success of the skills-building conference, NAN immediately began to plan a second conference, in Washington, D.C., in November 1989, which would attract more than eight hundred participants. Only a few months after the New Orleans conference, though, strange things began to happen within NAN. On February 18, 1989, Paul Kawata announced that he would resign as NAN's director. "The time has come to move on," he said. "When you've been involved with AIDS as long as I have, it's important to go on to new challenges within the epidemic." In his three years at NAN, Kawata had increased the agency's budget from its original $5,000 to $1.9 million and its staff from himself to twenty-one. GMHC's Richard Dunne, chair of NAN's board at the time, said, "All of us in AIDS are grateful for [Kawata's] pioneering efforts." Seattle activist Jim Holm—who was then cochair of the National Gay and Lesbian Task Force, and had moved from Seattle to Washington to be NAN's director of administration and finance—was appointed acting executive director.[12]

By the time Kawata actually left NAN, on April 15, it was common knowledge that he'd been forced out by the board of directors because the organization had outgrown his ability to manage it. That same month I was laid off from my own job at NAN with the explanation that funding for my position had been cut. This was the first clue I had that NAN's finances were far less rosy than the agency's director and development department had painted them. Bill Freeman, who was hired in 1988 as NAN's first development director, said that he raised "about $1.8 million" for NAN. But, he added, "Given the structure of the organization, it was a sinking ship."[13]

In his role overseeing NAN's income and expenses, Holm recalls, "We kept getting more optimistic projections from [the development department] than were realized until we got ourselves into a very tight position." Holm said that there was jockeying for position between Kawata and Freeman, because Kawata had been accustomed to using his persuasive charm to raise money for NAN and had a hard time relinquishing the fundraising role to Freeman, a professional fundraiser.[14]

Even more taxing to the organization was the change of its board chairs. Richard Dunne stepped down on June 26, 1989, and on September 1 he resigned his position at GMHC, because he was himself struggling with AIDS (he died on December 29, 1990, at age forty-six). In his place came Richard Keeling, a physician who directed the University of Virginia's student health department and was board president of the American College Health Association—but who had no experience running a nonprofit organization, as Dunne had. Beginning with Kawata's departure, NAN was rocked by a series of scandals that stunned AIDS activists and organizations throughout the country. In one way or another, they all stemmed from the organization's inept management—the very thing NAN was created to alleviate in AIDS organizations. Bill Freeman left NAN in the summer of 1989, and the agency was unsuccessful in attracting another development director, at least partly because the board couldn't agree on just how NAN ought to raise money. Holm tried to implement an austerity program but the board resisted, wanting to hold out until a new director had been hired. His impossible job was to preside over the shrinking of an organization that had expanded too rapidly under Kawata's enthusiastic, albeit inexperienced, leadership.

After the board finally conducted a national search for a new executive director, Holm seemed the candidate of choice. But a change of heart on the part of Keeling during the final round of interviews, in Chicago at the end of October 1989, ended Holm's—and every other—candidacy for the job. A member of the board's search committee, Eric Engstrom, director at the time of the Minnesota AIDS Project, suddenly expressed interest in the NAN position himself. As Jim Graham put it, "It was a highly unusual situation for a candidate to come from the search committee. I didn't know [Engstrom] was interested in the job." Holm said, "I knew something was very wrong. While I was enroute to the last interview, I was stopped in the hall by Rich Keeling, who informed me that he was not recommending me, but Eric Engstrom."

No one knew at the time that Engstrom and Keeling had become romantically involved. Keeling was ostensibly heterosexual, married to a woman. He and Engstrom denied that they were having an affair—although when Engstrom was fired by NAN's board only a few months later, Keeling's wife sued him for divorce and Engstrom decided to move to Charlottesville, Virginia, where Keeling lived. The two later moved together to the Midwest. Holm was, to say the least, extremely angry about being passed over for Engstrom in view of the egregious conflicts of interest that had propelled the Minnesotan into the director's chair.

As creditors barked outside NAN's doors, Engstrom's first move, according to Holm, was to deplete NAN's treasury by paying in full a $60,000 bill for the 1989 skills-building conference. Holm had suggested structuring the debt, paying it off in installments, but was overruled by Engstrom. "All of a sudden," said Holm, "we didn't have money for payroll."[15] In March 1990, NAN cut its already shrunken staff of seventeen by nearly a third. "We definitely have experienced revenue shortfalls since January," Engstrom understatedly told the *Washington Blade*. He reasoned that the $40,000 he expected to save each month on five unfilled staff positions would suffice to replenish the depleted cash flow and hire a fundraising consultant. The problem was that no combination of any five salaries at low-paying NAN would have totaled that amount of money.[16] Like NAN's development department, Engstrom was pulling figures out of the air.

Meanwhile, Engstrom and Keeling called upon foundations and large ASOs to try to bail out NAN. Holm said the pair "went to these foundations convinced that they were the team to save the AIDS effort in America." In a Minneapolis *Twin Cities Reader* article about "the rise and fall of AIDS activist Eric Engstrom," published six months after these events, Engstrom said his lawyers advised him to resign after NAN board members told him not to disclose to contributors the extent of NAN's financial crisis.[17]

As late as April 1990, Engstrom optimistically assured NAN's few remaining staff that the organization would endure. He didn't tell them that he was borrowing money against the NCAP funds simply to make the payroll, or that NAN was more than half a million dollars in debt. The money taken from the AIDS partnership funds technically belonged to NAN, but the fact was that the use of this money to meet NAN's operating expenses meant a diversion of funds that were meant for other purposes. In a fall 1990 article in the *Village Voice,* former GMHC director Rodger McFarlane referred to this as NAN's "fancy bookkeeping."[18]

NAN's board tried to put a positive spin on the situation, claiming in denial of the facts that the corporations and foundations that were contributing money to NAN and other AIDS organizations in increasing amounts were suddenly losing interest in AIDS. Engstrom warned that the federal government could not be counted on to increase its funding for AIDS. Finally, on May 15, NAN laid off its last eight staff members, and officially suspended operations on May 24, 1990. "Financial troubles" were blamed for NAN's demise. In a bizarre ending of the organization that had helped volunteers to become AIDS professionals, some of NAN's former staff donated their time as volunteers to assist in the agency's postmortem clean-up. After NAN closed, the *Chronicle of Philanthropy* noted, "In an ironic twist of fate, the national organization that helped hundreds of local AIDS groups raise money and manage their operations has shut down largely because it couldn't do either for itself."[19]

The dream that Paul Kawata and the six large AIDS organizations that initially backed him had seen materialize over the course of four and a half years had come to a troubled, troubling end. But even as NAN weakened and died, another, far bigger, force was gathering steam in the Congress of the United States. In many ways it would continue NAN's own efforts to forge cooperation among organizations with vested interests in AIDS and support a community-based response to the epidemic. NAN's goal of putting control of AIDS services into the hands of people in local communities would live on in the Ryan White CARE Act—far bigger and better funded than anyone ever thought possible.

*

In 1982, Pat Norman, the first director of the lesbian and gay health office in the San Francisco public health department, pulled together a group of five people to develop a plan (called simply the "San Francisco Plan") that would steer people with AIDS to the services they needed from the moment they walked in the door to the very end of their lives, which in those days tended not to be a very long space of time.

If the individual was worried about possibly having AIDS—and of course no one in 1982 knew what caused AIDS, and the HIV antibody test was three years into the future, so no sexually active gay man in San Francisco at the time could be certain he would not develop the disease—he was sent to the Mission Health Center, in the middle of the Castro area. The Shanti Project provided emotional support as well as housing, and the newly formed K.S. Foundation (now the San Francisco AIDS Foundation) offered supportive social services. If the individual had Kaposi's sarcoma, he'd be referred to Marcus Conant's K.S. Clinic at the University of California–San Francisco. For *pneumocystis* pneumonia he'd be sent to San Francisco General Hospital. Looking back to that time when everyone was trying to figure out how best to deal with AIDS, Norman said, "We hadn't been in an epidemic like this before. What book do you read in order to be able to do that? Now there are some books, but there weren't before."[20]

The organizations in San Francisco that were providing AIDS services in those early years were central components of what came to be known as the "San Francisco model" of AIDS care. That model, called a "continuum of care," comprised a number of services typically provided by various community-based agencies that serve to keep someone who has AIDS out of the hospital, living at home, and functioning as well and long as possible. These include case management, hotlines, resource materials, workshops, attendant care, a "buddy" program to assist with practical needs, centralized or home-delivered meal services, ambulette services to get to medical appointments, a skilled nursing facility, a health-related facility that combines residential and care needs, hospice care, support groups and peer counseling, recreation or activity programs, legal services, financial advocacy, and group or scattered-site housing.[21]

In November 1985, the board of the Princeton, New Jersey-based Robert Wood Johnson Foundation (RWJ), the nation's largest philanthropy devoted to health care issues, authorized a $17.1 million AIDS Health Services Program to stimulate the development of community-based AIDS services throughout the country. Paul Jellinek, RWJ's vice president for programs, told me that the foundation was unsure exactly how its money would be best spent. So they invited Dr. Philip R. Lee, then director of the Institute for Health Policy Studies at the University of California–San Francisco, and later the assistant secretary for health in the first Clinton administration, to meet with them in Princeton to talk about the San Francisco model of AIDS care.

"Phil described what happened in San Francisco," said Jellinek. Lee told them that a combination of out-of-hospital, community-based support services and in-hospital treatment not only cost less than hospital treatment alone, but it was more in keeping with the needs and wishes of people with AIDS. Said Jellinek, "We saw that we could play an important role by helping others to learn about what had been done in San Francisco, and testing the viability of the San Francisco model in other communities that were beginning to see increased AIDS cases."[22]

In addition to having at least a hundred AIDS cases, the most important requirement for the cities that received funding from RWJ's program was a willingness among medical, social service, and community-based organizations to cooperate in the development of systems of care.[23] In November 1986, RWJ made awards to nine projects serving eleven communities with the country's highest AIDS caseloads—Atlanta, Dallas, Fort Lauderdale, Jersey City, Miami, Nassau County (N.Y.), Newark (N.J.), New Orleans, New York City, Seattle, and West Palm Beach.[24]

To help replicate the San Francisco model of coordinated AIDS care in its eleven pilot cities, RWJ hired some of the architects of the San Francisco model itself. Dr. Mervyn Silverman came onboard to direct the AIDS Health Services Program, bringing with him as deputy director Cliff Morrison, from San Francisco General Hospital. Known as a bridge-builder since his days in the Peace Corps, Silverman was at home with RWJ's efforts to stimulate cooperation among various health care and social service providers in the participating cities. "I've always believed in getting people to sit around a table and reach consensus if possible," says Silverman. "I did the same thing when I headed up the Robert Wood Johnson AIDS services program." He noted that often the different care providers would come "kicking and screaming" to the table, but that it was important "just to have people talking to each other, which quite often they don't do."[25]

Morrison's job with the program entailed visiting the participating cities to help coordinate their AIDS services. Morrison said that although RWJ originally intended to replicate the San Francisco model, it soon became clear that would not be fully possible in other cities because of social, political, and financial differences. Recognizing the limited extent to which San Francisco's model could be replicated elsewhere, the RWJ program revised its goal to simply build on a community's existing service structures and networks.

Morrison recalls, "People would say, 'You can do those things in San Francisco that we can't do here.'"[26] Of course one of the biggest differences between San Francisco and virtually everywhere else in this country is the city's highly visible and politically influential gay community—with its many heterosexual supporters. Perhaps most importantly, the organizations that made up San Francisco's continuum of care—including the San Francisco AIDS Foundation, the Shanti AIDS Residence Program, the Visiting Nurses Association, and the AIDS unit at San Francisco General Hospital—were fortunate to have a large pool of volunteers to draw upon in the city's gay community. As early as 1984–85, volunteers in San Francisco had provided more than eighty thousand hours of AIDS-related social support and counseling services, responded to more than thirty thousand telephone inquiries and letters, and distributed nearly two hundred fifty thousand pieces of literature. Undergirding their efforts was an extremely supportive city government, which provided 62 percent of the funding needed by the volunteer-run service organizations, some $7.4 million in fiscal 1984–85 alone.[27]

Until the RWJ program ended in March 1992, both Morrison and his boss, Silverman—as well as RWJ's national advisory committee, chaired by Phil Lee, and his successor, June Osborn, who also chaired the National Commission on AIDS under President Bush—sought to keep the communities focused on one central thing, whatever their local efforts might be: the individual with HIV or AIDS. "We always had as our foundation the person afflicted with the disease," said Silverman, "not how can we save money, how can we cut corners."[28]

AID Atlanta was the only gay community-based ASO among

the eleven RWJ sites to be selected as the program's coordinating agency; in most of the other cities, the public health department administered the program. AID Atlanta's main role was to provide case managers who coordinated services with other subcontractors in the city's consortium of AIDS service providers. Grady Memorial Hospital, for example, provided HIV outpatient services as well as acute care services, and the Visiting Nurses Association coordinated home care for people with AIDS. Jesse Peel, a retired psychiatrist who was on AID Atlanta's board at the time, says, "It was a distortion in some ways because we were the young, inexperienced organization that didn't know how to do things—as opposed to the established entity [administering the RWJ program] in most cities. But it gave AID Atlanta a position of influence within the community. It gave us an enormous amount of leverage, especially with government funding, and a level of respectability we never would have had."[29]

After selecting the sites for the RWJ program, the next step was planning strategically for what services would be needed, and who or which organization would best provide them. In developing its RWJ program plan, Bea Kalleigh says the city of Seattle had an advantage in that service providers could look at and learn from the experiences of the first cities affected by AIDS. "It was clear by the mid-eighties," she said, "that Seattle was more likely to follow the path of San Francisco [with AIDS cases mainly among gay men] than New York [with equally large numbers of cases among injection drug users]. I hate to call it an advantage, but that's what made developing that kind of vision or plan easier for Seattle than it was for some of the first cities."[30]

The third and most difficult step in implementing the RWJ program was getting local agencies to cooperate with one another. Even in Seattle, which became a model of cooperation, the agencies that became key components of the city's early AIDS services network— Shanti Seattle, the Chicken Soup Brigade (which grew out of the Seattle Gay Clinic), the Seattle AIDS Support Group, and the Northwest AIDS Foundation—were initially competitive. But the Mayor's Task Force on AIDS, established in 1983, made it clear there would be more than enough work for each organization. The former three-term mayor himself, Charles Royer, said in 1989, "The private nonprofits must come to the city with a plan that shows how they are going to cooperate with other agencies, or they don't get any money from the [city]."[31] Fortunately, Seattle had a long history of cooperation between the gay community and the public health department, which helped to avert many of the problems faced by other cities where such a relationship didn't exist.

In 1989, the federal Health Resources and Services Administration (HRSA) funded four demonstration projects—in Los Angeles, Miami, New York, and San Francisco—modeled directly after RWJ's AIDS Health Services Program. By providing public funding, HRSA hoped to stimulate existing nonprofit community-based organizations to develop a comprehensive out-of-hospital service delivery system for PWAs.[32] Joseph O'Neill, a gay physician long involved in caring for AIDS patients and now director of HRSA's AIDS Bureau—the office that oversees Ryan White CARE Act funding—describes the HRSA demonstration projects as a "primordial" version of the CARE Act.[33]

In fiscal 1991, the first year Ryan White funds were available, the nation's hardest-hit state, New York, received nearly $63 million. By then, 42,548 AIDS cases had been reported in the state. The nation's second-hardest hit state, California, received a total of $44.7 million under all the titles and programs for which the state was eligible in fiscal 1991. At that point, 38,437 people had been diagnosed with AIDS in the state since the start of the epidemic. By fiscal 1994, California had nearly tripled its CARE Act funding to just under $123 million. In both states—as in all other states receiving CARE Act funding—Title I cities and counties accounted for the bulk of the federal AIDS services funding that was being received. Together, the two states had received more than half a billion Title I dollars by the end of the CARE Act's first five-year funding cycle in 1995.[34]

Among the AIDS services paid for by CARE Act funding are primary medical care, substance abuse treatment, food and nutrition services, housing services, and medications. As with the RWJ community consortia—and harkening back to Pat Norman's AIDS Coordinating Committee even earlier—the CARE Act mandates that states and communities receiving AIDS-services funding must pull together "planning councils" to assess the local need and determine how the funding should be apportioned among service providers.

At the national level, as well, HRSA has involved representatives of service organizations and people with AIDS—now referred to as "consumers"—in its planning processes. The AIDS program, now HRSA's single largest program, accounts for the bulk of its budget. Stephen Bowen, a physician and former CDC official who directed HRSA's AIDS Program Office (now the AIDS bureau) from 1990 until 1995, told me, "We've really attempted to make programs be responsive to the needs of communities, their wishes, and have actively emphasized and encouraged the involvement of people with HIV as part of the planning councils, technical assistance, and program oversight." In fact, said Bowen, a high percentage of HRSA's staff overseeing the CARE Act funding and recipients "are people who have been direct service providers." He added that a "significant cadre" of openly gay people work in HRSA's AIDS program and that the agency "actively recruit[s] HIV-positive people."[35]

One of HRSA's openly gay employees is Miguel Gomez, who started his AIDS career as the second employee of the AIDS Action Council, hired in 1985 by Gary MacDonald. After a few subsequent jobs working on AIDS issues—including three years at the National Council of la Raza, where he started an AIDS program for the nation's largest national Hispanic organization—Gomez was hired by HRSA to be one of its key spokespersons for the CARE Act programs. Reflecting on the CARE Act's debt to—and differences from—the original San Francisco model developed largely by gay people, Gomez explained that in the CARE Act the federal government was interested in replicating the model of integrated community-based services, rather than the particular services or organizations in San Francisco per se.[36]

Besides bolstering the already existing AIDS service organizations throughout the country, the availability of so much money under the CARE Act on a competitive basis brought many people and agencies that had never before been involved with—or necessarily even interested in—providing AIDS services to the AIDS "industry." By the mid-nineties, an estimated eighteen thousand organizations throughout the country were providing some kind of AIDS-related services—some two hundred different agencies in San Francisco alone.

How and why did all these organizations appear? Paul Kawata, the former NAN director and current director of the National Minority AIDS Council, echoed what I've heard from others: "There was so much rage and anger," he said. "And it felt like there was a lot of dollars. So if you weren't going to meet my needs, I'll go off and start my own organization."[37] Anger and large amounts of CARE Act money fueled a lot of activists—and a hell of a lot of AIDS organizations.

I asked HRSA's Joe O'Neill whether the country can sustain the multitude of AIDS service providers now drawing down CARE Act funding. "You can't, at least not on the public dole," he said. As an example, he referred to the extraordinary number of agencies providing AIDS services in San Francisco. "We can't pay two hundred executive directors out of Ryan White money," he said. To continue getting Congress's support of the CARE Act—which was in doubt between the time of its expiration in 1995 and much-delayed reauthorization in 1996—O'Neill foresaw a coming time of "painful discussions" and consolidation. "I'm not referring to the care and maintenance of organizations," he said. "I'm referring to the care and maintenance of sick individuals."[38]

No one who participated in Pat Norman's AIDS Coordinating Committee back in 1982, the NAN "AIDS Into the Nineties" conference in 1987, the Robert Wood Johnson Foundation pilot projects, or the HRSA demonstration projects in the late eighties, could have guessed how far-reaching their vision for AIDS services would prove to be. As they depended upon the kindness and donations of friends and strangers alike, those pioneers could only dream of something like a CARE Act. They never dreamed there would be so fantastically much money for AIDS services, or that so many organizations would become interested in providing them.

Nor could they have foreseen that there would often be so much ill will among AIDS "industry" advocates in Washington as they fought with one another for the biggest piece of the federal money pie they could possibly get. And how could they possibly have known the AIDS industry would "de-gay" itself, denying the proud heritage of the gay people who were its pioneers? Then again, the "de-gaying" of AIDS by the Washington lobbyists representing the AIDS industry had brought about the CARE Act in the first place.

*

Representatives of the AIDS "industry" spoke regularly of the needs—at least the needs as they were defined by the service organizations—of so-called "special populations." Strangely, somewhere in the discussions of what people with AIDS need, gay men no longer were considered a "special population." One could sit, as I have done, in meetings with AIDS advocates who speak of every possible type of individual affected by HIV—women and children foremost among them, followed by people of color, substance abusers, the homeless—and not hear the words "gay men" come up even once. You might wonder, as I have done, when gay men—whatever their race—had supposedly overcome America's antigay bigotry, effectively prevented new infections, and received all the AIDS services they might need.

You might wonder as well why the advocates weren't talking about gay men when they continue to account for the majority of AIDS cases and new HIV infections in most of the United States. Before the CARE Act, gay lobbyists in Washington, to win support and funding, encouraged politicians to feel good about doing something for the women and children, eagerly downplaying the vast numbers of gay men afflicted by AIDS. Now AIDS service providers themselves championed people with AIDS who were poor, female, ideally prepubescent ("innocent victims," they were called)—and definitely not white or gay.

As AIDS advocates pushed and pulled Congress in 1995 to reauthorize the Ryan White CARE Act for another five years, the internecine squabbling among them spilled onto the pages of the *Washington Blade.* What became starkly clear to those outside the inbred world of AIDS advocacy was that AIDS had become a big business. It was also apparent that those who lobby the federal government for AIDS funding speak of the "needs of people with AIDS" as though they are necessarily and always the same as the needs of their own particular organizations.

AIDS had become a special interest in the truest sense. And the advocates were interested in keeping AIDS as special as possible. Doing so ensured that the CARE Act's hundreds of millions of dollars would continue to flow to the legions of AIDS organizations, paychecks would be processed on time, and expense accounts would ensure the globe-trotting advocates' continued enjoyment of their favorite hotels and restaurants. The days were past when activists slept on one another's floors and couches to save money, and signed onto the "cause" because they were angry and committed. AIDS had become a career that offered perks, travel to interesting places, and the righteous sense that one was doing "God's work." Jean McGuire's vision of AIDS organizations putting themselves out of business by incorporating AIDS services into mainstream health and social welfare organizations seemed shortsighted; she hadn't foreseen the way the millions from the CARE Act would spawn a now self-perpetuating "industry."

The public battles among the lobbyists revealed just how far the AIDS industry had come since Gary MacDonald *was* AIDS Action Council and the only full-time AIDS lobbyist in Washington. The battles made it apparent that besides the traditional enemies of the AIDS "movement"—including price-gouging pharmaceutical companies and the federal government's lethargy—there was another enemy even closer to home. This enemy, dividing and coming perilously close to conquering the AIDS advocates themselves, was something as old and tainted as politics itself: greed and the lust for power.

Advocates used their respective versions of the "needs of people with AIDS" as bludgeons against one another for daring to disagree over political strategy in their joint—and frequently disjointed— efforts to get the CARE Act reauthorized by a Congress now controlled by Republicans. The Act's two most heavily funded sections were Title I, designed to provide funding assistance to the hardest-hit metropolitan areas, based on their cumulative AIDS cases since the start of the epidemic, and Title II, which provided grants to the states for AIDS services. In 1995, AIDS Action Council supported a new appropriation process being considered in the Senate that would have jointly funded AIDS services in cities and states, rather than separately as had been done in the CARE Act's first five years. The council touted this single appropriation as a way to address the growing numbers of AIDS cases outside the cities that were the first—and are still the hardest—hit by the epidemic. Other advocates, however, wanted to retain the original funding formula, fearing that a single appropriation would take money away from the hard-hit cities where most people with AIDS live, and would give a disproportionate amount of funding to rural areas and smaller towns.

Mark Barnes, then the executive director of AIDS Action Council, wrote in the *Washington Blade* in April 1995, "For the past several years, cities and states have lobbied separately for appropriations of funds under Title I and II. . . . What if, instead of lobbying separately for their own funds, the cities and states would need to lobby together for a common pot of money, so that each dollar won would be of benefit to PWAs in both cities and states?"[39]

Ernest Hopkins, a black gay man affiliated with a group called the Cities Advocating for Emergency AIDS Relief (CAEAR) Coalition, responded for the "other side." The coalition was formed in 1991 to lobby for increases in Ryan White funding for the nation's forty-nine eligible Title I metropolitan areas. Its supporters included the National Association of People with AIDS, Mobilization Against AIDS, and the National Task Force on AIDS Prevention. In an opinion article in the *Blade* a week after Barnes's own article, Hopkins wrote, "If changes in the funding formula shift money from urban to rural areas, and the pooling of funds for Title I and II leave urban areas vulnerable to further shifts in funds, a disproportionate number of those who will suffer will be those who depend on federal funds the most: the urban poor, including high percentages of minorities."[40]

Pat Christen, the nongay director of the San Francisco AIDS Foundation, had been one of the people who masterminded the legislation that became the Ryan White CARE Act as a way to provide "disaster relief" to hard-hit cities like San Francisco. But in June 1995 Christen resigned from AIDS Action Council's board, after serving on it for eight years, because she believed the council's support of the single appropriation measure would be harmful to her organization. In her seven-page resignation letter, Christen wrote that "the Council is advocating for a position that literally takes desperately needed resources away from people with AIDS in one community in order to give those resources to people with AIDS in another needy community."[41] Christen told me, "I felt that in good conscience I couldn't sign a $70,000 check over to an entity that in the end, were their positions to be implemented, would harm the city of San Francisco."[42]

On a political level, it isn't surprising that the executive director of San Francisco's leading AIDS organization should see the interests of her agency, the city, and people with AIDS as one and the same; in the game of politics, as Chai Feldblum put it, winning as much as possible is what it's all about. To some, however, the single appropriation that AIDS Action Council supported seemed to be a reasonable attempt to address the changing demographics of the epidemic and to loosen the grip that cities like San Francisco had on CARE Act funding because of their big caseloads and big, influential AIDS organizations.

As reasonable and fair as it might have seemed to those supporting it, the manner in which the council came to endorse the single appropriation concept raised serious questions about its own ability to see the interests of people with AIDS as being sometimes different from its own interests or those of its member organizations. The chair of AIDS Action Council's policy committee, Doug Nelson, was also the head of a group called the Campaign for Fairness. The campaign's goal was to increase federal funding for AIDS organizations in rural areas that felt "ripped off" because they were receiving less under the CARE Act than the cities that had tens of thousands of AIDS cases. For Nelson, it seemed a classic Robin Hood scenario: take from the rich, give to the poor. As he saw it, the "poor" naturally included the AIDS Resource Center of Wisconsin, of which he was executive director.

Nelson was able to use his influential position within AIDS Action Council to push his agenda, the single appropriation idea, under the rubric of "fairness." As director of an AIDS organization in Milwaukee, a second-tier city, Nelson's self-interest in advocating to change the CARE Act funding formula threatened to split the national AIDS advocacy coalition down the middle. To add further weight to what he and a number of others viewed as a supremely moral crusade, Nelson's Campaign hired former AIDS Action Council director Dan Bross—now employed by a lobbying firm run by two former members of Congress, both Republicans—to push for the funding formula changes on Capitol Hill. No one, except Pat Christen, seemed to see a conflict of interest in Nelson's simultaneously chairing the policy committee and steering AIDS Action Council—and the public debate—toward advocating a position which benefited the organization that paid his salary.

The Campaign for Fairness wasn't the only group to hire former

AIDS Action Council staff to represent their special interests. Tom Sheridan left AIDS Action Council in late 1990—not long after the Ryan White CARE Act that he was so instrumental in passing was signed into law, and not long after Jean McGuire left Washington because, as she saw it, the window of political opportunity on AIDS had closed. Sheridan formed a lobbying firm called the Sheridan Group, and in 1993 he formed the AIDS Political Action Committee to try to win favor among politicians the old-fashioned way: by donating money to their campaigns.

Like other AIDS advocates in Washington in 1995, Sheridan lobbied for reauthorization of the CARE Act—on behalf of the San Francisco AIDS Foundation, as well as for Ernest Hopkins' own CAEAR coalition, listed respectively as numbers 1 and 2 on the Sheridan Group's list of clients. Pat Christen had become a member of the honorary board of AIDS-PAC. "All the executive directors from the major AIDS organizations are on the honorary board," Sheridan told me.[43] Not unexpectedly, they strongly opposed the single appropriation being advocated by AIDS Action Council.

When the CARE Act was finally reauthorized, in May 1996, through fiscal year 2000, it seemed the best that could be said for the AIDS advocates who lobbied for it was that they had united to resist the cuts in funding that were rumored to be in the works by hostile Republicans. The rifts among them had been revealed for what they truly were: competing organizational interests, frequently masked in rhetoric about the "needs of people with AIDS." In actual fact, they spoke on their own behalf, which sometimes included the interests of people with AIDS, but at other times seemed to have much more to do with their board members' personal priorities and the expectations of their now-large staffs to be paid on a regular basis.

At the height of the acrimony and jockeying for position among the lobbyists on the CARE Act reauthorization, Cornelius Baker, then policy director of the National Association of People with AIDS, told the *Blade* that he couldn't think of another instance in which AIDS advocates had experienced "even half the amount of rancor as the one involving Ryan White reauthorization." Then again, Baker added, "none have had this amount of money attached to them."[44]

No one could deny that services for people with AIDS are vitally important. But an informed observer had to question why the AIDS lobbyists focused exclusively and tenaciously—ripping one another to shreds, if necessary, in the process—on services funding. They had never managed to find the same level of passion for mounting a major push to get the federal government finally to pay for prevention campaigns that were relevant to people's real lives. Might it have something to do with the fact that funding cuts would mean that they'd have to find a way to collaborate so that perhaps one or a few organizations could serve multiple populations—rather than there being a different organization for every possible variation on the theme of personal identity? Or, more to the point, might it mean that their own organizations, paychecks, and perks would have to be scaled back?

From where he sat in Dianne Feinstein's office in the U.S. Senate, Ralph Payne, then the senator's staffer for gay and AIDS issues, told me in late 1995 that the many AIDS advocates who called upon him had never talked, for example, about AIDS research. On the other hand, he estimated that he probably attended a hundred meetings about the Ryan White CARE Act. He said that while the activists were "blackening the sky with planes" to fly into Washington "to argue about minutiae and funding formulas in the Ryan White CARE Act," none of them seemed interested in other federal entitlement programs that provide support to people with AIDS, such as welfare and Medicaid. Yet in his home state alone, he said, "There's as much money flowing into California Medicaid dollars as in all Ryan White dollars; Medicaid is by far the biggest AIDS program in the country."[45]

In fact, 40 percent of people with AIDS end up on Medicaid as their sole means of support, according to Tim Westmoreland, an expert on Medicaid and AIDS. "Ryan White is a drop in the bucket compared to Medicaid," he said. Long familiar with the priorities of AIDS advocates from his years of being lobbied by them while he worked in the House of Representatives, Westmoreland cautioned, "If we fail to defend Medicaid, we will be doing a tremendous disservice to people with AIDS."[46]

Once it seemed the CARE Act would be reauthorized, AIDS advocates did turn their attention, at least partially, to Medicaid. In October 1995, AIDS Action Council director Barnes wrote in the

Blade, "While Ryan White provides more than $600 million a year to cities and states hardest hit by AIDS, *more than $3 billion* [my emphasis] in Medicaid funds are spent annually on medical services for the poorest and sickest people with HIV disease. In its role as a safety net, the Medicaid program finances clinic, hospital, and nursing-home care and lifesaving AIDS drugs for more than half of the Americans living with HIV disease."[47]

Since the survival of so many people with AIDS was quite literally at stake in the debates over Medicaid reform, one might reasonably ask why AIDS advocates were so late in focusing on the federal/state entitlement program. After all, they claimed that the "needs of people with AIDS" were their first priority. Could it have had something to do with the fact that Medicaid provides health care for individuals—and doesn't put money into the coffers of AIDS service organizations? As Ralph Payne observed, "The lobbying becomes about increasing funding for the organizations, and has very little to do with the people who need the services, very little to do with ending the epidemic."[48]

But there was something else at work, too. The years spent building the country's AIDS services infrastructure were years when the goal of AIDS lobbyists in Washington was to win as much as they could for AIDS alone, with little regard for people with other diseases or whose financial precariousness left them as dependent upon the government as many people with AIDS were. Reflecting upon the "exceptionalism" that underlies federally funded programs like the Ryan White CARE Act, Jean McGuire said, "I was deeply disturbed by difficulties we had having any kind of conversation about what did it mean in the Medicaid program I worked on so long to create different levels of access relative to the particular disease you have. What did it mean to say this particular disease elevates the status of your poverty above someone else's poverty?"[49]

McGuire said that AIDS advocates have resisted framing the struggle for protection from discrimination and against utter destitution in a broader "poverty discourse"—what it means to be both sick and poor in the wealthiest nation in history—because they view the broader systemic reforms that are so clearly needed in the nation's health and social welfare programs as beyond either the scope of their concern for AIDS or their ability to effect change. Yet, as McGuire pointed out, one can't really talk about AIDS without talking about issues of poverty, disenfranchisement, and the cracks in the nation's social welfare infrastructure that can swallow someone who is sick and poor. The more thoughtful leaders in the gay rights movement have said similar things about how the struggle for equal rights for gay men and lesbians is ultimately about the struggle for the dignity and freedom of all people.

Jane Silver, the public policy director for the American Foundation for AIDS Research, told me, "AIDS is a prism by which to look at all that's wrong with the social welfare system." For AIDS advocates, though, Silver said it's a question of whether to take their pot of money and run—or to work toward broader reform that will benefit people with AIDS as well as people with other compelling medical needs. She said, "It becomes a question of, do you take on the welfare system, and the social service system? Or do you carve out AIDS-specific services? It's the same dilemma of how much can AIDS advocates fix, and how."[50]

Before AIDS forced young white middle-class gay people to confront both mortality and the inequities of America's social welfare system, they, like most young white middle-class people, didn't think much about programs like Medicaid or welfare. But they were outraged and appalled when they saw professionally successful, sometimes affluent, gay men lose their jobs, their homes, and be forced to spend themselves into poverty in order to be eligible for federal assistance to pay for exorbitantly priced AIDS treatments and to get from gay community organizations the services they couldn't receive from mainstream health and social service providers. AIDS advocates successfully persuaded the federal government to fund special programs for people with AIDS under the CARE Act. But as the epidemic continued to spread among nongay, nonwhite, non-middle-class people, their arguments began to seem shortsighted, even selfish. What they wound up with is a parallel system of services created specially for AIDS, even as people who were poor and sick with the "wrong" disease (that is, not AIDS) continued to struggle with inadequate health care and social welfare programs.

One might reasonably expect that an important lesson from the gay community's experience with AIDS would be a recognition of the fact that everyone who is in need is equally deserving of assistance and support. But AIDS advocacy has gone well beyond the gay community that initiated it. AIDS service organizations now constitute an industry whose lobbyists in Washington work to make sure their employers get all they can. They play up or play down whichever subpopulation of people with AIDS suits their needs of the moment. If they are speaking to members of Congress, women and kids are still a sure bet to win support. If they speak to a group of gay people—who are still good for very generous donations—they might actually acknowledge that gay men continue to bear the overwhelming brunt of the epidemic in this country. As with the seasoned lobbyists in the halcyon days of the NORA coalition, whatever it takes to win is what they do.

They play within a system that rewards those with political and financial resources, even as those who lack them are forced to languish without a CARE Act to meet their particular needs. They talk a good line about race and poverty and all the "isms" and "phobias" that, for them, neatly explain the AIDS epidemic and the nation's response to it. But they don't ask the most obvious questions: Why should AIDS services now get more than $1 billion a year under the nation's only disease-specific funding measure? Is it because of the disease's infectiousness? Or because of the young age and productive years lost of its victims? Those are certainly compelling reasons to make AIDS a top priority. One final question, though, is avoided because of the discomfiting implications of its answer: Is AIDS an "exception" because of the political and financial resources of the AIDS industry, and because the CARE Act is now the largest budget item at the Health Resources and Services Administration, the biggest funder of the AIDS industry, and every bit as invested as the advocates in the CARE Act?

Perhaps such questions will be sorted out and answered in time. For now, AIDS advocates likely will continue fighting to keep their own piece of the pie, arguing that AIDS is exceptional and should continue to be treated as such by the federal government. "We may still be too scared to ask those questions," says Jean McGuire. "They are ultimately about giving up privilege."[51]

*

"This is like the campaign that has no election day," said Tom McNaught, who had been the communications director for Boston's AIDS Action Committee for more than four years at the time of our interview. McNaught had seen his share of political campaigns as a staffer for openly gay former U.S. Representative Gerry Studds (D-Mass.). But the campaign against AIDS is different from any McNaught had experienced before, and its interminableness was wearing on him. "I sometimes feel guilty," he said, "that I can't sustain the energy level I had when I was putting in seventy-hour weeks, coming in on weekends, and chewing Nicorette gum like it was going out of style." He asked, "How many rallies, how many national debates, how many get-out-the-votes, and how many clever efforts that you'd do in a campaign can you do when you don't even have an election date?"[52]

By the time I interviewed McNaught's boss in 1995, Larry Kessler, the executive director of AIDS Action Committee, had been at the organization's helm since its January 1983 inception. I asked Kessler whether he expected still to be doing in the mid-nineties what he was doing in the early eighties. "No," he said, without hesitation. "We originally thought we'd be out of existence in three years, that this was very short-term, there'd be a cure and treatment would be quick." Those expectations obviously needed to be revised as a cure and even effective treatments proved to be elusive. "By the fifth year," he said, "we started thinking more in ten-year terms. In the tenth year, we started thinking in twenty to twenty-five-year terms." The agency had just leased space for a thrift shop to help diversify its income. "We signed a ten-year lease that goes until the year 2005," said Kessler. "Now it seems like that's not enough."[53]

AIDS Action Committee was unusually fortunate to have a leader like Kessler, who brought with him not only many years of experience as a community activist, but also a willingness and ability to go with and manage the flow of organizational growth spurred by a burgeoning epidemic and, at least in the nineties, vastly increased financial resources. More typically, AIDS organizations that were born and reared in the early to mid-eighties experienced sometimes wrenching growing pains as they evolved from the jury-rigged volunteer organizations that sprang up in the epidemic's early years, into professionally run community institutions often with annual budgets now in the millions of dollars.

For most AIDS groups, the focus on the short term stemmed from the faith of virtually everyone in the early years that there would be a cure within a relatively short period of time. The San Francisco AIDS Foundation's former communications director Joe Fera said the agency had been reluctant to plan for the future. "We thought long-range planning implied that we have to be there a long time," he explained. "Our hope was that we would not be here in five years, or that in five years we would be dealing with a mop-up situation. And that has not proven to be the case."[54] In Chicago, Eileen Dirkin, director of the Howard Brown Memorial Health Center, said, "The fact that it's no longer 'until the cure,' but is now a permanent issue and a permanent disease, brings about a whole different set of responses and frustrations."[55]

Karl Mathiasen III is the founding director of the Washington, D.C.-based Management Assistance Group. Seventy years old at the time of our interview in 1995, Mathiasen has worked with many nonprofit, politically liberal organizations in his many years as a management consultant. Mathiasen's clients have included virtually all of the nation's largest AIDS organizations, and he is seen as something of a management guru among the leaders of those organizations. Each year since the National AIDS Network started it in 1988, Mathiasen has presented workshops on "the organizational life cycle" at the annual Skills Building conference.

As Mathiasen sees it, AIDS service organizations began as the campaign-like groups that Tom McNaught and thousands of others who ran and provided services through them expected them to be. But unlike political campaign organizations—dedicated to the specific, short-term goal of beating an opponent—the AIDS groups were faced with the prospect of a far longer and more arduous campaign than anyone imagined in the first few years of the epidemic. When it became evident that the campaign against AIDS was going to require a long-term commitment, it became equally apparent that the organizations created to serve those affected by AIDS were going to have to shape up if they were going to hold their place on the frontline of this particular war.

Mathiasen said, "We knew halfway through the eighties that this was not a campaign and the organizations had to settle down and create appropriate boards and set up systems." All organizations resist systems, he said, and this was particularly true with ASOs. "Part of the reason," he explained, "was resistance to bureaucracy and institutionalization, which was unattractive to AIDS activists who had felt put down by institutions in their lives before." He added that besides the usual nonprofit resistance to "shaping up," there was a fear of "creating monster organizations of the kind that are going to reject us." Although he didn't use the term, Mathiasen described the "internalized homophobia" that gay people working in ASOs turned upon one another and upon the organizations themselves. "Part of the reverberations and problems within ASOs is a result of gay politics," he said. "There's a lot of anger, a lot of putting other people down that seems to enter into the organization more thoroughly than in other organizations."

In particular, said Mathiasen, the leaders of AIDS organizations are favorite targets for this projected self-hatred. He illustrated his point by recalling the demise of the National AIDS Network. "When NAN folded," he said, "and some of the leaders were dismissed, it wasn't that they were dismissed as leaders. They were first not acknowledged as having been leaders, and were dismissed as not doing the right job without an acknowledgement that they were probably the right person for the job when it began." Not only was their work unacknowledged, but they were dismissed as people. Said Mathiasen, "They were banished in a way, put down, depersonalized. You were not only a bad leader, you were a bad person." He added, "That infuriated me."

On his first visit to GMHC, Mathiasen said he was fascinated by the "family atmosphere" of the organization. "ASOs created a sense of family for gay men in particular who did not have that," he said, "a place where they could be free about their sexual orientation, where they could be demonstrative." But he believes that some of the family feeling had to give way to the need for efficient and stable organizations, the lines drawn more clearly between the personal and professional. Bureaucratizing, institutionalizing—the business of running a business—"was really necessary for the work that had to be done," said Mathiasen. "Even if it wasn't a campaign, the business of getting organized was unattractive business. Some people got it and some people never did. People forced out felt they'd lost their families as well as their jobs."

One of the unique challenges for AIDS organizations has been what Mathiasen describes as their "telescoped growth." They have grown—sometimes explosively—because of both the burgeoning epidemic, and because of the increased availablility of funding, particularly through the CARE act. This has meant, said Mathiasen, that "things that took three or four years in other organizations had to be done in six to eighteen months."[56]

Torie Osborn, who was executive director of the Los Angeles Gay and Lesbian Services Center for four years, understands the need for gay and AIDS organizations to be professionally run. Osborn, who holds an MBA, notes that virtually all advocacy organizations in this country start out as volunteer groups before becoming "professional." "The only thing different about AIDS," she said, "is the impact of gay culture on the organizations, and the fact that because the epidemic has moved so quickly, and we've had to do the government's work for them, the growth has been compressed into a shorter period of time. Other than that, guys, we ain't no different from anybody else. Every Chinese community center, every YMCA, every nonprofit organization in this country started out as a small grassroots group." She added, "We've created an AIDS industry. How the hell else could we do it? You can't just keep running these [ASOs] out of your living room forever."[57]

Former GMHC director Tim Sweeney believes that the "industrialization" of AIDS is a good thing. "I can tell you I ran the biggest AIDS organization in America," he said. "I needed better management skills. I was in over my head at times and it was very frustrating." He added, "That's why I'm frustrated when people say that AIDS has become an industry. I almost want to say, 'Thank God,' if that implies experience, if that implies people who have taken risks, failed, and learned from them. I think that's okay. We're not innately intelligent about all these things."[58]

As the AIDS industry grew, questions arose as to just how well-compensated "AIDS professionals" ought to be. Former San Francisco AIDS Foundation director Tim Wolfred believes that those who work in AIDS organizations deserve to be paid, even well-paid. "There is work to be done," he said, "and people doing it deserve to make a decent living." An executive director responsible for running a multimillion dollar agency must have skills that, as Wolfred pointed out, are in high demand—and compensated with high salaries—in a competitive marketplace. "Despite what it might look like from the outside," he said, "I don't think there is a surplus of people who can manage something of that size. So part of what you're doing is paying a competitive salary to keep those skills in place. That's the heart of how our capitalist system works, whether we agree with it or not."[59]

Wolfred's successor at the San Francisco AIDS Foundation, Pat Christen, is clear about why she does the work—and why she deserves a salary commensurate with her skills and experience. Christen is one of the mere 7 percent of all the nation's executive directors of gay and AIDS organizations earning six-figure salaries—she received compensation totaling $176,742 in 1996.[60] "I believe strongly that I have considerable skills to lend to this effort and that they should be lent," she said. "I'm not independently wealthy, so I can't do this work and lend these skills unless I get paid for them because I have to pay the rent and I have a daughter to raise. I don't view that as a bad thing that people earn salaries to do good work."[61] Christen's salary regularly generated considerable protest by members of ACT UP/San Francisco, whose leftist ideology hasn't kept pace with the growth of the AIDS industry. In 1998 AIDS activist Michael Petrelis allied himself with antigay Republican members of Congress in criticizing the salaries of AIDS organization directors such as Christen. He failed to acknowledge, however, that even the best paid of them earns considerably less than what the American Society of Association Executives considers normal for executives of nonprofit groups of comparable size.[62]

The influx of a new generation of gay activists who cut their political teeth in ACT UP provided the growing AIDS industry with fresh troops to replace the first line of older activists who founded the AIDS organizations, many of whom were burned out by grief and politics or died from AIDS themselves. Although one of the canons of ACT UP's politically pure orthodoxy was that it was a mortal sin to be paid for working on AIDS issues, many of the group's members did in fact move into paying jobs in the AIDS industry.

Once inside the AIDS industry, the perspective of activists often changed as they realized how challenging it is to manage budgets, compromise, and negotiate—to be "professional." "There are times I really miss those hard moral lines I had as a street activist," said Jeff Graham, an ACT UP member who became director of Atlanta's AIDS Survival Project. "Sometimes I get scared that there won't be people keeping me on my toes and reminding me that this is not about careers, and not about jobs, and not about the creation of an industry, but about the elimination of an epidemic."[63]

Joe Fera, who, together with Pat Christen, started in the mid-eighties as a volunteer in the AIDS Foundation's speakers bureau, noted that managing the agency's growth to ensure that there will continue to be a San Francisco AIDS Foundation to serve people with AIDS requires skilled professionals. But like many "old-timers" in AIDS organizations around the country with whom I've spoken, Fera rues the loss of what he called the "activist urgency" that charged the foundation in its early years, as people have joined AIDS organizations because they see it as "a good career move." From being a "radical" group—"We used to put out posters of naked men with condoms on their dicks"—Fera said, "We've tended to grow into the center. It's kind of tough to swallow on some level because you want to be out there, and radical, but you find yourself more in the parochial center." He added wistfully, "That's an issue that organizations go through as they grow."[64]

When GMHC bought and consolidated its operations in one building in 1986, there was a hue and cry among staff and in the gay community as well: How could GMHC spend money that was intended for AIDS services on a building? The controversy over the purchase of the building—which actually proved a wise investment as it increased markedly in value, but which the agency outgrew before too long—is emblematic of some of the reasons for the ambivalence towards the AIDS industry felt by many in the gay community and among long-term staff and volunteers in AIDS organizations.

Derek Hodel, GMHC's former director of federal affairs, said, "There was a visceral revolt on the part of staff, who were upset with the new space." Although the new building provided the chance to move out of five separate, cramped locations, Hodel said that staff reacted negatively to the new space because it confronted them with the organization's—and the epidemic's—permanence in a way they never had anticipated. "All of a sudden this place looked like a bank," he explained, "instead of the slapdash, haphazard, on-the-fly kind of spaces they'd been using. When folks confronted that, it was very difficult for them. People didn't want to work there. It changed the quality of their thinking, the way that they felt."[65]

Suzanne Ouelette, the CUNY psychology professor, said that in her studies of GMHC volunteers, she found that most of the volunteers take a "really don't care" attitude towards the agency's bureaucracy as long as it doesn't impede their volunteer work. For the staff, though, Ouelette found that the bureaucratization could be alienating, forcing them at times to be dispassionate and "professional" when they might actually have been feeling the "activist urgency" that Joe Fera spoke of.

For Ouelette, too, GMHC's physical space provided a metaphor of the mixed blessing that is the AIDS industry. "In the original space," she said, "everyone was on top of everyone else, but you felt a kind of connection. You'd walk in and it was terrible and dirty. But there was a chair lift there. It was rickety, but the chair lift was a clear marker that there were folks coming into and leaving the building who needed help going up the steps. Right away, you knew where you were. Now in the new space, if there weren't the posters, and people didn't take time to decorate their cubicles, you almost could be anywhere."[66]

Like GMHC, AIDS service organizations throughout the country increasingly resembled the "mainstream" agencies for which they were intended to substitute when gay men were their main clients because mainstream organizations wanted nothing to do with them. Now they could pay their staffs on time, and sometimes quite handsomely. Now there were "AIDS professionals" whose entire careers were built from the epidemic. And now a parallel AIDS fundraising industry had become a profit-making venture for entrepreneurial capitalists, the "activist urgency" too often giving way to packagers, promoters, and profiteers whose "compassion" was available to the AIDS industry—at an often considerable financial and public relations cost.

With so many organizations invested in the continuation of the AIDS epidemic, it now seemed that "putting themselves out of business" was the last thing on anyone's mind.

WAR BONDS

I don't want you to give me your surplus.
I want you to give with personal deprivation.

MOTHER TERESA

As always, the efforts of individuals to elicit support—whether volunteer labor or financial contributions—made all the difference in the AIDS epidemic. Gay men hit up their friends for contributions, and gay staffers in the nation's private philanthropic organizations urged their employers to get involved at a time when the federal government still thought AIDS and gay people would just go away if they were ignored long enough. Eventually entertainers and socialites who were either gay themselves or had gay friends overcame their fear of bad publicity by lending their celebrity to the cause of fundraising for AIDS. But the stereotype of gay people as all having white skin, plenty of money, and access to celebrities often hindered their fundraising efforts—especially in the black community, where big check writers were scarce. But even the AIDS organizations formed by white gay people began to have problems with raising money when questions arose about how, exactly, the money was being spent. Learning about accountability seemed every bit as hard as learning how to raise money in the first place.

More than five thousand people gathered on the beach at the western edge of Fire Island Pines on Sunday, August 20, 1995, for GMHC's thirteenth annual Morning Party. GMHC flags rippled in the ocean breeze as costumed revelers—reminiscent of the famous summer parties in the island's heyday as a gathering place of the gay

Beautiful People—danced and sweated with others whose choice of apparel was merely fashion-forward swimwear. The *New York Times* reported the party among the various other charity events it noted in its Sunday "Styles" pages—including another AIDS fundraiser, a party at the Southampton home of theatrical producer Martin Richards to benefit Broadway Cares/Equity Fights AIDS. The Morning Party raised $350,000 for GMHC.[1]

Times had certainly changed.

When Larry Kramer and his friends canvassed the Pines and Cherry Grove, Fire Island's other mostly gay area, over Labor Day weekend 1981, they netted a mere $769.55 for the entire weekend. The Pines Pavilion, the hottest dance club in the island's trendiest area, wouldn't let them solicit donations on its premises. And an all-night vigil in front of the Ice Palace, the big dance club in the Grove, by Kramer and his friends Rick Fialla and Paul Popham, brought in a paltry $126. In the first four months of raising money for AIDS in New York during that first year of the epidemic, a total of $11,806.55 was collected—more than half of it at an August 11, 1981, fundraiser at Kramer's Fifth Avenue apartment. Even then, however, five people had given $1,000 each and two gave $500 each. "Which," Kramer noted, "means that the rest of the entire gay community in the city of New York has contributed to this cause the sum of $5,806.55."[2]

When GMHC cofounder and writer Edmund White's benefit dance committee received the ten thousand printed invitations for the new organization's first major fundraiser—"Showers," an April 8, 1982, disco dance benefit at Paradise Garage—board president Popham was furious that the return address said "Gay Men's Health Crisis." He didn't want the word "gay" to appear on anything sent through the mail lest it force open someone's closet door. "What about my mailman?" asked Popham, mortified to think the mail carrier might know something as private as the fact of Popham's homosexuality. "He's going to know I'm gay." An incredulous Kramer retorted, "What about your doorman? You drag tricks up to your apartment every night. Don't you think your doorman suspects something? Why aren't you worried about him?" Despite fears of being ignored by the many gay New Yorkers for whom being gay meant nothing more than clubbing in the discos on the weekends,

"Showers" raised $52,000 from the apolitical crowd of partygoers.[3] Kramer says, "We felt we had the support of the community to do what we were doing—whatever that was."[4]

A year after that first benefit, GMHC on April 30, 1983, hosted the largest gay event ever held to that time, and for the first time a charity event sold out Madison Square Garden's 17,601 seats in advance. The Ringling Brothers Circus event featured Leonard Bernstein conducting the circus orchestra in the national anthem, as well as a program that contained Mayor Koch's proclamation of "Aid AIDS Week" and page after page of memorial notices of men who had died of the still-mysterious disease.[5] The *New York Native* had helped to promote the event, ensuring its great success, while the *New York Times* ignored it despite the size of the crowd. The circus cleared $250,000, making GMHC one of the wealthiest gay organizations in the country. Still, the circus raised $100,000 less than the 1995 Morning Party, despite the fact that it drew three and a half times the number of people.

Rodger McFarlane, who became GMHC's executive director shortly after the circus fundraiser, recalls that when GMHC signed the contract with Ringling Brothers to sponsor the event, the group had to come up with an initial $100,000 payment within three weeks. Where else would they get the money but from their circles of upper-middle-class gay friends? "We went through our phone books of people who could loan us a thousand dollars," recalls McFarlane. A hundred people agreed. "Is that grassroots?" he asked. "It's very green grass." McFarlane attributes the circus's success to the fact that, as he puts it, "We had a bunch of white faggots who knew people." Nevertheless, he added, "Considering the disposable income of that group, we were shocked by the stinginess of it. Everybody thinks it was a groundswell of support, but it wasn't."[6]

Meanwhile on the other coast, a June 23, 1983, fundraiser for San Francisco's K.S./AIDS Foundation brought out the first entertainment stars to participate in an AIDS benefit. As Randy Shilts noted, most celebrities at that point, "including many who had built their careers on their gay followings, were not inclined to get involved with a disease that was not . . . fashionable."[7] Actress Shirley MacLaine pulled down the top of her strapless gown to show the audience that she had more than the great legs that host Debbie

Reynolds mentioned in introducing her. For her part, Reynolds lifted the back of her own gown to reveal her skimpy black underwear. Television actor Robert "Benson" Guillaume and singer Morgana King joined the others in the symphony hall—which was filled only because the AIDS foundation had given away free tickets.

Cleve Jones recalled Marcus Conant's directness when the doctor first approached him with the idea for the K.S./AIDS Foundation, and the fact that millions of dollars would have to be raised to support the effort. "When Harvey Milk ran for supervisor," said Jones, "his total campaign budget was $30,000. I'd never raised that much money." Looking back at the foundation's beginnings, Jones added, "Within a matter of years it became routine for gay community-based organizations to raise and spend millions of dollars every year."[8] By the time of my interview with Jones, the San Francisco AIDS Foundation was operating on an annual budget in excess of $15 million.

Gay people throughout the country in the early eighties solicited donations from their friends to pay for AIDS services that couldn't be provided by volunteers—and that most certainly were not paid for by the federal government. In Atlanta, Jesse Peel threw a fundraiser at his home in July 1984 that raised $5,000 for the newly formed AID Atlanta. "That was big bucks in 1984!" Peel said with a chuckle.[9] In Miami, Health Crisis Network's first director, Sally Dodds, remembers a fundraiser in someone's home in Coconut Grove at the end of 1984 that featured singer Barbara Cook and raised about $8,000. "It was a lot of money," she said. "We thought we were rich." One thing that struck Dodds as peculiar, though, was the fact that the gay men at the party wouldn't sign a check to Health Crisis Network, choosing instead to make cash contributions. Of course that way the bank clerks who processed the checks, like Paul Popham's mailman, wouldn't know the men were gay or had given money to a gay organization—or, more to the point, that they were associated in any way with the "gay disease."[10]

In February 1985, AIDS Project Los Angeles (APLA) asked actress Elizabeth Taylor to lend her name to its "Commitment to Life" fundraiser to be held in September (as it happened, only weeks before Taylor's friend Rock Hudson succumbed to AIDS on October 2). Bill Meisenheimer, who was APLA's executive director at the time, says that Taylor was the first "really big name" star to get involved with raising money for AIDS. Meisenheimer, who counts himself a personal friend of Taylor's, said, "She had been very angry at people not wanting to get involved, because she had friends who were getting sick and dying, and she couldn't understand why people wouldn't get involved. She'll tell you she was very angry about people sitting on their butts."[11]

On Sunday, July 28, 1985, a huge crowd turned out for an AIDS walkathon that raised $630,000 for APLA. Los Angeles Mayor Tom Bradley joined movie stars in praising Rock Hudson's announcement three days earlier that he had AIDS as a main reason for the walk's success.[12] The AIDS walks had begun a year earlier in Boston, after Mayor Raymond Flynn agreed in 1983 to participate in a cross-state run to raise money for AIDS and suggested that in 1984 the event should be a walk through the streets of Boston "to educate everyone," as Ann Maguire, Flynn's liaison to the city's gay community at the time, recalls.[13] The walks continue throughout the country, raising millions of dollars—in some cases the bulk of their funding—for local AIDS service organizations.

Other events that have become mainstays of AIDS fundraising include dance-a-thons—Boston also pioneered the AIDS dance-a-thon—and, since 1993, the various AIDS bike rides. Dan Pallotta, a Los Angeles fundraising consultant, began the California AIDS Ride, from San Francisco to Los Angeles, to raise money for AIDS service providers in the two cities. The rides have been extremely successful, at least in terms of raising awareness of AIDS and grossing large amounts of money. The total amount of pledges has increased each year from the first ride's $1.6 million, to more than $9 million raised in the San Francisco to Los Angeles ride in 1997—the largest-ever AIDS fundraising event.

Most AIDS fundraisers created by gay people didn't have the large corporate sponsors and national promotion of the AIDS rides, because most were done on a small scale at the local level. In Atlanta, for example, Tony Braswell, is the executive director of AID Atlanta—by day. By night, though, at least on Sunday nights, Braswell becomes "Maytag," a drag queen, camping it up at the Armory, one of the city's gay bars. But not in the Ru Paul mold of pseudo-feminine glamour and curvaceousness. "I'll wear a $200 ball gown and tennis shoes," said Braswell. "We don't shave, don't cover our arms. It's very camp." Braswell, whose lover of twelve and a half years died of AIDS, performs at the Armory in weekly benefits—he and his costars are called the "Armorettes"—that grew out of their efforts in the mid-eighties to raise money for the bar's softball team. "As people began to get sick," explained Braswell, "we put a bucket out that said 'This is for people with HIV/AIDS.'" The bucket evolved into weekly fundraising drag shows to help people meet their medical bills and house payments. The shows further evolved into a more coordinated effort with social service organizations, like AID Atlanta.

Each November, Atlanta's drag queens compete for the crown in the city's annual AIDS fundraiser, called "Homecoming," by raising money for different AIDS service organizations. Braswell was homecoming queen in 1993 because he raised the most money for the Grady Memorial Hospital infectious disease clinic he directed at the time. The event, he said, "is very mainstream." After local television anchorwoman Angela Robinson helped Braswell and his friends organize "West Hollywood Squares"—featuring a Hollywood-Squares-like set, participants' names drawn from a hat, and "fabulous prizes"—Braswell said the fundraiser was moved "to a whole new level." He explained, "When she lent her name to it, one of our city council members said 'I want to do it.' The mayor's office called and said they would talk to us. We had several key business people. Now we're 'drag queens to the stars,' as we say."[14]

In Atlanta, it took the willingness of a local TV news anchorwoman to get other nongay people involved in raising money for AIDS. Nationally, it took Elizabeth Taylor's announced commitment in 1985 to spur others to follow her lead. Taylor's commitment to AIDS has continued unabated, and at the 1996 International Conference on AIDS, in Vancouver, she received eight standing ovations during her moving speech to the assembled scientists and AIDS activists. As National Minority AIDS Council director Paul Kawata put it, "When Elizabeth stood up with Rock and said, 'I will give my life to fighting this disease,' it became okay."[15] In the years after 1985, celebrities practically tripped over one another to get their names on honorary program committees for AIDS fundraisers and to speak and receive awards for their "compassion" from grateful AIDS organizations.

In 1993, when HBO filmed *And the Band Played On,* based on Randy Shilts's 1987 bestseller about the early years of the AIDS epidemic, stars flocked like lemmings to be cast in the made-for-TV movie—but only after Richard Gere agreed to play the small role of a Michael Bennett-like choreographer with AIDS.[16] Suddenly Steve Martin, Angelica Houston, Alan Alda, Glenne Headly, B. D. Wong, and others found the $7 million film irresistible. Matthew Modine headed the cast in the role of Don Francis, the CDC scientist who was thwarted at every turn in his efforts to get the federal government to do something to stop the epidemic when it first began. Openly gay actor Sir Ian McKellen played the part of San Francisco gay political activist Bill Kraus, who succumbed to AIDS in 1986. Lesbian actress and comedian Lily Tomlin played Selma Dritz, the infectious disease specialist in the San Francisco Department of Public Health who, after looking at the extraordinary rates of STDs among gay men in the city just before the epidemic started, warned, "Too much is being transmitted."

It was also in 1993 that Hollywood finally produced a major motion picture that dealt with AIDS, despite the involvement of individual actors and the movie industry's professed concern in its October 1991 formation of Hollywood Supports, an organization intended to assist those in the film business affected by AIDS. Tom Hanks starred as AIDS-stricken gay lawyer Andrew Beckett in *Philadelphia,* one of the most successful dramatic films of 1993, earning $125 million at the box office worldwide before being released on video.[17] When he was asked whether it was a difficult career decision to portray a gay man with AIDS, Hanks said, "I'm greatly pleased and very, very honored to have been a part of the first mainstream, big budget, American motion picture to deal with the subject matter."[18] I wept along with Hanks—and my ex-lover Bill, who entered the hospital two days later for what proved to be his own last round with AIDS—as the actor recalled his gay theater-teacher heroes in a tearful acceptance speech for the "Best Actor" Oscar during the Academy Awards presentation on March 21, 1994.

One of the worst-kept celebrity "secrets" ended in 1994 when singer Elton John finally admitted publicly that he is gay. To his credit, John at that point was already using his popularity to raise substantial amounts of money for AIDS causes, channeled through the Elton John AIDS Foundation he formed in 1992. That year he contributed all the proceeds from his singles sales in America of "The Last Song," a moving song about a young man with AIDS making peace with his father before the son dies. Once he finally committed himself, John raised millions for AIDS. But, he noted, "I didn't really get involved until I spent some time with Ryan [White's] family and met Ryan and saw the injustices that his family had to endure because of AIDS."[19]

The biggest celebrity athlete AIDS story after Magic Johnson's 1991 announcement that he was HIV-positive, and Arthur Ashe's April 8, 1992, press conference to confirm rumors that he indeed had AIDS, was the 1995 revelation by four-time Olympic gold-medal diving champion Greg Louganis that not only was he gay but that he was HIV-positive as well, and had in fact already suffered several AIDS-related bouts of illness. Louganis immediately became the highest-profile gay man ever to go public at one time about both his homosexuality and his HIV infection. In his autobiography *Breaking the Surface*—which premiered at number one on the *New York Times* best-seller list on March 19, 1995—Louganis says he decided to write the book after a health scare made him realize he might not have long to live. "I didn't want to wind up like Rock Hudson or Liberace," he (and coauthor Eric Marcus) wrote, "Rock Hudson only came forward with the truth at the very end of his life, long after he was in a position to tell the public himself. Liberace died hoping to take his secret with him. I want to be able to do this with dignity, to stand up with a sense of pride in who I am, to say, 'This is who I am and this is what I have and this is what I've done.'"[20]

By the end of 1995—a decade after Rock Hudson went public about having AIDS, and his friend Elizabeth Taylor made the epidemic "okay"—many celebrities and other wealthy and socially prominent people had jumped on the AIDS bandwagon. Singer Deborah Harry, whose song "The Tide Is High" set the whimsical but determined tone of the 1990 AIDS film *Longtime Companion*, played a benefit concert on September 3 at the Town Hall in Provincetown, Massachusetts, to benefit the Provincetown AIDS Support Group. "It fit my schedule, I thought it would be fun, and it's P-town," said Harry, adding, "And of course it's AIDS."[21] That year, pop singer Cyndi Lauper and jazz singer Dianne Reeves performed at the closing ceremonies of Whitman-Walker Clinic's ninth annual AIDS walk in the nation's capital, led by Tipper Gore.[22] And comedian and talk-show hostess Rosie Perez walked a ten-kilometer "act of penance" in the AIDS Walk Colorado to raise money for AIDS services and to assuage her conscience after not visiting a friend in the hospital with AIDS until the day after the man had died.[23]

Blaine Trump got involved with God's Love We Deliver, New York City's meals program for people with AIDS, after losing friends and "because she's a caring soul," as executive director Kathy Spahn put it.[24] Others of her wealth and social standing also got involved because they knew someone affected by AIDS, or because they knew someone who knew someone with AIDS. Either way, there was a personal connection to the disease—typically far fewer than six degrees of separation. They volunteered time, contributed money, and urged their friends to do the same because the epidemic had become real for them.

To the dismay of AIDS fundraisers, though, the unwillingness of many closeted, wealthy gay men to be open and honest prevented their wealthy heterosexual friends who may have been willing to contribute from knowing how they might help or how much they might be able to donate. In Washington, D.C., I have reported on the segregation between gay and heterosexual people that for years was a major handicap for AIDS fundraising efforts in the city. The lack of connections by AIDS service providers to Washington's charity-ball set hindered the providers' ability to procure for their own work some of the money those wealthy people contribute to other charities. But it was more than that. In a city where A-lists are predominantly political (with a handful of real estate developers and media celebrities thrown in), the arts crowd—the artists, fashion designers, and entertainers who were hit by AIDS early and hard because of the large number of gay men among them—doesn't have the same social cachet with the fashionable party throwers that it has in cities like New York and Los Angeles. The lack of social cross-pollination meant that for many years, prominent Washingtonians often remained isolated from AIDS, the epidemic being nothing more to them than the background noise among "the masses."

Many of the gay men who move among Washington's wealthy and high-powered—even men whose own lovers were known to have the disease—were loath to speak about AIDS with their heterosexual colleagues for fear of being associated with the stigmatized disease. Whitman-Walker Clinic board member Riley Temple, a black gay lawyer, told me that "There are [gay] people who would ordinarily move in those circles who for many reasons feel it's risky even to bring the [AIDS] topic up. They're afraid their business or social colleagues would associate them with a disease that is usually associated with the kinds of people who would not frequent those events." Gay men whose primary need was to be accepted by heterosexuals—to be insiders in a city populated by people who crave insider status—could not bring themselves to associate in any way with a disease that, above all else, has been, in this country, a disease of "outsiders."

Jennifer Phillips, a trustee of her family's modern-art museum, the Phillips Collection, described a "voluntary segregation" between Washington's gay and heterosexual communities. "I don't think there's a tremendous amount of interaction," she said. "The gay community is not very 'out' in Washington, as it is in Key West, for example, where I have spent the last several winters and where there is integration of the homosexual and heterosexual communities." It was her gay friends in other places who spurred Phillips to get involved with AIDS causes in Washington. Even when she and her husband, Laughlin, signed up for an Art Against AIDS committee, it was because they were asked by professional New York fundraisers. Local AIDS fundraisers—from Whitman-Walker Clinic, for example—hadn't approached them or others like them who had money and the desire to give it. "I've been amazed," said Phillips, "that the AIDS community is not doing as much reaching out to people like me." Even the clinic's Riley Temple admitted, "I don't think it's that [society] people are not willing to get involved—we just haven't asked them."[25]

Throughout 1990, Michelangelo Signorile, in his weekly *Out-Week* "Gossip Watch" column, hammered at David Geffen, one of the wealthiest men in Hollywood and at that time still a closeted homosexual. "I don't care how much blood money you've given to fight AIDS," wrote Signorile in a typically histrionic column. "You slit our throats with one hand and help deaden the pain with the other." In September of that year, Geffen's name appeared on the benefit committee of APLA's annual "Commitment to Life" fund-raising event. After seeing the event's guest list, a Los Angeles group, Artists Confronting AIDS, sent a protest letter to APLA saying, "Commitment to Life?! Honey, next year call it what it really is: Commitment to the Closet." After sticking a tentative toe out of his closet in a February 1991 *Vanity Fair* interview—he claimed he was "bisexual"—Geffen finally came out fully as a gay man at the end of 1992, when he received an award from APLA for his contributions.[26] In March of that year, Geffen had given $1 million to APLA for new office space.[27] He has since given millions more to other AIDS organizations, including GMHC and AIDS Action Council.

The undeniably important contributions of time, money, and lucrative connections that people like David Geffen, Elizabeth Taylor, Blaine Trump, and many others made to support AIDS services, raise one troubling but important question: Where were these people before AIDS? Why weren't they there to assist gay people as they struggled to achieve equality and to lessen the hatred and violence towards them? Some of them, like Geffen and Elton John, were hiding their homosexuality in closets lined with vast amounts of money. But the others? Elizabeth Taylor? She was widely known to have a number of gay friends, including Rock Hudson, yet it wasn't until they were diagnosed with a fatal illness that she saw the need to speak out on their behalf. As Tim Wolfred, the former director of the San Francisco AIDS Foundation, put it, "Who would speak out for us before AIDS? Who would publicly defend us? America wasn't ready until we were dying, when we had this epidemic. Before then, all the public images of us were twisted, perverted, and nobody spoke up against that—not even gay people themselves."[28]

Indeed, heterosexuals and wealthy but closeted gay men weren't the only ones to avoid gay community organizations and fail to speak out on behalf of gay people before AIDS. Most of the gay and lesbian rank and file also weren't involved in, or did not give money to, gay political and social service organizations until the AIDS epidemic showed them their connections to one another and the political implications of their personal lives. Also like many heterosexuals, many gay people didn't contribute or get involved with AIDS until someone told them it was acceptable to do so. As Urvashi Vaid points out, "As AIDS activism and fundraising developed a social cachet—through the involvement of straight celebrities and wealthy individuals—more gay people felt comfortable getting involved."[29]

By staying in the "closet" about their sexual orientation or concern about AIDS, many gay people hoped to avoid being labeled and stigmatized by disapproving heterosexuals. But this attitude also prevented heterosexuals from seeing gay people as real human beings. As efforts to raise money for AIDS showed time after time, whether for an AIDS walk or a corporate contribution, the willingness of gay people to be open and honest about their lives, fears, and pain, has enormous power to heal them—and to win allies who share their humanity and concern. As with everything else gay people accomplished in the AIDS epidemic, being honest and having integrity took courage and a refusal to buy into the shame that many heterosexuals want to impose on gay people and on AIDS. Which goes to show that love, concern, and the drive for survival eventually win out over fear and even the need for approval.

*

Before AIDS, Atlanta psychologist Don Smith said his city's gay community "wasn't enormously visible except on the bar circuit." In the early eighties, though, Smith wasn't part of the bar scene, and was just coming out as a gay man. "Once I saw the AIDS epidemic was going on," he remembers, "it was like this was far too important for me to worry about what the public thought of my sexual orientation." In March 1983, Smith got involved with AID Atlanta as a volunteer support-group leader. The organization had no paid staff, and in fact, said Smith, "To call it an organization at that point was an overstatement; it was more like a disorganization." Raising money for services was tough going, especially because the bar owners thought that talking about AIDS was "bad for business." That changed, though. Said Smith, "When the bartenders and owners started to die, fundraising became very successful in bars." Suddenly, the bars that were for many gay people the center of their social lives said it was okay to talk about AIDS, and this even made AIDS fundraising fashionable.[30]

The history of private-sector AIDS fundraising is a collection of stories like Smith's. Just as Elizabeth Taylor made AIDS a legitimate cause for celebrities—both heterosexual and gay—by her own example, others with money to give or fundraising skills to offer came forward only when someone they respected said it was not only necessary but that it was okay to do so. That's how it happened not only in the gay bars and among celebrities and the wealthy, but also in the nation's philanthropic foundations and charitable organizations. Typically a gay man who either had AIDS himself or knew someone who did, or a sympathetic heterosexual—most often a woman—would call attention to the epidemic and point out how his or her employer could provide funding assistance to a struggling community AIDS organization.

In 1986, the Ford Foundation asked Michael Seltzer—a gay man long involved with philanthropy and, at the time, cochair of Lambda Legal Defense and Education Fund—to survey the landscape of foundation giving for AIDS and advise them on how they might respond. Seltzer published his findings in a 1987 report titled *Meeting the Challenge: Foundation Responses to Acquired Immune Deficiency Syndrome*. He also spearheaded the 1987 formation of a Council on Foundations affinity group, called Funders Concerned About AIDS. The group was formed to educate those in the foundation world about AIDS, and the role that private philanthropic funding could play in responding to the epidemic. Seltzer, who shortly after our interview left his position as the founding executive director of Funders Concerned to join the staff of the Ford Foundation, said, "When AIDS dropped like a bomb into the foundation world, people didn't know about it unless they knew somebody who was gay."

At Funders Concerned, Seltzer's job was to educate foundations about the ways in which AIDS was relevant to their areas of concern. For a program on AIDS and black women's health, for example, Seltzer brought in the executive editor of *Essence* magazine to speak about why funders should be interested in black women's health. For foundations interested in the arts, Funders Concerned showed them why AIDS is an arts issue. Rather than encouraging foundations to create AIDS programs per se, Seltzer said, "Our goal is to help them understand the links between their interests and the opportunities to respond to AIDS."[31]

The lessons that Seltzer and Funders Concerned attempted to impart to the nation's private foundations were long overdue by the time serious money finally began to be channeled to AIDS prevention and services. Although the AIDS epidemic was designated as such in 1981, it wasn't until 1983 that four foundations made five small grants. Despite the fact that AIDS was being called the greatest public health crisis of the century, it was only in 1987 that two dozen of the more than thirty-two hundred foundations nationwide actually made grants for AIDS.

Like the federal government, most foundations took a wait-and-see attitude toward AIDS in the early years. Briefly, it went something like this: "Let's wait until we know whether predictions come true about AIDS 'breaking out' into the 'general population'"—that is, into the white heterosexual middle class. "In the meantime let's see just how long gay people can foot the entire bill for 'their' epidemic." As for many individual Americans, the 1985 death of Rock Hudson was a turning point in the awareness of AIDS by foundations, according to Seltzer's 1987 report. "The heightened visibility of AIDS in the country at large also had a notable effect on foundation funding efforts," it said.

A year after the Ford Foundation report, another study of philanthropic AIDS funding, by the Foundation Center, noted that by August 1988 some 157 foundations had awarded 593 grants for HIV/AIDS programs, totaling $51,599,545. Thirty-one million of those dollars had been allocated in the 1987 funding year—not coincidentally the first funding year after Rock Hudson's October 1985 death. Still only 3 percent of the nation's foundations that make awards larger than $100,000—to wit, the wealthy ones—had given money to AIDS causes at that point. At the time of the Foundation Center report, there were 73,000 AIDS cases in the United States.[32]

Of the private foundations that had given money for AIDS by 1988, the Princeton, New Jersey-based Robert Wood Johnson Foundation (RWJ) was far and away the largest single funder, having given nearly $27 million—more than half of all the private foundation funding for AIDS to that point. RWJ's single largest AIDS grant was in 1988 for $4 million to WGBH, the public television station in Boston, to produce *The AIDS Quarterly,* an educational series hosted by Peter Jennings. But to be able to contribute money for AIDS, RWJ, the nation's largest health care philanthropy, had to find a way around its policy of not making grants for particular diseases. Paul Jellinek, RWJ's vice president for programs, explained how the foundation came to see AIDS as relevant to its interests. "We actually had a very interesting internal debate about whether or not to get involved with AIDS," said Jellinek. "In part it was because we were not focused on specific diseases, but also it was not clear what our role would be if we got into this. At that point, fewer than 20 percent survived more than two years after diagnosis. From a health care standpoint, there was little to do other than palliative care. Our major emphasis had always been health care." Jellinek said that RWJ didn't see basic research as a needy area because it was (presumably) being handled by the National Institutes of Health. Epidemiology was the bailiwick of the Centers for Disease Control. And public education was supposed to be the province of the surgeon general.

"So it was not clear what role, if any, we might play," Jellinek continued. When Dr. Philip Lee, from the University of California–San Francisco, told RWJ about the "San Francisco model" of coordinated AIDS care, it was a revelation. Said Jellinek, "We recognized that there are service needs here, a real need for home and community-based services. If those services were not available, people with AIDS might wind up being hospitalized inappropriately, or sent home without adequate support services."[33] RWJ responded by establishing its $17.1 million AIDS Health Services Program, the pilot projects intended to replicate the San Francisco model of coordinated AIDS services. In March 1988, the foundation solicited proposals from community-based organizations for AIDS prevention and service projects focusing on those at highest risk. RWJ didn't specify the level of funding it would make available for the projects—and was overwhelmed by more than a thousand proposals requesting a total of $537 million. The foundation ultimately selected fifty-four projects, totaling $16.7 million.[34]

How did RWJ's example affect other foundations? The federal government? Jellinek said, "We were somewhat disappointed that the size of the response wasn't greater. There was a broad response, with a lot of foundations [giving money], but not always at the level we had hoped given the severity of the situation." As independent entities, Jellinek explained, foundations have an advantage over, say, the U.S. Congress, in that they can pick an issue or organization they're interested in funding and move on it relatively quickly. In an odd twist, though, RWJ found itself not only pointing the way for a hesitant federal government but actually trying to fill a gap that should have been filled by the Feds.

Though he didn't speculate as to why the federal government took so long to make an appropriately substantial financial commitment to AIDS, Jellinek tactfully said that "We were pleased that in fact some of these programs made it easier for the federal government to move forward. The HRSA [AIDS services demonstration] program was modeled after RWJ, which in turn was modeled after San Francisco, which subsequently laid the groundwork for [the] Ryan White [CARE Act]. The AIDS Prevention and Services projects made it easier for CDC to open their funding directly to community organizations."[35] For decades privately funded groups were looking at the kind of long-term care that infectious or chronic diseases would require. But with AIDS, "a foundation program served as a surrogate for, rather than as an example to, the federal government," as Daniel M. Fox puts it in *AIDS: The Burdens of History.*[36]

The Ford Foundation responded to Seltzer's 1987 report by launching the National–Community AIDS Partnership (NCAP) the following year, with an initial $2 million, to be housed at the National AIDS Network. Seltzer said, "I suggested we needed to create an entity that would be respected by foundations and corporations at the national level. That was the genesis of the National AIDS Fund [as NCAP is known today]." The National AIDS Network folded two years after the philanthropy was established, but Paula Van Ness remained the Fund's president. She could have been speaking for AIDS-related causes in general when she said of her own experience, "What could have been a short-term job has turned into a long-term job."[37]

The National AIDS Fund took the concept of community-wide planning—RWJ used this in its local planning consortia, and the Ryan White CARE Act continues to use it in distributing the federal government's hundreds of millions for AIDS services—to make

funding awards on a matching basis. Money from national foundations channeled through the Fund is matched with money generated
by the Fund's thirty-two "community partners" around the country.
Van Ness explained that if, for example, the Fund has $75,000 to
give, a grant is awarded to an interested community only after it
forms a local advisory committee, conducts a community needs assessment, and uses the $75,000 to leverage an additional $75,000
from local charitable funders. In its first decade, the Fund raised
more than $70 million for organizations providing AIDS prevention
and care, and its community partners gave a record $10 million in
1997 alone.[38] Since 1993, the Fund has administered money raised
by Elton John through his Elton John AIDS Foundation. As Van
Ness put it, "Elton John is the money machine; we're the distribution
department."[39]

The first national philanthropic foundation focusing exclusively
on AIDS was formed by people who were seeing young gay colleagues get sick and die, and wanted to do something to help. The
design and fashion industries were hit hard by AIDS because of the
disproportionately large number of gay men who work in them. The
growing toll led a group of industry people to join textile designer
Patricia Green on April 25, 1984, to form the Design and Interior
Furnishings Foundation for AIDS. At its tenth anniversary in 1994
the foundation changed its name to the Design Industries Foundation Fighting AIDS, though it continued to be known most commonly as DIFFA. Green recalled the reason others responded so
readily to the letter she had sent around to colleagues in the industry.
"There was a sense of desperation among us," she said, "that we had
to do something, right now, that nobody was listening while all around
us, our friends and colleagues were disappearing and dying."[40]

Like many people involved in fighting and raising money for
AIDS, DIFFA's organizers were struck by the firsthand experience
of someone actually living with AIDS. At an early meeting of the
group at the Manhattan offices of the American Society of Interior
Designers, Richard Medrano, a young Mexican-American designer,
stood and addressed the group forthrightly about his illness. Mathilde Krim, who in 1983 had formed the AIDS Medical Foundation
in New York, was there, as was Rodger McFarlane, then director of
GMHC. For many it was the first time they'd heard someone with

AIDS talk without shame about what it was like to live with the highly stigmatized disease.[41]

In its own first decade, DIFFA had raised and distributed nearly $19 million to more than six hundred community-based organizations across the country to support their efforts to provide direct care, education, and prevention. Twenty affiliated chapters and organizing committees throughout the U.S. raised funds and awareness largely through special events that drew from their local design industries. As *Art & Understanding* put it, "By capitalizing on the talents and products of top artists, designers, corporate leaders, and celebrities, DIFFA produces events that seem almost magical when compared to many others."[42] Almost equally magical was the fact that DIFFA seemed to be an efficiently operated charity, at least until a substantial loss on a series of fundraising parties in 1994 forced questions about the group's overhead costs—because it had found ways to raise money that relied heavily on volunteers and donated goods and services, as did AIDS service organizations in the early years.

To think that DIFFA began because Pat Green had been affected by the death of a friend is to be reminded of the power of one: one life lost, and one person's commitment to make a difference. As Green put it, "People get involved with organizations like DIFFA not because of the huge amounts of numbers of people that have died, because you can hear that ten thousand people died last year and still not have it seem real. It's not until you have it happen to you—until you lose one person, know one person who has died of AIDS—that it really changes everything."[43]

Not one death, not even tens of thousands of deaths, could move the Reagan administration to assert authority in the nation's response to the growing AIDS epidemic, and it was left to Congress to appropriate more funds than the administration requested for research into the mysterious disease. A 1985 report by the congressional Office of Technology Assessment noted that "increases in funding specifically for AIDS have come at the initiative of Congress, not the administration."[44] At least partly because of the administration's reluctance to fund AIDS research during the first few years of the epidemic, Daniel Fox notes, "voluntary contributions and state appropriations for laboratory and clinical investigation have been more important than in other recent epidemics."[45]

This was where the American Foundation for AIDS Research (AmFAR) came in. In 1983, Mathilde Krim, a Ph.D. research scientist whose now deceased multimillionaire husband Arthur was chairman of Orion Pictures, was alarmed by news from her colleague Joseph Sonnabend about the strange symptoms that were afflicting his gay patients in Greenwich Village. With more than $100,000 of her own family funds, Krim formed the AIDS Medical Foundation in New York. In 1985, the foundation merged with a similar Los Angeles-based organization called the National AIDS Research Foundation—which had been started by Michael Gottlieb, Rock Hudson's personal physician, among others—and AmFAR was born. Krim's scientific credentials and, even more importantly, social cachet among the rich and famous, brought substantial attention to AIDS and contributions to AmFAR. A quarter-million dollars from the estate of Rock Hudson helped launch the foundation, and the role of Elizabeth Taylor as its national spokeswoman brought the foundation immediate prominence, glamour, and "mainstream" acceptability.

Bill Meisenheimer, who left his job as director of AIDS Project Los Angeles in October 1985 to become AmFAR's first executive director, explained that the foundation's mission "was to promote development of research through seed grants so people could go get real grants." AmFAR had a significant advantage over other AIDS groups in that it was not seen as a "gay" organization, which was intentional. Said Meisenheimer, "A more mainstream organization could perhaps appeal to people who wouldn't relate to a grassroots—gay—organization."[46] To further enhance both its credibility and visibility, AmFAR brought on Mervyn Silverman, the former health chief from San Francisco who was later hired by the Robert Wood Johnson Foundation to direct its AIDS Health Services Program, as president of its board. Silverman, who was still AmFAR's president in the mid-nineties, told me, "By being private, rather than government funded, AmFAR could be creative, flexible, and fast. Few of those words apply to government. The government hadn't demonstrated the capacity to make a difference. AmFAR could be a catalyst for young researchers to try ideas. In the early years, every dollar we put into research germinated twenty-seven times that amount."[47]

It was almost six years to the day after Michael Gottlieb's first published report of mysterious cases of *pneumocystis* pneumonia among five gay men in Los Angeles that President Reagan finally spoke publicly about the AIDS epidemic. It was not surprising that he chose to do so at a May 31, 1987, AmFAR benefit dinner in Washington, because the presence of Elizabeth Taylor and other heterosexual actors and celebrities ensured that Reagan would feel at home. Of course the death of the president's friend and White House guest Rock Hudson two years earlier hadn't inspired him to speak about AIDS then, even as America shuddered with fear of the disease.

Reagan's call for "routine" HIV antibody testing of certain groups of people was booed by the $250-a-head AmFAR crowd in the tent that had been erected for his sideshow before the actual dinner. Meanwhile, outside the tent I marched and shouted with the hundreds of others who had come to protest Reagan's years of negligence on AIDS and draconian, politically motivated measures against unpopular groups. Stephen Beck, then director of the National Association of People with AIDS and an organizer of the protest, said, "People with money, let's call them the elite, can go to dinner and they can feel comfortable thinking about AIDS as an issue. What we're trying to demonstrate is that when we're talking about AIDS, we're talking about people." The people I was talking about as I marched in the protest that night were my friend Allen in New York, bedridden and blind from cytomegalovirus, and my then twenty-eight-year-old friend Gregg in Chicago, who had just learned he was HIV-positive and referred to himself as "damaged goods."[48]

The "power of one" inspired people and organizations to take action and contribute money. The power of many—and of their money—was amazing to witness. Unfortunately, the good will and generous donations couldn't keep the viral enemy at bay. What's more, the fallout of its assaults included the breakdown of good will between concerned people. Even in this war, "officers" too often pursued their own agendas, dividing the ranks and hindering the cause to make a point. Even in this war, American racial politics too often hindered the battle against AIDS.

*

One of the most insidious stereotypes about gay people is that they are all affluent and white. Of course no one can deny that the first people in this country to be afflicted by AIDS were the relatively affluent white gay men living in the gay ghettos of the large coastal cities in the seventies and early eighties. At the same time, though, no one can deny that those men also were the first to rally in response to AIDS by caring for the afflicted, raising money to provide services, and educating others about the disease. Unfortunately the public image of gay men has tended to focus less on their compassion and generosity in the epidemic than on the fiscal wherewithal of a small but highly visible segment of the community.

This image has worked against gay people at the highest levels of government by giving the impression—though of course people see what they choose to see, no matter how selectively incomplete the picture—that the gay community could take care of its own, without assistance from the federal government, despite the fact that gay people pay taxes to support the government, like other Americans. In fact, the Presidential Commission on the Human Immunodeficiency Virus Epidemic, created by President Reagan in 1987, observed that part of the reason for the government's failure to fund AIDS programs at a level commensurate with its own declaration of AIDS as the nation's top health priority was the belief that AIDS was limited to a well-organized, affluent segment of the population.[49] Even conservative Supreme Court Justice Antonin Scalia implied that gay people are all affluent—they "have high disposable income," he wrote—in his dissent from the court's 1996 decision striking down Colorado's antigay Amendment 2.[50]

To dispel the myth of universal gay wealth and skin tone, all you need to do is talk with people who provide AIDS services and health care in cities throughout the country. At AIDS Action Committee in Boston, for example, executive director Larry Kessler says, "We seldom get the yuppie gay man. It's more of a lower-class issue, poor white or black. It's more like the crowd you'd see in a soup kitchen. Someone with lots of insurance, a housemate, lover, or family, isn't likely to be at our Monday night dinner as they once were."[51] In Chicago, Howard Brown Memorial Health Center's clientele still are mostly gay. But director Eileen Dirkin says, "We see a lot of people come in here for primary care who are service workers—waiters, for example—who are amongst the working poor; they don't have health insurance."[52] And in Baltimore, Dr. Joe O'Neill said, "Amongst the maybe 20 to 30 percent of gay patients I have, most of them have been medically indigent, or have drug use problems—problems that aren't significantly different from anybody else living in a housing project or inadequate situations in the inner-city of Baltimore."[53]

The misguided perception of all gay people as wealthy and white has had major ramifications for the ways in which AIDS service organizations receive funding, whether from the federal government or private sources. Frank Pieri, chairman of Howard Brown's board at the time of our interview, said the city of Chicago's attitude toward gay organizations such as the health center, is that "they have more money and more resources, and they should support themselves—they shouldn't rely on city dollars." Increasingly, however, even the organizations that were founded by white gay men in the early years of the epidemic serve nonwhite, even nongay clients. But that hasn't necessarily translated into more funding to provide those services. Echoing remarks I have heard across the country, Pieri said, "For the most part, they are funding minority organizations, or organizations that are willing to go into the minority neighborhoods. And they're not funding what they perceive as gay white male institutions."[54]

Tim Sweeney, who for four years directed GMHC, the nation's largest and wealthiest AIDS service organization, said, "People have looked at the gay community and said 'You have access to private dollars.' But if and when those private dollars aren't there for the gay community, then what happens? Because they're not always there. And just because they're there in New York or San Francisco or Los Angeles doesn't mean they're going to be there in Omaha." He noted that the vast majority of gay Americans don't have access to organizations like GMHC that can pull in rich movie stars and classical musicians to do fundraisers. He added, "I get really uncomfortable with those broad generalizations that are based on a handful of organizations."[55]

Urvashi Vaid attributes the image of gay homogeneity and disposable income to surveys that have been conducted of the readers of gay and lesbian magazines—a typically more educated and affluent group of people—and the visibility of upper-middle-class gay people. Lorri L. Jean, executive director of the Gay and Lesbian Community Services Center in Los Angeles, the nation's largest and wealthiest gay social services organization, concurred with Vaid's assessment. "It worries me," she said, "when a lot of us claim that the gay community is wealthier, has a higher per-capita income—all those things—because I think they're only surveying a certain slice of our community. In fact many in our community are barely above the poverty level or below it, just workaday blue-collar folks."[56]

Again, to dispel the myth of universal gay wealth and skin tone, all one needs to do is talk with the Reverend Carl Bean, the black gay minister who founded the Minority AIDS Project. Based in the impoverished South Central area of Los Angeles, the project is the nation's largest AIDS service provider for African-Americans. Yet the agency has struggled for its life since its 1985 birth. A lack of interest by wealthy white gay people, the furtiveness of many black gay people, a shortage of wealthy, openly gay blacks willing to give money, and an ever-growing caseload have kept the Minority AIDS Project close to the edge. "We're still struggling," says Bean. "We struggle to pay payroll. We struggle to keep the doors open. We struggle to keep the pantry full. Most of the time it isn't full, and payroll is late, and we borrow from Peter to pay Paul."[57]

In many cities, including Los Angeles, the AIDS service organizations established by white gay men expanded as the epidemic expanded, providing services to any and all who needed them. At GMHC, the progenitor of all AIDS organizations, the drive to "be all things to all people" led to what Linda Campbell, the heterosexual African-American director of New York's Minority Task Force on AIDS, described to me as a kind of colonialism. Although nearly half of GMHC's clients today are not white, and the agency provides training on "multiculturalism" to staff, questions persist as to whether GMHC—or any one agency, for that matter—should be the preeminent agency to serve everyone affected by HIV and AIDS. Campbell noted that among AIDS service providers in New York, the expansion of GMHC to serve nonwhite, nongay communities "brings a lot of tensions for us that have more to do with issues of race and power in this country than they do with the fact that you're white and gay and I'm a heterosexual female."[58]

Black gay and AIDS activist George Bellinger, Jr., said, "You can't blame them completely," as he spoke of GMHC and other large AIDS groups founded by, and still perceived as "belonging to," white gay men despite racially mixed staffs and very high numbers of clients who are neither white nor gay. "You have to also blame the funding streams because they pick out the best proposals, and the evaluation of what looks the best. We fund them rather than the group that really knows the community and is struggling."[59]

In fact, the struggle faced by the newer AIDS organizations founded by and for people of color is similar to that of the older gay organizations in that a lack of experience in writing successful grant proposals has often hindered their ability to compete with their more seasoned counterparts in the gay community. In an example too familiar to minority-run AIDS organizations, it was at least partly because of a lack of staff capable of writing a highly technical grant application that IMPACT-D.C., a Washington, D.C., organization that provides services to black gay people with AIDS, missed its chance at a $130,000 federal contract in 1994, according to Keith Fabré, the group's deputy executive director.[60]

But this experience is not unique to AIDS organizations nor to people of color; in the early years of the epidemic, it was familiar to the agencies established in the white gay community as well. In an article I wrote for *10 Percent* magazine about the competition for funds between white gay and people-of-color AIDS groups, I quoted Bill Freeman, then director of the National Association of People with AIDS, as saying, "It's not correct to say that gay-identified organizations early on had capability; they didn't. They were always on the brink of going out of existence because of fear, prejudice, outright discrimination, and the constant challenge of fundraising. The minority community is now experiencing what the gay community experienced early on."[61]

To attribute the expansion of the so-called white gay organizations to nothing more than a kind of plantation paternalism is to grossly simplify the situation. There certainly has often been that sense that "We've been there, done that, and can either do it for you or show you how to do it our way." But at least as forceful in the groups' expansion was the pressure by funders—particularly the city, state, and federal governments—to require that the gay agencies serve everyone. Judith Johns, a former director of Howard Brown, and at the time of our interview the director of AIDS programs for the city of Chicago, said, "What we found in Chicago is that many of our agencies that historically were considered gay are no longer designating themselves as gay."[62] She said that as grants and contracts became available to provide services to nongay, nonwhite people, the gay-identified organizations went after them—at first because no one else wanted them, but then because they were able to write the strongest proposals.

But Johns failed to mention the role that the city's funding requirements played in forcing the gay groups to shift their focus. Frank Pieri explained it this way: "It's kind of odd," he said, "because here you're doing not-for-profit, significant work. Nobody denies that who you're serving needs the care; it's not like you're serving people who don't need it. But you're almost made to feel like you're doing something wrong because you're *not* all things to all people, or your mission is what your mission has always been. Howard Brown has never changed its mission from gay and lesbian health care." He added, "Minority groups and women and children need care; I don't deny that. What I'm saying is that I think the gay community has been lost in this. So many gay dollars are being donated to organizations that are losing touch with their gay and lesbian roots because the federal funding is not going there, the state funding is not going there, the city funding is not going there. You won't get it if you say we're just a gay and lesbian organization."[63]

While there have been tensions over money in cities throughout the country between the older gay AIDS organizations and the newer agencies serving people of color, a situation developed in Washington, D.C., during the summer of 1993 that was every bit as hot, sticky, and uncomfortable as the city's summertime weather—and took the competition to a whole new level. While AIDS ravaged the nation's capital (Washington has the highest per-capita incidence of AIDS in the U.S., particularly among blacks), the tensions between AIDS service providers reached a boiling point.

Those involved, or who wanted to be involved, in providing AIDS services battled one another with a fierceness that *Washington Post* columnist Richard Cohen said made the war in Bosnia "seem like TV's old Nelson family."[64] The opponents were black and white, and either openly or at least known to be (but denying they were) gay. Their weapons were crude but extremely hurtful: charges of racism, homophobia, and intimidation tactics that would rattle the steeliest nerves. The ostensible "prize" they were fighting for was a $2 million AIDS services contract funded by the federal government and channeled through the District's AIDS office.

The real issue dividing them, however, was the same as that in communities across the country: Who should provide AIDS services to the gay and bisexual men of color who account for such a disproportionately high percentage of the city and the country's AIDS cases. Should it be the "white gay" AIDS organization that had been providing services for years? Should the funding be used to buttress the fledgling AIDS program of a minority-run agency? Or should the money go towards creating a new AIDS organization altogether?

The bickering between the white and minority gay AIDS groups was not new. Whitman-Walker Clinic director Jim Graham said, "The [District's] first AIDS controversy was racial." He explained that when the District government in 1983 awarded its first AIDS contract, "We spent the summer of 1983 arguing whether the money should go to Whitman-Walker Clinic or to some undesignated black organization."[65] That first contract was for $17,500—pocket change compared to the millions now at stake. As the funding available for AIDS increased over the years, so did the decibel level of the arguments over who should get it. The only thing that plummeted in the city of escalating AIDS cases was the depths to which some would sink in trying to procure or protect their own slice of the AIDS funding pie.

When the AIDS epidemic began, Whitman-Walker had already been in existence for a decade. AIDS services were a natural extension of its work in the gay community. For its part, the city was only too happy to award its first contract—and many subsequent contracts— to the clinic. "Whitman-Walker took the city off the hook," said Jane Silver, who at the time of the first contract award in 1983 was the AIDS adviser to D.C.'s public health commission and later was the city's first AIDS chief. "We were trying to know what to do while the clinic was serving patients," she added.[66]

Between 1983 and 1993, Whitman-Walker had become the District's leading AIDS service provider by growing and expanding to meet the ever-increasing demands of the epidemic. While it started out as an essentially white gay organization, director Graham proudly pointed out that the clinic now was what is commonly called "multicultural." Gay white men now made up less than a third of its staff, which in 1993 numbered nearly two hundred, and its clients were more than two-thirds black and Hispanic. In 1992, Whitman-Walker opened a satellite clinic in Anacostia, an area of the city that is 96 percent black. And in the fall of 1993, it opened the Elizabeth Taylor Medical Center, to provide primary care services to people with HIV.

In 1993, the District government decided that, instead of automatically awarding the AIDS services contract to Whitman-Walker, as it had done for a decade, it would invite competitive bids. But the District's expectations were high after the tremendous return it had gotten on its investment in the clinic over the years. In fact, the requirements of the "soup-to-nuts" contract, as Graham described it, read like the clinic's own service directory: primary care, medical evaluations, STD treatment, on-site HIV antibody testing, case management, referrals for at least three thousand patient visits a year, dental and pharmacy services, legal services, and the training and supervision of at least fifteen hundred volunteers. Quite simply, no other organization in Washington, black or white, could match Whitman-Walker in terms of AIDS experience, ability to deliver the services required by the contract, and skill at writing grant-winning funding proposals. After all, none of them had the clinic's level of funding or years of building the kind of organizational infrastructure needed to support the level of services the city expected.

One organization emerged, however, represented by a belligerent and gay-baiting consulting group called URBAN (United Response to Black America's Needs), Inc. URBAN was formed by several black gay men to go after the $2 million contract after they left their jobs in Whitman-Walker's own grant-writing department, where they were privy to the clinic's funding information. URBAN's client, the Abundant Life Clinic, is run under the auspices of the Nation of Islam. Its director, Abdul-Alim Muhammad, is the Nation of Islam's "health minister" and a national spokesman for Louis Farrakhan, the controversial leader of the Black Muslim group known for his support for racial separatism, hateful views of whites, Jews, women, homosexuals—and his belief that AIDS is a "white plot" against the black race. The involvement of the Nation of Islam in the city's AIDS funding dispute gave the issue "a whole new spin," as Whitman-Walker's Graham so understatedly put it.

When the city awarded the Abundant Life Clinic only $213,000, about a quarter of the amount it had requested, URBAN went ballistic. The group's president fired off a vitriolic letter to the director of the city's human services department, which oversees its AIDS office, in which he claimed racial discrimination; demanded that the city's AIDS chief, Caitlin Ryan, be fired for what he claimed was her favoritism toward white gay groups, such as Whitman-Walker; and, for good measure, threatened to sic Louis Farrakhan on the District's then-mayor, a black woman. Courtland Milloy, a black *Washington Post* pundit, published a column about the situation that sent shock waves through the city's AIDS services community and further escalated the racial tension. In the column—later described as an "unfortunate event" by the *Post*'s ombudsman when it warranted an exceptionally long follow-up correction[67] and a two-part critique because of its many lapses in both fact and logic[68]—Milloy characterized Ryan as "a fierce lesbian warrior" who had turned the city's AIDS office over to a "loyal gay cabal."[69]

In her own defense, Ryan told me that during her two years as D.C.'s AIDS chief, she had overseen a 93 percent increase in Ryan White CARE Act funding to minority-operated organizations—as well as a 542 percent increase to nonminority organizations, including Whitman-Walker, that served between 70 to 99 percent minority clients. She pointed out that, in view of the District's black majority population, "It is important to realize that in a city like this, most public money goes to serve minorities," regardless of the real or perceived skin tone of the service agency's staff.[70]

In this superheated atmosphere, Ryan was eventually fired from her job. Once she was effectively out of the way, URBAN organized a new coalition of primarily black organizations to go after the $2 million contract when the city decided to repeat the bidding process. Called the "Sankofa" (after a Ghanian symbol representing the healing arts) Community Coalition of HIV/AIDS Services, the alliance included a number of the city's leading minority-run organizations. URBAN announced on behalf of the coalition that Abundant Life

Clinic would be its primary service provider. But newspaper head-lines in the *Washington Post* and *Washington Blade* betrayed the sharp disagreements among the city's black gay AIDS service providers over whether the clinic could effectively serve black gay men who repre-sented more than half the AIDS cases in D.C.'s black community, in view of the antigay views of the Nation of Islam.[71]

URBAN published bizarre editorials and letters to the editor in the *Washington Blade,* disavowing any connection to the gay commu-nity and beating the same drum of racial separatism for which Far-rakhan is known. In one, the group's "chief of staff"—who refused to answer my faxed questions and repeated telephone calls after agreeing to be interviewed—wrote, "We are not allies of . . . 'gay liberation' and don't claim the 'rainbow flag' as ours. We are mem-bers of a community with a history in this nation rooted in struggle against white injustice, racism, and oppression."[72] Trying to play the voguish game of out-victimizing other victims, URBAN was roundly condemned by both blacks and whites.

When the District government finally stopped its hand-wringing a year later, it awarded the AIDS services contract to Whitman-Walker Clinic after all.[73] While URBAN bitterly challenged the "le-gality" of the contracting process, others in the black gay community recognized the need for conciliation and cooperation between blacks and whites. Carlene Cheatam, cochair of the D.C. Coalition of Black Lesbians, Gay Men, and Bisexuals, said, "We have confidence the clinic, in receiving the award, will do its share of serving African-Americans who are affected by the disease."[74]

Even apart from the challenges of grant-writing and competition for funding with more experienced gay AIDS organizations, black AIDS groups have had a hard time generally in raising money among African-Americans. In a 1995 *New York Times* article, Minority Task Force on AIDS director Linda Campbell was quoted as saying, "I don't have a single black major donor over $1,000. There are no David Geffens in the black community."[75] At least not among the black gay people who—as white gay people have done among whites—lead the African-American community's efforts on AIDS. Geffen had recently donated $1.5 million to God's Love We Deliver, the New York agency that provides meals to homebound people with AIDS, and $2.5 million to GMHC.

As a result, the Task Force, like other minority-run AIDS organizations, was forced to rely on government funding for the bulk of its annual budget—which, as Dennis Altman warns in his book about community-based responses to AIDS throughout the world, is a precarious position to be in because of the potential for pressure to compromise the organization's identity. "It is necessary to be cautious about the embrace of the state," writes Altman, "like that of the cobra, it can be fatal."[76] At the 1995 Gay Men of Color AIDS Summit, held in San Francisco, groups representing African-American, Latino, Native American, and Asian/Pacific Islander gay people resolved that organizations that are run by or serve gay men of color "must diversify their funding base to ensure program flexibility and continued viability."[77]

Describing the black community's hesitant response to AIDS, Campbell said, "We're still at war with ourselves about AIDS in a way. What we see in the epidemic—like the drug use—reminds us of all the evils that have torn us apart. It's not what we imagine ourselves to be in this country. I've been told blacks give our money to other things: churches, black colleges, fraternal organizations." Keith Cylar, the codirector of Housing Works, a Manhattan agency founded by ACT UP members to house people with AIDS, said he was having better luck raising money from blacks than the Task Force, but not much better. "It's kind of like a lot of black families have a cousin who is a drug addict, but you don't embrace him," he said. "And if I'm going to write a check to a cause, does it go to something that might kill me in ten years like AIDS, or to stopping stray bullets?"[78]

Such a question goes to the heart of much deeper racial and socioeconomic problems that are well beyond the ability of AIDS service organizations to solve and this book to discuss. But the effect of tensions that stem from those problems in distracting, even derailing, efforts to provide AIDS services to those who need them has been a constant source of strain for everyone involved. Clearly there are no easy answers. But as questions about racial attitudes are sorted out in the kinds of national "conversations" called for by President Clinton in 1997, other questions demand answering by AIDS service organizations and the for-profit businesses that have been established to raise money for them. The willingness (or lack of it) of AIDS fundraisers to account for the proceeds of their efforts has brought its own challenges to the continued viability—and credibility—of all AIDS organizations.

*

As the AIDS industry grew and became more professional because of funding from the Ryan White CARE Act, another industry grew up alongside it. From the earliest events organized by volunteers— the walkathons, dances, silent auctions, and so on—emerged for-profit companies run by entrepreneurial former volunteers whose business is raising money for AIDS. Just as AIDS service organizations dislike the suggestion that their self-perpetuation is at odds with their original mission of putting themselves out of business by ensuring that sensitive AIDS services are "mainstreamed," these well-paid pros respond angrily when asked to account for the money they spend on sometimes outrageous overhead costs. But like the AIDS service providers, their discomfort with being scrutinized by the gay community that has so generously funded AIDS services is necessary if they expect to have continued support.

During the 1994 "Stonewall 25" events commemorating the Stonewall uprising in New York City, the usually successful DIFFA lost $30,000 on a series of sixteen parties called "Out in New York '94" that it cosponsored with Broadway Cares/Equity Fights AIDS and *Out* magazine. The group had anticipated profits of $1 million. "There were just too many damn events," said DIFFA's director Rosemary Kuropat, who left the organization a year later. "I think our community perceives itself as sort of having an insatiable desire to party. There was too much going on."[79] To cope with the actual and projected losses, DIFFA laid off six employees, postponed salary increases, and sought voluntary pay cuts of up to 25 percent.[80]

AmFAR, by far the wealthiest national AIDS organization in the country, saw its budget shrink from a high of $24.8 million in fiscal 1993 to a fiscal 1996 budget of only $16 million. In a press release, AmFAR president Mervyn Silverman said, "It is becoming increasingly difficult to raise money for AIDS research programs because of growing complacency and a sense of resignation about the epidemic."[81]

When the AIDS Action Foundation, the financial muscle behind AIDS Action Council, the Washington, D.C., lobbying group, reported a drop of $342,000 in 1993 donations, then director Dan Bross told the *Washington Blade,* "People are getting tired and getting burned out on AIDS issues. We're thirteen years into the AIDS epidemic. What we're seeing from a lot of AIDS organizations is that it's increasingly difficult to raise money."[82]

What was happening? AIDS, which had gone from being the gay community's private burden to become a more than $1-billion-a-year publicly funded federal program and cause célèbre, was, once again, having trouble attracting private dollars. In an article about the challenges to gay and AIDS groups in raising money, *Outlines,* a Chicago gay community newspaper, noted that corporate givers are more interested in other social service programs than in AIDS. While foundations are often good sources for seed money to start a new project, they balk at paying the operating expenses of an established but still-struggling organization. High overhead costs eat up the profits of fundraising benefits. And finally, said the article, "Individual donors, long the lifeblood of gay and AIDS-related organizations, are feeling the tug of literally dozens of organizations vying for the attentions of their wallets."[83]

Therein lies the rub, says Michael Seltzer: There are far too many AIDS organizations vying for the same limited pot of private dollars. For him, the solution is "a large, broad-based national AIDS organization that represents all the voices of people affected by AIDS, and has the integrity of representing everyone affected as a large, visible force—just like Planned Parenthood or the Children's Defense Fund." He contrasted the multitude of organizations throughout the country providing some kind of AIDS services with the single organization associated with fighting another, earlier epidemic. "In the thirties," said Seltzer, "there were not all these multiple organizations concerned with polio; there was one national organization with local chapters. And guess what? They beat polio. Everyone in the U.S. knew that polio equaled the March of Dimes."[84]

A survey by the American Association of Fund Raising Counsel, Inc. (AAFRC) estimated that, in 1992, between $575 million to $850 million of privately raised money went to AIDS causes. This seemingly large amount of money pales in comparison to, say, the

$1.4 billion raised by the Salvation Army in 1995 alone. In the mid-nineties, a scandal in the national office of the United Way and other factors suppressed Americans' charitable impulses. Boston's *Bay Windows* noted, "Fundraising experts blame a range of causes: skepticism about waste and fraud in larger charities, uncertainty about the economy, and a 'compassion fatigue' that burned out potential donors. AIDS fundraisers say this burnout has a new, terrible dimension for them: Many of their strongest advocates and donors in the gay community have died. Others have given all they can."[85]

Still others had begun to question just where, exactly, the money they gave to help fund AIDS services is going. In 1995, *POZ* magazine published the first of its now-annual assessments of AIDS fundraising. What it revealed was jarring. Kiki Mason, a journalist who covered parties and served as a publicist and event planner for New York's Community Research Initiative on AIDS (Mason died of AIDS on June 19, 1996), noted in his hard-hitting article "Black Tie Lies" that the money-losing parties during Stonewall 25 were neither the first, and have hardly been the only, AIDS fundraising fiascos.

The *Los Angeles Times* reported on an AmFAR fashion show that cost $715,000 and raised $750,000—not exactly efficient fundraising. And despite its claims of fundraising efficiency, DIFFA was spending 50 percent of the money it received from events to produce them. In contrast, Broadway Cares spent only 8 percent of the nearly $2 million it raised in 1994 on event production. As Mason concluded, "AIDS service organizations have to make themselves responsible to the community. They must begin dissuading mounting fears by coming clean with their figures. If they have nothing to hide, they have nothing to fear."[86]

It wasn't, however, only the AIDS service organizations that needed to come clean and be held accountable. What Mason called a "shadow industry" has grown up to raise money exclusively for AIDS. Now even the AIDS walks are run by professionals. And the costs merely to produce the events are, in some cases, hundreds of thousands of dollars more than the early AIDS fundraisers ever made. Like AIDS services, fundraising for AIDS has become a big business. But for years few questioned the disposition of the money raised in the walks and dances and, more recently, in the AIDS rides. Those raising money for AIDS were seen as doing "God's work," and so, apparently, were accountable only to a heavenly authority. More earthly minded people, however, began to ask, "How much of the money I contribute actually goes to the AIDS service providers for which it is ostensibly raised? How much goes to cover the 'overhead' of producing the event and paying the salaries of the full-time staffs? Finally, how much of it lines the pockets of the for-profit producers of the event?"

Is it reasonable for Whitman-Walker Clinic to spend $450,000 to earn $2 million? That was what the clinic expected to spend on and earn from its 1996 AIDS walk. For the first time, Whitman-Walker had hired a group called Walk the Talk Productions, a Los Angeles-based firm run by AIDS walk organizer Richard Zeichik. Zeichik and former partner Craig Miller cofounded Miller, Zeichik and Associates, which produced the first AIDS walk in the city of Los Angeles in 1985. The agency has produced many subsequent walks in a number of other cities, including those in New York and San Francisco, two of the largest in the country. Whitman-Walker laid off two of its own staff to make way for Zeichik, who would be paid an "agency fee" of $65,000 for six months of full-time work. That's well over $10,000 a month simply to plan the AIDS walk that for the previous nine years had been organized by Whitman-Walker staff and volunteers.[87]

By 1996, the AIDS bike rides had become a full-fledged money-making industry in their own right, with rides not only from San Francisco to Los Angeles, but also from Boston to New York, Philadelphia to Washington, D.C., Minneapolis to Chicago, and Orlando to Miami. The rides were promoted by the makers of Tanqueray gin and vodka, whose rascally character, "Mr. Jenkins," touted both the rides and the liquor in clever print advertisements in magazines, aimed primarily at the gay community and young people.

Paid staff of the 1996 Philadelphia to Washington, D.C., AIDS Ride drummed up contributions by giving pep talks and showing a tear-jerking promotional video in the homes of people who had signed up to ride. The message repeatedly was to "give the riders the experience of their lives" by donating enough money—fairly large contributions were strongly encouraged. Underscoring the fact that the ride was more than just an effort to raise money for AIDS services by welcoming all who wanted to participate, each rider—as it were a proxy for the actual contributors—was required to raise at least $1,400 if they hoped to enjoy the "once-in-a-lifetime" experience offered by the AIDS ride. Riders in the San Francisco to Los Angeles ride had to generate $2,500 each.

In the Philly-to-D.C. ride, 1,901 riders raised a gross of $4.5 million. After the congratulations to the returning "heroes" who had ridden from Philadelphia to Washington, D.C., had died away, some of the participants and sponsoring organizations began to ask bottom-line questions about the efficiency of the ride's actual fundraising. In a letter to the editor in the *Washington Blade,* published shortly after the ride, a rider named James F. Smith wrote, "Of major concern to me and many other riders I spoke with was the production cost." He described the large paid staff, frequent mailings to the riders, and rented (as opposed to donated) vehicles to accompany the riders as examples of what seemed to add up to excessively large overhead expenses. Smith continued, "I am sure I will have several critics who will, as usual, scream about my questions, and argue that the event is totally justified and worthwhile at any cost. It is not. Cost containment is the first and primary goal to funnel the maximum cash to needy organizations."[88]

When figures were released after considerable delay by Pallotta and Associates, the for-profit company that organizes the AIDS rides, the AIDS organizations in Philadelphia were told they would share a total of $330,740 from the $1,661,173 raised by the Philadelphia contingent of 786 riders. This meant that seventy-nine cents of every dollar raised by the Philadelphians went to "overhead"—including $417,628 for staff salaries and another $180,000 in "production fees"—to cover Philadelphia's share alone. Washington fared somewhat better. Its 1,300 riders pulled in $3,034,840, of which $1,565,544 was eventually split between Whitman-Walker Clinic and Food and Friends, a meals program for people with AIDS. Still, this meant that for the D.C. contingent forty-eight cents of every dollar raised went to "expenses."[89] The organizations were grateful for the money, and praised the ride without qualification, giving no public indication that they were concerned about the high cost of raising it.

In April 1996, the Pennsylvania attorney general launched an investigation of the Philadelphia–D.C. AIDS Ride, when AIDS groups in Philadelphia feared that the cost to produce the ride would eat up a considerable portion of the money they raised.[90] After the ride, Dan Pallotta, founder of Pallotta and Associates, remained mysteriously "out of the country" and didn't return phone calls to concerned AIDS organizations and the media scrutinizing the situation. When the company finally released the figures, it did so with a volley of blame for the Philadelphia AIDS groups themselves. Pallotta said there were "too many" AIDS organizations in the city, "fighting with one another over the shrinking pie, instead of coming together to find solutions." What he failed to address, however, was why the "pie" itself had shrunk so drastically. An editorial in *Philadelphia Gay News* observed that the words "accountability and arrogance . . . come to mind" in reviewing Pallotta and Associates' preliminary figures. It concluded, "Maybe [Philadelphians] expect people and organizations to take responsibility for their actions. Maybe Philadelphia and the AIDS Ride are incompatible in that way."[91]

When all was said and done, the AIDS groups in Philadelphia had pulled out of the AIDS Ride for 1997. Within weeks, Pallotta and Associates were advertising a 1997 ride to begin in a then-undetermined site in central North Carolina and terminate in Washington. This time only the groups in Washington would benefit. "As a rider in the Washington, D.C. AIDS Ride Presented by Tanqueray, you can participate in the most successful AIDS fundraising effort in history," promised the ad for the reconfigured ride.[92] Of course it didn't reveal that overhead costs, to be borne by the D.C. groups alone, were expected to be even greater in 1997.[93]

As the 1997 AIDS rides got underway, the bad press continued to mount. In April, the Pennsylvania state attorney general concluded his yearlong investigation into the 1996 Philadelphia to Washington ride. Pallotta and Associates, together with three of the Philadelphia AIDS organizations that participated in the 1996 ride, were fined $134,000 for misleading the public over how much of the money raised from the Philadelphia portion of the ride would go to the charities as opposed to "overhead." The agreement reached between the attorney general and the organizations charged that the organizations had "misrepresented" to the public that they expected to earn a 60 percent profit margin for the event, even after "unforeseen circumstances" before the ride that they knew would make that kind of profit impossible. Under the settlement agreement, the three AIDS organizations each paid $8,000, and Pallotta and Associates paid $110,000. Attorney General D. Michael Fisher said his office would donate $112,000 of the fines to AIDS organizations—though not to the ones that paid the fines.[94]

An investigative article in a Minneapolis newspaper in July 1997—aptly titled "Taken for a Ride"—noted that seventeen hundred bicyclists were expected to ride in the second Twin Cities to Chicago AIDS Ride, raising more than $2 million. Yet public documents filed by the AIDS organizations that were to benefit from the ride indicated that a mere 31 percent, or $627,843, would actually reach the organizations after "expenses." After similar "expenses"— including $403,136 for salaries and commissions, and 16 percent of the money going toward ambiguous "other" costs—only 38 percent of the more than $2 million raised in the 1996 Twin Cities ride actually reached the AIDS service organizations. In contrast, Minnesota's Charities Review Council noted that the Minnesota AIDS Project's annual AIDS walk spent only 7 percent on overhead costs. A bikeathon sponsored by Habitat for Humanity typically spends 20 percent of its proceeds on overhead. A ride coordinator for Pallotta and Associates was quoted as saying that the "personal life-changing experiences" of participating in the rides made the AIDS rides unique. But Tom Sullivan, of Pro Events International, who organized the Habitat for Humanity ride and other biking-for-charity events in Minnesota and nationally, called the AIDS ride expenses "simply ludicrous."[95]

In Florida, six AIDS service organizations in 1997 severed their ties with Pallotta and Associates after receiving only eighteen cents of every dollar raised in the Florida AIDS Ride for two years in a row. The remaining eighty-two cents on the dollar went to "overhead." John Weatherbead, an official with CenterOne, a Fort Lauderdale AIDS organization involved with the ride, said the Florida groups were considering organizing their own bike benefit ride in 1998.[96] And in Philadelphia, plans were underway for "Ride for Hope," which organizers said wouldn't be as elaborately produced as the AIDS rides. "Everything will be very low-key and grassroots," said Nurit Shein, director of Philadelphia Community Health Alternatives, the sponsor of the event. "Expenses will be kept to a bare-bones minimum."[97]

Pallotta and Associates' "national director for logistics," Kevin Honeycutt, told the *Washington Post* that the company is forthright with AIDS organizations about the risks and benefits of being involved in the AIDS rides. "We come to an agreement with our client," he said, "about what is an achievable—sometimes aggressive but achievable—registration number and performance rate. We investigate what the market can pull, how much the incidence of HIV is in the market, and we look at how we can market the ride to recruit enough riders so it's a win-win for everyone." The *Post* noted—apparently this was meant to assuage critics of Pallotta and Associates—that "public records confirm that Pallotta, thirty-six, lives in a modest home and does not own an airplane, boat, or exotic car."[98]

The 1997 North Carolina to Washington AIDS Ride generated $3.8 million. Whitman-Walker Clinic and Food and Friends, the two D.C. groups to benefit from the ride, received about $1 million each. The remaining money—nearly $1.7 million, forty-four cents of each dollar raised—went to "overhead."[99] Just as the ride got underway, an AIDS service group in Raleigh, N.C., pulled out of plans for a 1998 ride and another group announced it would probably not be able to pay Pallotta and Associates' up-front $180,000 fee. A number of riders reported that they had difficulty getting contributions from people who were upset that so much of their contribution would be going to the ride's overhead costs.

Could anyone *really* be surprised? At a time when American charitable giving has been affected by scandals and embezzlement at mainstream philanthropies, why did AIDS ride organizers believe their particular effort was an exception? When they weren't coldly calculating about "markets" and "what is achievable," like Pallotta and Associates' Kevin Honeycut, they waxed rhapsodic about the public relations value and "life-changing experiences" of the rides. But they didn't seem to understand that even generous people expect accountability where their money is concerned. The days of giving money for AIDS services that winds up lining the pockets of those profiting off of AIDS were numbered. What about that $1 billion-plus in Ryan White CARE Act funding for AIDS services? It is paid for with our tax dollars—yet, as Larry Kramer always pointed out, we're still paying twice for AIDS services when we donate money. And now we're being asked to pay for hefty salaries and bonuses for profiteers. What about trying more cost-efficient means of fundraising than the special events, like the AIDS rides, that make some people feel good and other people rich? Surely not all those volunteers who used to organize the bikeathons and walkathons at minimal cost had become money-grubbers?

For years, AIDS organizations relied on what Paula Van Ness calls "black-tie bake sales," special events—the walks, the dance-a-thons, the fashion and drag shows, and now the AIDS rides—to raise substantial portions of their annual revenue. As the epidemic stretched on, though, they had to develop more fundraising savvy and turn to more traditional forms of fundraising, such as planned giving, estate bequests, marketing, and the cultivation of major donors who renew their pledges each year. Like many other nonprofits, they also had to learn to use direct marketing to target fundraising solicitations at individuals known by traits such as their spending habits and magazine subscriptions to be sympathetic to the AIDS cause.

Among gay and AIDS groups, *POZ* magazine publisher Sean Strub is looked to as a guru of direct mail fundraising because of his impressive success in making money for himself as well as a number of causes and organizations he supports. In 1996 alone, Strub anticipated gross earnings of $11 million from the four enterprises that comprise his Strubco. Drawing upon his "national community master file" of six hundred thousand names, Strub helped to raise $400,000 for GMHC from one fundraising appeal alone, and contributed heavily to ACT UP/New York's $1 million budget at the height of the protest group's short but dazzling life. But he was now feeling weary of the inefficiency and lack of accountability. As he put it, "In general, I'm kind of disillusioned with the institutionalization of the community organizations. Dollar for dollar, I don't think they're as effective today as they were ten years ago."[100]

Yet gay community dollars continue to flow into AIDS organizations and high-priced fundraising events like the AIDS rides. As the epidemic stretches into the foreseeable future, some in the community have begun to demand an accounting of how their contributions are being used—and who, exactly, is benefiting from them. It is an understatement to say that gay people have been extremely generous with their time, talents, and money in the interest of caring for people with HIV and AIDS.

But as the epidemic continues to move beyond the gay community, and as organizations that were created by gay people when AIDS was an overwhelmingly gay problem continue, rightfully, to serve all who are affected by the disease, the nagging of one question becomes louder with each fundraising event and direct mail solicitation: Why should gay people, estimated at most to be 10 percent of the population, underwrite the costs of AIDS services for everyone? Certainly the AIDS service organizations originally founded by and for gay men have gone far beyond the call of duty by serving many others affected by AIDS. But should gay community money continue to pay for services for nongay people? And, at a minimum, aren't there more efficient ways of raising money than, say, an AIDS ride that consumes as much as 82 percent of the money raised, as it did in Florida?

Michael Seltzer says, "The story that hasn't been told about our community is that the philanthropic, charitable response of our own people has been overwhelming." He adds, however, "We, our lesbian and gay community, have carried this responsibility almost single-handedly—the entire burden of addressing *the* major health threat of the last part of the twentieth century worldwide. We can't do it alone anymore."[101]

"Alone" is precisely how gay people have had to face the AIDS crisis too much of the time. "Alone" is never so solitary a state as it is in facing death. Behind the appeals for money and support, behind the politics and posturing—behind everything gay people have done in response to AIDS—there is the death. Gay people have been so extraordinarily charitable because they have been hit so extraordinarily hard by the massive numbers of gay men who have died from "complications associated with AIDS." More than anything else, gay America has come of age by being forced to confront mortality, by being cruelly disabused of the illusion that sustains Americans who foolishly believe their diets, pills, plastic surgeries, and transplants will somehow keep the Grim Reaper at bay. Oddly, in confronting death at such a young age, gay people have learned the "secret" of living that most people don't learn, if ever, until old age. What an expensive gift.

IN MEMORIAM

Here pause: these graves are all too young as yet
To have outgrown the sorrow which consign'd
Its charge to each . . .

PERCY BYSSHE SHELLEY, *ADONAIS*

Gay people have been devastated by the AIDS epidemic. Fortunately, not even all the death and destruction to our community could obliterate our gay spirit that has helped us and our forebears throughout history to survive regular attacks of one kind or another. Yet many gay people struggled to believe that their losses mattered, that their grief was as real and every bit as significant as that of nongay people. The politics of mourning were as volatile in the gay community as the politics of AIDS were in Washington. Refusing to accept the social message that their lives and loves somehow didn't matter, gay people insisted that their losses would indeed count. With creativity, humor, and a great deal of pain, gay people confronted the nation with the fact that we were suffering—and it didn't seem to care. Our mourning often turned to militancy as we raged against the darkness—and against those who hid in the dark from what was happening in their beloved America.

On Friday the thirteenth of March 1987—the morning after ACT UP was officially created in a meeting at New York's Gay and Lesbian Community Center[1]—the *Wall Street Journal* reported on page one, "AIDS has been cruel to Greenwich Village and its homosexuals."[2] The Village was being devastated by AIDS. The *Journal* noted that at least seven hundred of the more than nine thousand AIDS cases in New York at that point were reported among the Village's estimated eighteen thousand homosexuals. One of every twenty-five gay men in the Village was living with or had already died of AIDS. Life continued in the Village. "But," noted the *Journal*, "more young men these days get around with the help of canes or walkers. Wartime metaphors spring to people's lips. And the keeping of lists has become a grotesque commonplace."

Police officials reported that weekend pedestrian traffic on Christopher Street—the street that gave birth to and symbolized Gay Liberation—had dropped as much as 40 percent. Rob Kilgallen, owner of a candle shop on the street, said that because of the withering of the street's life he now closed shop at eight rather than ten or eleven as he used to do. He noted that on the same street the owners of a flower shop, card shop, and a store selling movie memorabilia had already died. And at least three gay bars in the Village had closed for lack of business.

While AIDS laid siege to the Village and other gay communities around the nation that March, the Reagan administration announced that it was finally forming a commission to look into the disease that by then had grown to 51,000 cases in 113 countries—six years into the epidemic.[3] AZT was reported that month to halt the spread of the virus in the body. And on the last day of the month, polio vaccine inventor Jonas Salk successfully mediated a settlement in the rancorous debate between the French and Americans over who actually discovered the AIDS virus. One of the biggest steps forward in the nation's halting response to AIDS also was made that month in the Supreme Court's decision in *School Board of Nassau County v. Gene H. Arline.* The court ruled that someone with a contagious disease—school teacher Arline had recurring tuberculosis—is considered "handicapped" under federal antidiscrimination laws. Urvashi Vaid, then the media director for the National Gay and Lesbian Task Force, said, "Now people with AIDS will have a leg to stand on."[4]

In San Francisco that spring, Cleve Jones and a group of strangers met in the Castro district to discuss their idea for creating a memorial quilt, a huge patchwork whose individual three-by-six-foot panels would commemorate those who had succumbed to AIDS. Jones says,

"We wanted to illustrate the enormity of the AIDS crisis by revealing something of the lives behind the statistics, to provide evidence of the calamity that we saw unfolding."[5] The Castro at the time was shrouded in gloom thick as the city's famous fog. Men speak today of the "dark years" in the mid-eighties, when so many gay-owned businesses in the Castro closed—sometimes because the owner had died; other times because the clientele were dead. Thousands would gather for candlelight vigils, then quickly disperse afterward, retreating to the safety of home. The hilarity that had sparkled in the air and sparked the westward migrations of gay men to the city in the seventies had given way to a stunned, mournful silence.

In an op-ed article in the *New York Times* published on Christmas Eve 1994, San Francisco novelist Fenton Johnson captured the shattering losses he and other gay men had suffered, as well as their attempts to make some kind of sense of so much senseless destruction of their lives and community. "The intertwining of death and life is something I have been given much cause to contemplate across a decade of helping friends greet their deaths," he wrote.[6] A 1994 report by the San Francisco public health department predicted that by 1997, more than 26,700 AIDS cases would have been diagnosed in San Francisco, mostly among gay and bisexual men. An additional 18,000 gay men would be infected with HIV, though not yet diagnosed with AIDS. All told, the first sixteen years of the epidemic would find 45,000 residents infected with HIV, diagnosed with or dead from AIDS—nearly two-thirds of the estimated 75,000 gay men in San Francisco at the start of the epidemic.[7]

Considering these numbers, it seemed nothing short of astounding when the *San Francisco Examiner* noted in a page 1 story that AIDS no longer ranked among the nation's urgent worries.[8] Then again, a local right-wing "shock jock" in San Francisco—one of the world's hardest-hit cities, and the city famous for its compassionate handling of the AIDS crisis—was still calling for the quarantine of people with AIDS.[9] In some ways it seemed the only thing that had really changed from the early years of the epidemic was the now-huge numbers of deaths. Since the earliest calls like that of this troglodyte, nearly 15,000 San Franciscans had died of AIDS—almost all of them gay men.

As we sat outdoors on the last night of January at the Castro area's Café Flore, Johnson offered a poignant image from his own life that provided a glimpse of what life is like now for so many in the city by the bay—and far beyond. Strains of "Where the Boys Are" drifted across the cool night air from a nearby bar. In a Kentucky-accented voice as resonant as his prose, he told me, "No one I knew in San Francisco around 1978 to 1980 is alive. That was when I first came to the city, and first came out." Although not HIV-positive himself, Johnson gave voice to the speechlessness of the horrors we all have witnessed. He described men who had renovated houses in the city's worst neighborhoods, just for the experience. "It was immaterial to them whether the house had any value ten years from now because they're not thinking in terms of ten years from now." Not only was it painful to witness, but it shook up one's personal moral categories. Johnson explained, "You talk about lessons and grace and words like that, then you come face to face with someone who is talented and handsome and sweet and charming and intelligent and clearly a wonderful force in society and you learn they're grappling with this terrible thing. It really challenges your ability, our ability, to find things like grace and lessons and joy—those necessary facts of life."[10]

"April is the cruelest month," wrote T. S. Eliot in *The Wasteland,* "breeding/lilacs out of the dead land, mixing/memory and desire, stirring/dull roots with spring rain." The cruelest month in 1994 claimed the life of my own ex-lover, friend, and influential AIDS lobbyist Bill Bailey. It also claimed the life of John Preston, a former editor of the *Advocate* and a prolific author. In an anthology of reflections on AIDS that Preston had edited, he captured in one sentence the shock, bewilderment, and bereavement that had descended upon America's gay communities by the late eighties. Describing his reaction to the unexpected news of the death of one of his own first loves, Preston wrote, "Now he was gone, and it wasn't just that he was gone, but that all these men I loved were dead and their connection with me was left hanging in the air, their spirits unresolved, the possibilities left unrealized."[11]

Eric Rofes says the gay community has become a "death-saturated culture." He notes that most gay men, when asked about the impact of the epidemic on their lives, naturally respond by counting the number of friends and lovers they've lost. But their losses go to the very depths of their being as gay men. As Rofes sees it, "[F]or many gay men, the epidemic has mutilated our identities, profoundly warping sexuality and intimate relations, and reaffirmed bigoted subconscious linkages between homosexuality and contagion."[12] The loss of life the community has suffered is staggering. But how do you measure the loss of so much joy and affirmation and possibility that were among the legacies of Stonewall?

"In modern times, no other single constituency has lost so many as a result of epidemic illness," observes English writer Simon Watney. "Outside of wartime or great famine, mortal illness and death on this scale is unknown, marking our experience as unique."[13] Of course the experience of suffering and loss is not unique to gay people. But in terms of the sheer volume of sickness and death—of mostly young people—the experience of gay Americans is unprecedented, particularly in an age when we thought medical science had virtually conquered infectious disease. As Sandra Jacoby Klein, a therapist in Los Angeles who has worked with bereaved gay men since the early eighties and is the author of *Heavenly Hurts: Surviving AIDS-Related Deaths and Losses,* has put it, "There is simply no equivalent to this experience in the nongay community."[14]

Besides the loss of life itself, the deaths from AIDS of gay and other men have taken a statistical toll. The *New York Times* reports that "despite two world wars, the Depression and epidemics, nothing in this century has affected the life expectancy for New Yorkers as greatly as AIDS." The city's cumulative 81,500 AIDS cases at the time of the article's 1996 publication—80 percent of them among males—have compressed the average life expectancy of males born in New York City, even as the average life expectancy for women in the city continues to rise. Just behind the city's leading killers, heart disease and cancer (whose rates declined between 1980 and 1990), AIDS "has become so pervasive in New York City that it is affecting the statistical chance of babies and men under forty to make it to old age, because AIDS mostly kills men in their thirties, while the other diseases kill older men." In a grim twist on New York's penchant for starting national trends, the *Times* noted that similar trends were likely in other cities where those most affected by AIDS tend to live.[15]

Psychologist and epidemiologist John Newmeyer, who has

worked with AIDS since late 1982 at San Francisco's Haight-Ashbury Free Clinic, offers a sobering assessment of the impact of AIDS on gay people and on America. Because AIDS mostly affects young people, he said, the years of potential life lost far surpass those lost to the nation's other leading causes of death, which mostly afflict older people. He explained that if a man dies at thirty-five who would otherwise live to seventy, thirty-five years of life are lost. Said Newmeyer, "When the cancer people say we have four hundred thousand people dying of cancer a year and AIDS kills only eight thousand a year, that doesn't account for years lost. Added up over all the gay men who've lost their lives to AIDS, the number is staggering."[16]

Andrew Sullivan, the openly gay and HIV-positive former editor of the *New Republic,* has said that for gay people, "Death is less an event than an environment."[17] The toll of living in what has seemed to many gay men in the nation's cities like a battlefield on which they witness the protracted and brutal deaths of so many of their young comrades has scarred them for life. One of the first articles ever to assess the psychological impact of AIDS upon gay men said that it was "omnipresent and profound."[18] That was hundreds of thousands of deaths ago.

While preparing a sermon to commemorate the bombing of Hiroshima, Chris Glaser was struck by the parallels between the ways that the city's survivors coped with their horrific devastation and the gay community's coping with AIDS. Acknowledging the obvious differences between the two disasters, Glaser also pointed out the truly striking similarities. Survivors of the atomic blast felt as though "the whole world is dying," noted Glaser. "As gay men, our encounter with death from AIDS seems endless," he said. He likened the lingering threat of invisible contamination from radiation to the long incubation period of HIV in the body, "which may strike at any time."

Describing the way Hiroshima's survivors would continue to associate any kind of physical ailment with the atomic bomb, Glaser said, "The similarity to the experience of gay males is stunning. If we feel fatigued, experience any ailment from a cold or flu to an infection, our thoughts immediately turn to AIDS and death." Finally, he observed that the atomic blast survivors are stigmatized as "a tainted group" because of a lifelong identification with death and dying. Even worse, they questioned their own right to live "because of an unconscious perception of balance which supposes one's survival has been made possible by others' deaths."[19]

This "survivor guilt" is widespread among gay men, particularly those who are not infected with HIV. There is a feeling that one somehow doesn't deserve to live when so many good and wonderful others "who did the same things I did" have not survived. To ameliorate this guilt, many gay men get involved with gay or AIDS organizations.[20] Many others downplay their feelings, devalue the importance of their personal losses, and try to carry on as though they really don't feel that their heart has been wrenched out of their chest and an aching wound left in its place.

What's more, there has been something of a conspiracy of silence among many gay people who have experienced the most loss, a hesitation to speak about their losses, even among themselves, because they don't want to remind those living with HIV that, barring a stunning breakthrough in medical research, they too are likely to join those who are mourned. Walt Odets writes in *In the Shadow of the Epidemic*, "[I]f a man feels guilt or unworthiness for having had the good fortune to survive when another has not or will not, he will find it very difficult even to recognize his own distress and almost impossible to talk about it."[21]

Before the wider use of the HIV antibody test in the late eighties and nineties, all gay men were told by AIDS educators to presume they were infected. But the ability to know whether or not one is infected has had profound implications for the ways that gay men experience "survival" and bereavement, as demonstrated in a study by Columbia University researchers John Martin and Laura Dean.[22] They found that the psychological impact of AIDS-related losses is diminishing among gay men who survived the first decade of the AIDS epidemic. They pointed out, however, that this may be due to the fact that all gay men are becoming habituated to the experience of AIDS-related loss. That is to say the deaths of young men have become so commonplace as to make this inversion of the natural order seem "normal."

Men who are infected still experience great psychological distress as they witness the disease and deaths of others like themselves; they know the chances are high that they will experience a similar fate.

Men who are not infected, on the other hand, are distressed as well; they may have depression and traumatic stress, use sedatives, and even think about suicide. But their distress is less acute nowadays because they don't see their friend or lover's death as a portent of their own.

Some HIV-positive activists have protested that HIV-negative men shouldn't complain about the psychological burden they bear. No matter how heavy it may be, they say, it's still not the same as the utterly shattering impact of being infected with HIV. Atlanta physician Stosh Ostrow speaks frankly about living with HIV and about his belief that those who are not infected cannot fully understand what it's like. "Those of us who live in the shadow of the epidemic have a whole different perspective on life," says Ostrow. "HIV negative gay men don't have a clue what it's like, nor am I capable of explaining what it's like to live with HIV." Like many gay men with HIV, Ostrow said that living with the virus "made me become conscious." He speaks of "living each day as a gift," adding that for most people, "life, longevity, is an illusion."[23]

Apart from the indisputable difference between having and not having HIV infection, though, the line dividing the experiences of loss and sorrow of gay men who are and are not infected is a bit less distinct than the activists' hostile denunciations of what they call "viral apartheid" would make it. As Eric Rofes puts it, "We love to talk about 'viral apartheid,' but in daily life positive and negative are involved with one another."[24] Still, Rofes, like other uninfected men with whom I've spoken, is offended by the efforts of some to challenge the emotional impact of the epidemic on the lives of gay men who happen not to be infected with HIV. "What galls me about this," he said, "what I find remarkable about this, is no one talked to survivors of Nazi death camps and said, 'Well, you're a survivor, you have no problems, what are you complaining about.' No one talked to survivors of the dropping of the bomb on Hiroshima and said, 'You're one of the ones who lived, not one of the hundred thousand who died, what are you complaining about.'"[25]

Many remark that they feel much older than their years. In an essay called "Friends Gone with the Wind," Arnie Kantrowitz observed, "We are aging before our time. When we meet old friends in the street, we remember to be glad they are still with us. Our conversation sounds like my grandfather's did when he was in his eighties."[26] One of the most arresting illustrations of this sense of premature aging and bereavement is in a poem by Michael Lassell called "Pietà":

> A man who is ill
> visits his mother
> in her nursing home.
>
> You don't look well, she says.
> Neither do you, he says.
>
> My friends are all dying, she says
> My friends are dying, too.
>
> I'm afraid that when I die
> there will be no one left to
> say prayers at my grave, she says.
> It's my fear, too, he replies.
>
> And they sit and weep,
> each dropping tears onto
> the hands of the other,
> waiting for the after
> that follows hard
> the heels of time.[27]

For gay people in America today, "imminent loss is to our time what industrial optimism was to the times of out parents and grandparents," as *Angels in America* author Tony Kushner puts it.[28]

Still, many are afraid to really feel and express their losses. As Eric Rofes puts it, "We fear that if we open up, we'll never stop crying."[29] A gay man who shares his stories with others, who actually describes what he has witnessed and felt, risks admitting his sense of impotence in the face of an overwhelming disaster like AIDS. He risks having to let down the guard with which he's had to protect his emotions simply to survive. Fortunately, many gay men realize they must take these risks if they are *truly* going to survive. Again, Rofes: "By underplaying or denying the full range of impact of the epidemic and its power to transfigure emotions, memories, and psyches, the souls of gay men are kept locked in a perpetual winter."[30]

If gay people have downplayed their losses because they are so overpowering, nongay people too often have downplayed the gay community's losses because they have refused to recognize the humanity they share with homosexual people. Even so, homophobia alone doesn't account for the disdain and neglect shown to gay people with AIDS and their survivors; what does account for it is a fear of death that pervades American culture. To acknowledge that so many have died at such youthful ages of a disease that science to now has been unable to cure carries an expensive cost: you must surrender your denial that you will eventually die. As John Snow, an Episcopalian priest and professor of pastoral theology at the Episcopal Divinity School, put it, "Is it any wonder that AIDS has brought such a mixed and confused and at times almost insane response from our society? A society that thought it might have death on the run has discovered or uncovered what we suspected all along and tried so hard to deny. We have discovered that human beings are irretrievably mortal."[31]

Many heterosexuals have long associated homosexuality with death, at least partly because the traditional absence of children in many gay people's lives affronted the belief that one achieves a kind of vicarious immortality through children.[32] Jeff Nunokawa writes that even before the AIDS epidemic American culture regarded homosexuals as "marked men," doomed because of their homosexuality to early death. Despite worldwide evidence to the contrary, he notes that in the eyes of many, gay men with AIDS are "not only people with AIDS but *the* people with AIDS." The connection between AIDS and gay men, he adds, "encourages our culture's sometimes lethal distaste for, and anxiety about, homosexuality."[33]

Ben Schatz eloquently describes the tenuous place of gay men in an American society bent on denying their humanity and ignoring AIDS. "I sometimes feel like gay men are dangling by their fingers from the edges of a roof," he says, "and every minute or so you can look over at the man next to you just in time to see him let go and drop. But up on top of the roof, the rest of the country is having a cocktail party—and except for those people who are walking around stepping on our fingers, they're not even aware we're hanging there. Yet man after man lets go and falls, and you're dangling there and thinking, 'Can I really hang on? How long can I hang on? This seems impossible.' And man after man loses his grip and falls to his death, and up above you hear ice tinkling in the glasses, but the pile of bodies down below is just getting higher and higher."[34]

Nongay America relegated the massive deaths of gay men in the AIDS epidemic to the sidelines of its collective consciousness by discounting the lives of those who, in this country, still constitute the largest share of the epidemic's victims. For many, AIDS offered a return to the debunked view that homosexuality is a "disease," and that homosexuals, somehow other than full human beings, actually have their "own" diseases.

In a powerful collection of photographs of 302 people who had died during one year of the AIDS epidemic—a fraction of the estimated 4,000 who actually died during that time—*Newsweek* in August 1987 noted, "Some commentators have found a degree of comfort in the statistics, as if AIDS had been satisfactorily contained in an alien population. It has not been; it has struck to the quick of American life." The magazine continued, "Each face in the album stands for a life cut short too soon; each represents a death in the American family."[35] We are then presented with twelve pages of snapshots. The overwhelming majority of the photos are of young men, and we are led to assume, through veiled references to their personality or work, that they are gay. Below the photos of the fifteen women and two children pictured in the collection—one of them for every eighteen men—are explanations of how they became infected with HIV. We have little choice but to conclude that the men pictured without such explanations contracted AIDS merely by being gay, that AIDS is a "normal" end of a gay life.

Even in its admirable attempt to show "the face of AIDS," *Newsweek* perpetuated the myths that comfort heterosexual Americans: that gay people are somehow different from "normal" human beings, and that AIDS is a "gay" disease that afflicts only sexual deviants and drug addicts (and their unfortunate offspring). But even nongay people who contract AIDS aren't allowed to be really "innocent": the caption beneath one woman's photo actually says, "She was a drug addict." This is presumably *Newsweek*'s version of a sympathetic epitaph. As Cindy Patton has put it, "[T]he huge stigma of contracting HIV continued to make every individual person living with the virus suspect of having 'done something wrong.' "[36]

The American family, as *Newsweek* represented it, seems clearly to have its favorite members as well as those whose "private" behaviors and sorrows must be kept out of sight (and out of mind) lest they reveal the family not to be nearly as loving as it would prefer to see itself. By dying so young and in such vast numbers and of such a horrific, incurable disease, gay men have audaciously pulled the mask off the mysterious guest at the nation's party, revealing that in fact Death has been among us even as we believed ourselves safe.[37]

*

John had passed in and out of lucidity since being admitted to George Washington University Hospital the day before. Pain shook his frail body one moment, morphine appeased it the next. His mother, father, and brother were down from Baltimore and would stay to the end—which would come in a matter of hours, the nurse said. Manny waited with John. For three years he knew this moment would come. Now this was it. Goodbye. Nine years of togetherness was ending in this hospital room. John, his thirty-nine-year-old lover, was dying of AIDS.

John was never a "patient," Manny said. He demanded nothing. In fact, Manny worried that one morning he would wake up to find that John had died in bed next to him, not wanting to disturb his sleep. But on John's last morning—the morning after Gay Pride Day—he called Manny's name over and over again. Manny had left the hospital at two, seeking much-needed rest. "Manny will be here soon," John's mother assured him. Manny returned at seven. The nurse gave John another shot of morphine to soothe the now-incessant pain. They called in a priest from nearby St. Stephen Martyr. John's mother sat at the foot of her son's bed, quietly saying her rosary. Manny held John's hand.

A final gasp and he was gone. It was over now for John. And just beginning for Manny. Manny was single again. And not just a single man but a man whose lover had died of AIDS—which, even in the frightened gay community, stigmatized him by association. Manny would still attend Dignity, the weekly gay Catholic masses where he and John had met and sung in the folk group. The next Sunday, Dignity would offer a memorial service for John, the one

John had planned for himself in such detail. John's parents would come. His friends would turn out in number to pay their last respects to the former seminarian, the man who had led them as Dignity's president, who in loyalty to his church had taken a lesser job with the National Catholic Conference rather than leave altogether when they learned he was gay and wanted him out. The service was simple, a folk mass. John's favorite homilist spoke, his favorite songs were sung. "That made it easier," said Manny. "It wrapped up the whole week."

Manny hadn't cried in the three months between the time of the memorial service and our interview, although he said there were teary moments. Mostly he wondered what grieving is. Is it being sad? Crying? Feeling helpless? Is it anger? "I've read a book on coping," he said. "But I don't even know what I'm supposed to be coping with." Back home in the Philippines, Manny said there are traditions surrounding a spouse's death. There is the novena, the nine days of prayer. On the ninth day there's a big party to celebrate the dead person's passing. Then there's a whole year of formal mourning to be observed. But Manny wasn't sure whether this applied to his mourning John's passing. After all, John hadn't *really* been his spouse, had he?[38]

When I wrote about Manny and John, in 1986, there was precious little information in the psychological literature about the bereavement of gay men. Laura Dean, director of the AIDS Research Unit of Columbia University's School of Public Health, recalls that one of the first papers she and her research partner John Martin (Martin himself died of AIDS in 1992) wrote on bereaved gay men was rejected by a journal. She told me, "One of the reviewers said, 'This is ridiculous, why would you expect a gay man to grieve over a lover?'"[39]

Before AIDS, though, even gay men didn't think about their partners' deaths. Nor, for that matter, did they think much about death in general. Like their fellow Americans, gay men simply didn't want to think of death as anything more than a vague abstraction, something that would take place in a far-off old age—a time that, for young gay men, was like a netherworld somewhere beyond their "real" lives. In 1981, the first year of the epidemic, psychiatrist and *The Joy of Gay Sex* coauthor Charles Silverstein published

Man to Man, the first book devoted to the subject of gay male love-relationships. He noted how gay men in the pre-AIDS years were at least as resistant to confronting their mortality as were their nongay counterparts. "Gay men don't die," he wrote. "The word 'death' never appears in gay newspapers or magazines unless it is related to the assassination of a civil rights leader. Fashionable bodies, lately adorned with beards and a narrow piece of studded leather around the wrist, fill the slick magazines that fuel our ever-present fantasies of seduction and sex. No room for death here."[40]

Although widespread death became a harsh fact of life for gay men in the eighties and nineties, death at a young age is still considered an "off-time event," because one ordinarily expects to confront it only in old age. But AIDS altered many of our expectations as it became the leading cause of death among twenty-five to forty-four-year-old Americans.[41] The AIDS epidemic reversed the natural order of life as the old buried the young and the young buried one another. Still another bizarre twist with AIDS was that a surviving partner himself was often infected with HIV, something that rarely happens with other life-threatening diseases.

In the decade-plus since I wrote about Manny's uncertainty of how to mourn his lover's death, somewhat more attention has been paid to the bereavement of gay men who have lost partners to AIDS. Unfortunately, Manny could not benefit from whatever comfort the new information might offer because within five years after our interview he, and virtually every other man I interviewed for the article, was dead from AIDS.

Despite the increased interest of researchers in the bereavement of surviving partners, the greatest single issue with which gay men must grapple is the same today as it has always been: the lack of recognition of their love relationship with the dead man. The efforts to gain such recognition are the very cornerstones of the gay rights movement, says Ginny Apuzzo. "We still fight for the right to love," she told me. "The one thing that we are told we can't do is the thing that makes us most human—that is, to love. You can't grieve what you didn't love. You can't be in this much pain and not have had love. How can you be a widower and not have had a spouse? How can you bury the single most important person to you, with whom you've lived for x-number of years, and not have had a relationship? What the hell was it?"[42]

The absence of society's approval—and especially the overwhelming disapproval—of gay relationships has led some gay men to disavow their partners at the moment of their greatest need. Telling themselves "it wasn't *really* a marriage anyway," some abandoned the man they professed to love because they were unable to confront the horrors of an AIDS death; or because they didn't have the fortitude to confront the internalized homophobia they have turned against themselves and their relationships. Gerald Soucy, then a mental health consultant at Chicago's Howard Brown Health Center, told me in 1986, "In order to avoid dealing with grieving, the hole, the emptiness left by death, you minimize to yourself the amount of intimacy that was in the relationship. You try to minimize the gap left in your life."[43] You convince yourself that even your own feelings of love are suspect and somehow inferior to those of a heterosexual spouse, so it's okay to leave—after all, you're not legally bound to stay.

Tony Kushner captured this self-hatred and abandonment in the character of Louis, who deserts his boyfriend Prior Walter, the central character in *Angels in America*, who has AIDS:

> LOUIS: Rabbi, what does the Holy Writ say about someone who abandons someone he loves at a time of great need?
>
> RABBI ISIDOR CHEMELWITZ: Why would a person do such a thing?
>
> LOUIS: Because he has to . . . maybe that person can't, um, incorporate sickness into his sense of how things are supposed to go. Maybe vomit . . . and sores and disease . . . really frighten him, maybe . . . he isn't so good with death.
>
> RABBI ISIDOR CHEMELWITZ: The Holy Scriptures have nothing to say about such a person.
>
> LOUIS: Rabbi, I'm afraid of the crimes I may commit.

Louis eventually attempts, unsuccessfully, to return to Prior, but only after complaining about being tormented by his guilt as symbolized in mental images of "Biblical things, Mark of Cain, Judas Iscariot and his silver and his noose, people who . . . in betraying what they love betray what's truest in themselves."[44]

Most gay men whose partners had AIDS did not leave them the way Louis left Prior. They toughed it out as best they could in the face of a hideous disease and the hatred of others who couldn't imagine "gay grief" because they couldn't imagine the love of two men for one another. Remarking on the support she observed gay men giving their partners and friends even early in the epidemic before we knew how AIDS was caused, Elisabeth Kübler-Ross, the world's best-known authority on death and dying, said, "They were willing to hold those young dying men in their arms so they would not feel unloved and deserted at the end of their lives. In those days they were unaware that one could not catch the disease by sheer proximity, yet they were still willing to risk their young lives to ease their friends' suffering."[45]

But even survivors who stuck around had to make their way through the emotional minefield of bereavement, largely unguided, because there are no established norms for mourning the death of a gay partner: A surviving lover isn't called a widow or widower. Rarely do financial benefits—a widow's pension, for example—accrue to him upon his partner's death. Typically he can't take time off from work. If he does, and if he wasn't "out" about being gay with his coworkers, they'll wonder about the intensity of his feeling for someone who was "just a friend," or "just a roommate."[46] This lack of recognition of the relationship, the loss, or the griever has been described as "disenfranchised grief."[47]

The surviving partner's disenfranchisement was often felt most acutely with respect to the family of the dead man. One of the first studies of surviving lovers noted that although some families accepted the lover, many did not. There were arguments over funeral arrangements, financial settlements, and disposal of possessions. "These problems are, of course, not unique to the AIDS situation," noted the authors. Nor did they originate in the 1980s. In fact, gay male partners were being pushed aside by biological families long before the AIDS epidemic. In the seventies, Howard Brown observed that "Relegated to the status of mere friend, the surviving partner must watch helplessly as members of his lover's family move in and establish their claim as next of kin, as they make funeral arrangements their own way, possibly shipping the body out of town."[48]

In *My Own Country,* Abraham Verghese describes his years as a physician who became, of necessity, the AIDS doctor in rural Johnson City, Tennessee. There he tended to HIV-infected gay men who had mostly grown up in the area and whose experience of gay life consisted largely of dancing at the one local gay bar, and furtive sexual encounters with one another and with the interstate truckers who passed through on their way north or south. Because of his personal experience as a foreign-born, albeit heterosexual, doctor, Verghese knew what it was like to be cast in the role of the "outsider." He poignantly captures the shattering effect of a gay man's being pushed aside by his dying lover's biological family when decisions are made as to whether or not to put the man with AIDS on artificial life support, something the man himself was adamantly against:

> The oldest brother spoke again. His tone was matter-of-fact and determined:
>
> "*We* are his family. *We* are legally responsible for him. We want you to do everything for him."
>
> *We are his family.* I watch Bobby's face crumble as he suddenly became a mere observer with no legal right to determine the fate of the man he had loved since he was seven years old. He was finally, despite the years that had passed and whatever acceptance he and Ed found together, an outsider.[49]

Of course there were families that respected their adult children's relationships, though their support may have been largely unspoken. Jim Halloran, a registered nurse in Houston who has drawn upon his training in oncology nursing to care for people with AIDS, describes the trying time he had in dealing with a lover who didn't want his family to know he had AIDS—even though they accepted the two men's relationship. The family was present when Halloran's John died. The word AIDS was never used. Legally, Halloran held power of attorney, though, as he pointed out "a piece of paper doesn't matter to family dynamics."

After the funeral, Halloran and John's sister were standing outside on the porch. "I was talking with Carmen, John's oldest sister, the matriarch of the family aside from Mama," he recalls. "I said, 'Carmen, there's something I want to tell you. In a week or two I'll send you all death certificates because you might need them for something. And on it, it's going to say that John died of AIDS.'" Halloran expected a blowup. But Carmen just nodded, said it wasn't a problem, and added that she probably would have gone about things the same way. Said Halloran, "Talk about a lesson. Here we are with our doctrine and dogma of here's how you do things—when the basic, simple truth is that within a family, family members know best how that family operates."[50]

In the late eighties, Randy Shilts reported that while some families abandoned their "leper" children, many others experienced a renewal of family ties after what may have been years of estrangement. "For many families," wrote Shilts, "news of a Kaposi's sarcoma or *pneumocystis* diagnosis rendered a dual diagnosis, informing the parent both of the child's disease and sexual orientation."[51] Families that had struggled to understand and accept their son's sexual orientation now were confronted by a disease that many in this country believed was either a result of or punishment for homosexuality. For parents of gay men, the question "What is the risk for AIDS?" became a terrifying addition to the usual concerns about having a gay child, such as "What will our neighbors say?" and "Where did we go wrong?" An April 1987 survey of 402 parents who were involved with the group Parents and Friends of Lesbians and Gays (P-FLAG) found that AIDS had reopened old wounds even for parents who had already come to terms with their child's homosexuality.[52]

Some parents reacted with hatred and anger, rejecting their gay sons at their moment of direst need because the sons were gay and had contracted the so-called "gay disease." John Paul Barnich recounted a particularly loathsome incident in Houston. "We had a little munchkin from L.A.," he recalls. "Joey, a street hustler. He had lymphoma of the brain." Given the gravity of Joey's condition, Barnich, then on the board of AIDS Foundation Houston, called Joey's father in Los Angeles. The father said he had no interest in seeing his son. When Barnich offered to raise money to pay the man's airfare, he still resisted. Barnich recalls asking, "What would you like us to do with the body?" To which Joey's father replied, "Put the little son-of-a-bitch in a Hefty trash bag and leave him out by the curb."[53]

People like Joey's father notwithstanding, many other parents responded with love, as outraged as their gay sons by the cowardice and neglect of the federal government and their fellow Americans in dealing with the epidemic. Suzanne Benzer is the consummate New York woman—slim and attractive, outgoing, energetic, and determined. Benzer is a board member of Mothers' Voices, a group founded in 1991 by five mothers who had lost a child to AIDS. The group's main purpose is to channel the mother's and other family members' grief into a movement aimed at changing public attitudes and policies. As we sat in the Manhattan office of Mothers' Voices, Benzer described what it has been like for her to see her twenty-eight-year-old son Bobby living with HIV.

"About four years ago," she said, "we suspected that my son was gay. He was involved with a boy, and the boy got AIDS." Benzer immediately called GMHC because she didn't know much about AIDS. "I raised my boys myself, so I'm pretty tough," she said. "But I was out of control. I couldn't make this better for him, and I still can't—either emotionally or physically, I can't. I can be there, but I'm completely powerless to make my child better." Benzer started going to a support group sponsored by the PWA Coalition. Downstairs were all the mothers who had children with AIDS; upstairs were mothers whose children had died. She said, "It was metaphoric because you went up the stairs when your child died."

Like other mothers and family members involved with Mothers' Voices, Benzer's grief over her son's condition turned into anger as she learned more about AIDS and about the government's stumbling efforts to address the epidemic. She joined ACT UP, "doing actions" such as sitting in the middle of the Brooklyn Bridge to protest, which helped her get through some of the anger and rage. "I never thought I'd see myself sitting in the middle of the Brooklyn Bridge," said Benzer. "I was an upper-middle-class lady. This was not what I thought life would hold for me. But my son. . . ." She doesn't complete the sentence.[54]

Other mothers joined ACT UP for the same reasons Benzer described. They called themselves "ACT UP in sheep's clothing" because, as mothers, they were able to appeal to heterosexual politicians on the basis of their shared "family values." ACT UP and Mothers' Voices board member Eileen Mitzman, whose daughter Marni died of AIDS at age twenty-six in 1991, typically set a picture of her daughter on legislators' desks, near their own family photos. "That's the only way to get them," she said. For years, she pointed out, they didn't identify with anyone who had AIDS. It wasn't their disease, so they did nothing. "Now, said Mitzman, "we show them pictures of children who look like their children, and they gulp."[55]

Because many gay people live far from their families, often in the nation's large cities where they feel more comfortable living their lives openly, they often regard their circles of close friends as the kind of family that Armistead Maupin said was common in San Francisco in the seventies. These gay family networks have been invaluable for gay men with AIDS, providing both practical and emotional care and support. Traditionally, parents, spouses, and adult daughters have been the informal caregivers of people who have an incurable disease.[56] But in these "chosen families," gay men have broken the mold of the traditional roles that men are expected to play in caring for ill family members. For the first time ever, American men have actually become primary caregivers.

When she was supervising buddies and crisis intervention workers at GMHC, Sandi Feinblum says she heard many gay men say "I never thought I was capable of doing this." One man in particular stood out in her memory, a man in his forties who became a crisis worker. Feinblum recalls, "When he would tell his friends and family—he was fairly well-to-do, kind of a fancy queen—they all laughed and said, 'You? We'll give you four days!'" She added, "It was so striking to him that people thought he was superficial and that nobody took him seriously. He realized that this was a big test to himself of who he was." Even gay men, often accustomed to being more comfortable than heterosexual men with the "feminine" aspects of their personalities, had to learn to be comfortable in caregiving roles traditionally assigned to women. Typically women didn't struggle over whether they were comfortable in such roles because, as Feinblum put it, "they've accepted that they're going to be helpers."[57]

The losses of professional AIDS helpers—particularly doctors, nurses, and psychotherapists—have often been overlooked. Those who aren't in the health care professions assume that the severe illness and death these people confront in their patients are simply a kind of occupational hazard, easily handled by trained professionals. But even trained health care professionals weren't prepared for the ghastly diseases and deaths of young people they confronted repeatedly in the AIDS epidemic. Like the surviving lovers of gay men with AIDS, the late Washington, D.C., bereavement expert and therapist Judy Pollatsek said that the grief of professional AIDS caregivers is "disenfranchised" because it is so typically unrecognized. If they are gay themselves, it is magnified by the fact that even in their personal lives they are likely to have dealt with AIDS in friends, the community—or themselves. And it is profound: shell-shocked doctors, nurses, social workers, therapists, and others were forced to confront death after relentless death. As Pollatsek put it, "We have not been trained to lose so many battles with so many people who are just like us."[58]

Even health care professionals sometimes had to step back from their work with AIDS patients because the stress and grief overwhelmed them. Washington, D.C., psychiatrist Jeff Akman said he had to limit the number of people with AIDS he sees in psychotherapy. "There's a certain number I can tolerate without destroying my own psychological health or my relationship or ability to work," he told me. Akman said he was able to keep working with AIDS patients, as he had been doing since AIDS first appeared in Washington, by focusing on the rewards of his work. He explained, "You have to think about the unbelievable gallantry of people who face this day in and day out, who deal with this awful illness and suffering and pain and death. I think in many ways it's the gallantry that sustains me, that makes practicing as a physician who mostly sees AIDS patients and people with HIV very rewarding."[59]

For a person with AIDS, grief begins at diagnosis. Like people with other life-threatening illnesses, such as cancer, people with AIDS go through a bereavement in which they mourn for themselves. Besides mourning their very real losses—the loss of health, of an attractive appearance, of a job and financial independence—people with AIDS experience a kind of "anticipatory grief" for their own potential death.[60] For gay men with AIDS who never confronted their internalized homophobia, diagnosis could unleash feelings of unacceptability. The disease could reactivate feelings of self-loathing even in men who had come to terms with being gay years earlier. This often had profoundly negative effects on gay people with AIDS. If they accepted and internalized the stigma that American society attached to AIDS, they might feel such extreme shame that they felt unentitled to live, in which case they might not seek or adhere to their medical treatment.[61]

University of Miami psychiatrist Karl Goodkin became interested in exploring the relationship between the bereavement of gay men with HIV infection and AIDS and the functioning of their immune systems, after observing that men who had a hard time dealing with their losses seemed to become clinically ill faster. There is a strong belief in the emerging field of psychoneuroimmunology that an intimate relationship exists between an individual's psychological health and the functioning of his immune system. Goodkin, a proponent of this view, describes what he calls "active" and "passive" coping, personal styles of dealing with loss that are respectively either hopeful or hopeless. Active copers are realistic about their health and the impact of the AIDS epidemic on their lives and community. Rather than feeling helpless, though, these people look at their HIV infection as an impetus to take control of their lives, to become politically involved, or to work with local AIDS organizations. Goodkin was intrigued by the fact that these active copers seemed to do better with their disease and to live longer than passive copers. They had higher CD4 counts and positive changes in natural killer cell function, another immune measure believed to be important in later HIV disease when these cells take over from the vanquished CD4 cells in defending the individual against viral illnesses and cancers.

Goodkin felt that loss was perhaps one of the most stressful events that people with HIV—particularly gay men—had to cope with on a chronic basis, both individually and in the community. In fact, Goodkin found a strong correlation between the loss of a significant other in the prior six months and decreases of CD4 counts up to a full year afterward. These observations led him to pilot-test a support group intervention in 1990 whose goal was to equip bereaved gay men with the psychological skills they needed to cope actively with their losses, thereby, Goodkin hoped, bolstering their immune systems. In its fifth year at the time of our interview, and now funded by the National Institute of Mental Health, Goodkin's bereavement support group at the University of Miami included 240 men, grouped separately according to whether they were HIV positive or negative, who had lost a close friend or lover within six months prior to entering the study. Participants were randomly assigned to either an actual support group, which met for ten weeks, or to a control group that didn't meet but did get called every three weeks to see how the men were coping with their loss.

Each session of the support group was devoted to a particular topic intended to elicit responses from the group members. The first set of topics made the individual conscious of his loss through questions such as, "What is bereavement?" and "What responses have you had from the medical care community?" The next sessions explored the implications of the loss for the individual's own mortality and spirituality. Finally, the group's last stage was the "moving on" phase, when members assessed how the intervention would help them deal with the particular loss that brought them to the group, as well as with future losses, including other losses besides death, such as the loss of a job or a relationship.

After the support group's ten weeks were up, Goodkin and his colleagues followed up with all the men every six months for two and a half years to assess their psychological and physical health. Goodkin found "significant buffering" against a decline in CD4 cell count and increased natural killer cell counts in men who were HIV positive and in the intervention. He said it would be some time before he could determine whether the intervention had attained its ultimate goal: deterring progression to clinical AIDS. In the meantime, he noted that even the men in the control group who received only phone calls seemed to benefit merely from being part of the study. Like the men who participated in the earliest studies in the epidemic, these men felt "validated" merely by having their losses recognized. As Goodkin put it, "Just being assessed about their loss and their loss burden was giving them self-affirmation that was important for them."[62]

New York's St. Vincent's Hospital was a welcoming neighbor to gay men in Greenwich Village long before the AIDS epidemic. In fact, the hospital is literally the next-door neighbor of the Gay and Lesbian Community Services Center, on West Thirteenth Street. So it was natural that when gay men in the Village began to get sick with AIDS in the early eighties, many of them went to St. Vincent's to be treated or to die. The families of these men, many of whom traveled long distances to be with their son or brother at the end of what may well have been a life of estrangement, often didn't know the men were gay. Still other survivors included articulate young friends or lovers, in touch with their feelings. The staff at St. Vincent's realized that the bereavement program they had in the hospice could be expanded to assist these people who were losing loved ones to AIDS. They trained volunteers to work, like "buddies," with AIDS patients until they died. And they established the first bereavement support groups anywhere in New York for people who had lost some-one to AIDS.

Sister Patrice Murphy, a registered nurse and Roman Catholic nun, directed St. Vincent's Supportive Care Program from the time the support groups began in 1983 until 1990. In an interview on Ash Wednesday 1995 at her home in the hospital's staff residence, Sister Patrice explained how the support groups operate. The first of the weekly meetings was to get people to tell their stories. "That was always a weepy session," said Sister Patrice. "Sometimes people felt they couldn't come back after that." The rest of the meetings followed no formal agenda because people would inevitably bring up the kinds of feelings and issues that Sister Patrice and her coleader hoped they would address. She told me, "I think once they knew they were accepted, that what was said in the group was confidential, that we cared about the fact that they were suffering, that we could cry with them—those kinds of things I think engendered a spirit of trust."[63] Men talked about feeling that a part of them had died with their lover or friend. Some talked about parents. Others talked about not wanting to be left behind when everyone they knew was dying. Most all of them asked, "Who's going to take care of *me?*"

When I first interviewed Sister Patrice, in 1986, I was curious to know how welcome gay men were at St. Vincent's, a Catholic hospital, in view of the Catholic Church's official condemnation of homosexuality, reiterated by the Vatican that very year.[64] She assured me that gay men were most welcome and had in fact been "always part of the scene" at the hospital because of its location in Manhattan's gayest neighborhood. "My role here is a nurse, a caregiver," she said. "I'm not here as a moralist or a judge." She noted, however, that one of the important issues confronting the gay men who were dying of AIDS at St. Vincent's was religion. "There is a searching," she explained, "a grasping for spiritual comfort, a desire to discuss and grapple with issues."[65]

Richard A. Rasi, a psychologist and Catholic priest in Boston who often celebrates mass for the gay Catholic group Dignity, described the spiritual issues he has helped gay men and their families confront in the AIDS epidemic. For many, he said, AIDS made them ask the same question they asked when they "came out" as gay: "What's wrong with me?" There were those whose thoughts turned to eternity when it seemed clear their future would be abbreviated. And then, said Rasi, there were the spiritual dimensions of the gay community's support, care, and love for those with AIDS. In doing memorial services or liturgies for gay men, Rasi dealt with families he often had never met. "A lot of the work that gets done in those situations," he explained, "is really the effects of the disease on the families—holding them and letting them know that they're okay, that their loved one is okay and that they didn't die because God hated them."[66]

The support groups continue to meet at St. Vincent's. By now thousands have gone through the eight-week program, meeting once a week to talk with others who understand about the losses they have suffered in the AIDS epidemic. There is a monthly memorial service for all who died in the month. Once a year there is a large memorial service that brings together all the past group members. As in any alumni gathering, they reunite to compare notes about how far they've come and gone since the time they shared a formative experience. These alumni share a deep bond, forged in the fires of anguish and loss. As Sister Patrice said, "I don't think anybody can really understand grief who hasn't been through it. But you can't even be hard on them because if they haven't felt the pain, how could they imagine it?"[67]

*

Since Harvey Milk's assassination in 1978, gay San Franciscans have mourned their dead in large candlelight marches that move like a dirge from the Castro district to City Hall. On the night of May 2, 1983, a dozen people with AIDS led the first of what would become an annual candlelight march, hoisting aloft a banner whose message would forever encapsulate the struggle that confronted each of them, as well as all gay people: "Fighting For Our Lives," it said. Gary Walsh, one of the city's first to be diagnosed with AIDS and the one who thought of the idea for the candlelight march, held the banner between Bobbi Campbell, the "K.S. Poster Boy," and Mark Feldman, an old boyfriend.

Some of the thousands who joined the march brought snapshots of friends who had died, while others carried signs that read like gravestones:

> Ken Horne
> Born July 20, 1943
> Died November 30, 1981

Six thousand people stood in United Nations Plaza to listen to speeches by people with AIDS. Mark Feldman told the crowd, "Our president doesn't seem to know AIDS exists. He is spending more money on the paints to put the American flag on his nuclear missiles than he is spending on AIDS. That is sick." Earlier in the day, Mayor Dianne Feinstein had met with a group of men with AIDS at her office after she issued a proclamation of AIDS Awareness Week. Also that day the Centers for Disease Control had released figures showing that the number of new AIDS cases in the United States had increased by 36 percent to 1,366 cases; 520 people were already dead.[68] Candlelight marches were held the same night in Boston, Chicago, Dallas, Houston, and other cities, sparking some of the first local media coverage of the epidemic. The *New York Times* buried its own few paragraphs of coverage inside the paper, and didn't even make reference to the fact that most of those who had participated in the marches were gay men, instead describing the crowds as "mostly male."[69]

The newly formed PWA Coalition of San Francisco had asked Paul Boneberg to help them organize the candlelight march in San Francisco, and to get other cities to hold similar marches. Boneberg still marvels at the drive of the men with AIDS who led that first march. He says, "I can't think of another community on earth that would think that the logical response to being stricken with an unknown disease is to come out, say your name on TV, and organize a march! It directly flows from Harvey Milk, and [his saying] 'Come out, come out! Organize, organize!'"

Although a candlelight march wasn't held in San Francisco in 1984—everyone was busy organizing the big march at the 1984 Democratic National Convention being held there that year—it was resumed in 1985, and organized by the newly formed gay-AIDS political group Mobilization Against AIDS. This time the PWA Coalition wanted candlelight marches not only in San Francisco and other American cities, but in other countries as well. Boneberg, who was then director of Mobilization, initially resisted getting the group involved with the candlelight march. He recalls, "I basically said I'm here to organize demos; I don't know anything about international organizing."

But the people with AIDS persisted. "And they did it," said Boneberg. "Richard Rector and Dean Sandmeyer and others organized candlelights in something like eighteen countries." Boneberg seems to wonder how he ever doubted the determination of those early PWAs when he adds, "And that's how it was done." While he still maintains that his role with Mobilization was political, Boneberg now understands that even the candlelight march was a kind of political art form. "When I look at the candlelight and what it's done," he said, "I think maybe I was actually doing mass art. What I really was engaged in was an artistic, cultural phenomenon. In hindsight, I tend to think the cultural response of the candlelight is amazing, and speaks to the depth of soul of our community."

The candlelight march's political impact has been felt in small American towns and around the world. Said Boneberg, "The most important candlelight is not the one that's occurring in San Francisco or New York, because they are organized. It's the one that's occurring for the first time in Lynchburg, Virginia, where you've got a mom, somebody else's lover, and they get together and they're doing this thing. That is the beginning of organizing." Internationally, this ritual created by gay Americans had profound effects. Within two years after Boneberg received a letter from a doctor in Tokyo, saying that in Japan people were ashamed of AIDS and he didn't think a candlelight would ever occur, the gay movement had started in Japan and they organized a candlelight memorial. All the Japanese networks showed people carrying candles down the street. Boneberg noted that during the 1994 international AIDS conference in Yokohama, an openly HIV-positive person addressed the prime minister. As Boneberg put it, "It was astute to provide this tool to people around the world and to say, well, we have found this to be useful. The more repressive and closeted or fascist a country is the more useful that tool is to them."[70]

In 1995, the twelfth International AIDS Candlelight Memorial and Mobilization was observed by 250 cities in 45 nations. In Washington, D.C., fifteen hundred people processed from Lafayette Square—across the street from the White House, where candles were placed in the windows facing the square to observe the occasion—to the reflecting pool at the U.S. Capitol. Underscoring the political nature of the march, AIDS "czar" Patsy Fleming spoke to the crowd about the cuts in AIDS funding then being considered in Congress. With her back to the Capitol, Fleming told the crowd, "We have to shine some light on what is being proposed in the building that stands behind me, because those of us who have experienced the kind of losses we have seen in the last fifteen years cannot stand still while the programs that help the people we love are decimated."[71]

Shining a light on the lives of people who died from AIDS was the task of obituaries. The final news reports of people's lives have been as politically charged a venue as any in gay people's efforts to mourn their dead and mark the community's losses. "After the recent bombing, our papers are filled with obituaries," said Oklahoma City psychiatrist Larry Prater in an interview a month after the April 1995 bombing of the Alfred P. Murrah federal building. "With the bombing it's been harder to tell who died of AIDS recently."

Even before the tragic bombing, though, it was hard to tell who in Oklahoma had died of AIDS by reading the newspaper obituaries. That's because there in America's heartland, AIDS means gay— which means gay men with HIV tend not to tell their families either that they are gay or that they have the virus. Prater said, "They're so closely linked there that to tell them they're HIV-positive is about the same as saying they're also gay." So many Oklahoma families— just like the families Shilts described years earlier—often don't know the son is gay or that he has AIDS until it's too late. Prater noted that things had improved somewhat because now at least sometimes an obituary will mention an AIDS death, or even the name of the "special friend." Still in others, he added, "there will be no clue whatsoever."[72]

Urban sophisticates might scoff at such provincial reticence. Unfortunately, they can't. Even the highbrow *New York Times* at the start of the epidemic refused to use the word "AIDS" in an obituary, and eventually mentioned a dead gay man's surviving lover only as a "long time companion"—as though he'd been a paid geriatric assistant or a pet. It was only in December 1995 that the *Times* agreed to change its policy against using the word "lover" in the death notices that survivors pay to have published. When New York's Gay and Lesbian Community Services Center paid for a death notice for its deputy director's lover, the *Times* ran the notice without the word "lover," as the center had requested. The center's executive director, Richard Burns, wrote in a letter to the paper, "Despite Mr. Woodworth's expressed intention and the Center's protestation, the *Times* inserted 'life partner' when referring to Mr. Woodworth's seven-year relationship with Mr. Vilanueva in the death notice which ran Saturday, December 9th." The *Times* responded to the center's letter by saying it had changed its policy. It reprinted the death notice, at no charge, on December 12—with the word "lover." Clearly the policy change didn't apply to the *Times'* obituaries because the newspaper of record's obituaries still do not use the word "lover."

In contrast to the obituaries in mainstream newspapers, which usually read like a résumé of the deceased's education and work life, gay newspapers tended to provide a more personal view of the individual. Typically a photograph of the man accompanied an affectionate description of his hobbies, names of actual pets, close friends, a lover if there was one, and remembrances of his charms and interests along with a description of his schooling and professional accomplishments. Since so many gay people are immigrants to their home city from somewhere else—typically a small town—these obits also often mentioned the reasons the individual moved to the place where he lived and died.

The eloquence of the June 1997 obituary for thirty-nine-year-old John Howard Martindale, Jr., in San Francisco's *Bay Area Reporter*, was typical. "John Martindale," it said, "died peacefully in his sleep in San Francisco on June 13 of AIDS. John's sweet nature and strong character were as present in his long battle with the disease as they were throughout his full life before it. Born in Newport Beach, Calif., John was a bighearted soul right from his youth. He moved to his beloved San Francisco just after high school and just in time to take part in the wonderful rise of the city's gay culture. As waiter and manager, John was a popular fixture at Vanelli's restaurant on Pier 39. He earned a bachelor's in business and became fluent in Spanish, enjoying long stints in both Mexico and Spain. As a hotline volunteer for Project Inform, John showed characteristic generosity with his knowledge and sensitivity. It was probably in the beautiful world of plants and animals, though, that John's gentle passions came through best. His gardens radiated his joy, and the love he shared with his Chihuahua, Carly, was truly endearing. John is survived by his devoted parents, John Sr. and Ann, and his loving sister, Lisa. There will be a memorial garden service at two-thirty p.m. on Friday, June 27."[73]

For years, the *BAR* each week included upwards of two full pages of obituaries, virtually all of them of gay men struck down by AIDS. Michael Bronski has observed, "Reading *BAR* is like walking through a graveyard, or viewing the Vietnam Veterans' Memorial Wall—the only difference is that you knew these people and may have seen them only a week ago." Describing his own experience of writing obituaries for Boston's *Gay Community News* in the early and mideighties, Bronski said, "Despite the terrors of writing and reading obits, there is also the satisfaction, however incomplete, that something is being done. Someone's life has been noted. Some attention is being paid. Someone else may read and understand a little more of how large, how inclusive and diverse the gay world is." He added, "[I]n taking action—as well as in remembering and mourning, which are part of each obituary—the pieces ease both the terror and the pity, and they become politically inseparable from the personal."[74]

It is precisely this linkage of the personal and political that distinguished many memorial services for gay men who died of AIDS, especially during the eighties when the fear and stigma associated with the disease reached hysterical proportions. On a political level, as the *New York Times* has noted, the gay community's memorials often have been "platforms for grief and celebration and the politics that surround AIDS. Participants not only cry and reminisce but rail against the government, push for more medical research and raise money to fight on." At the same time, "The friends and colleagues who plan the services make them highly personal, saying that one of their goals is to prevent a friend or relative from turning into one more statistic."[75]

Gay memorials served to affirm the value of gay lives, and of the deceased individual to the life of the gay community. By insisting that the word AIDS was named openly as the cause of death, gay people sought to remove the sting of what society considered a shameful death. Frequently there was more than one memorial tribute for the same man, generally because the man's family either couldn't make it to the memorial his friends organized in the place he lived as an adult, or because the family refused to attend a "gay" event. Even in his death, a man's family too often continued to deny the fact of his gay life. Judy Pollatsek said, "I remember early on with one family there were two funerals, a funeral for the friends and a funeral for the family in a traditional church." She noted that, particularly in the early years of the epidemic, "there was a real need to change the ritual, to stamp it in a different way. It became important that AIDS got mentioned one way or another, and that the person was gay. There was always some effort in those days, such a sense of people being on the outside, of banding together, of a community of PWAs."[76]

Many gay men are known to be exceptionally creative in their lives; they certainly have been creative in the ways they've memorialized their own and one another's deaths. Often men will plan their own memorial services in advance, permeated with the camp humor that has sustained gay people through the worst of persecutions, including that of a viral enemy. Pollatsek, who was not gay but had worked with and attended memorials for hundreds of gay men, recalled one memorial service that typified the untraditional, highly personal rituals often used to mark many gay men's deaths. "I remember Steven Chase's funeral in 1986," she told me. "Steven gave us elaborate funeral instructions that said things like 'By hook or by crook, my cat Sasha will be there,' and 'You will all drink a toast to me and throw your glasses in Tom's fireplace.' Tom was sweeping glass for weeks." She said that another treat at Chase's funeral was the batch of "Alice B. Toklas brownies" baked specially for the occasion.[77]

Randy Miller recalls the memorial service that black gay filmmaker Marlon Riggs planned in detail for himself. "He was really a control queen," said Miller, "so he had it choreographed down to the last minute. You could hear him in different parts. He had Aretha Franklin singing 'Young, Gifted, and Black.' You could hear Marlon considering himself young, gifted, and black. So it was all about him and odd things that he had put together himself. You could almost hear him chuckling. There were little things like that all through the service. It was really powerful."[78]

Power—specifically, personal and communal empowerment— was precisely the point of the memorials and other rituals gay people created in response to the thousands upon thousands of deaths in the community. After publishing a 1992 study of 207 bereaved gay men in the *American Journal of Psychiatry*,[79] Richard Neugebauer, a psychiatric epidemiologist at Columbia University, told the *New York Times*, "The gay community has helped people deal in a more constructive way with their grief. Rather than becoming incapacitated, they became politically and socially active and put their energies into that."[80] AIDS activist and cultural critic Douglas Crimp has noted that in fact many gay people transformed their grief into AIDS activism. "For many of us," he said, "mourning becomes militancy."[81]

The "militants" of ACT UP/New York had their own unique ways of memorializing their fallen comrades, empowering themselves, and pushing the political envelope all at the same time. The late ACT UP member and author David Feinberg described the group's private memorials in *Queer and Loathing*. During the group's Monday night meetings, members would take the floor for "mini-memorials" during which they offered personal reminiscences of the deceased. Feinberg wrote, "These are always contained, confined within the three-and-a-half hour agenda of the meetings; they generally last no longer than fifteen minutes. We end these memorials by chanting 'ACT UP, fight back, fight AIDS!' three times."[82]

Besides its "mini-memorials," ACT UP sponsored several "political funerals" in which the remains of one or more of its members were paraded about—either within a casket or as cremation ashes—in an effort to push the group's agenda. The most infamous of these "actions" was the attempt by ACT UP members to conduct a funeral ceremony in front of the White House for member Tim Bailey, whose body they carried in a casket. After the police struggled with the ACT UP pallbearers and arrested Bailey's nongay, nonactivist brother for assaulting a police officer, the group retreated and held their ceremony from atop the van that would return Bailey's body to a funeral home in New Jersey. Though not otherwise known for understatement, Feinberg concluded of ACT UP's political funerals, "The concept is unfathomable, incomprehensible, as difficult to grasp as death."[83]

The art that gay people created in the AIDS epidemic attempted precisely to fathom the depths of their suffering, comprehend the vastness of their loss, and grasp for meaning in what seemed the pointless tragedies they experienced. In essays, films, novels, poetry, plays, performance art, photographs, and symphonies, gay people sought to tell their stories to one another and to the world, and to connect their suffering to the loss that all who share "this mortal coil" will, at some point, experience. As Armistead Maupin puts it, "The bigger the calamity, the higher the art." He notes that the art of AIDS is "a healing and strengthening force," adding, "It's not a wishy-washy, airy-fairy affectation. It's a very gritty, gut-level, potent thing that not only strengthens the artist, but strengthens the recipients of the art."[84]

Many gay artists who were working before the epidemic applied their talents to the telling of the community's woeful tales. Andrew Holleran, author of *Dancer From the Dance,* devoted his attention mostly to the AIDS epidemic. But unlike Larry Kramer, who turned his post-*Faggots* "exile" to political ends by becoming an independent, chastising voice, Holleran seemed to retreat in a despair much deeper than what he expressed in his first novel, in 1978. In his third novel, *The Beauty of Men,* Holleran described the pervasiveness of AIDS in gay life and the denial that not having it elicits in many. When Lark, the novel's middle-age gay central character, and his friend Sutcliffe are told by an acquaintance in New York that a mutual friend had just died in San Francisco, they were relieved to know the man had been run over by a taxicab rather than dying "of it."

Holleran writes, "That was where AIDS stood in the hierarchy of misfortune, somehow; in a class by itself—so grim its aura extended to the fact . . . that people who don't have AIDS imagine somehow they're not going to die."[85]

The disproportionately large number of gay men in the arts meant there was a correspondingly large number of AIDS deaths among the artistic professions. Many in the arts feared that the loss of so many gifted young choreographers, dancers, musicians, novelists, painters, playwrights, and poets within such a compressed time period would continue to reverberate well into the future. When ballet legend Rudolf Nureyev died from AIDS in 1993, Gordon Davidson, artistic director of the Mark Taper Forum in Los Angeles, where Tony Kushner's *Angels in America* was first performed in a 1990 workshop, said, "The impact on the arts and culture is incalculable. The problem, aside from the horror of the deaths, is that the system by which we encounter art is a system of passing things down, and when you break the circuit the way it is being broken by AIDS, the damage may be irreparable."[86]

Although not every work of art by a gay person in response to AIDS had the bite of Larry Kramer's 1985 play *The Normal Heart,* such works typically demonstrated just how political one's personal experience can be. By illustrating the humanity of people with AIDS and showing the excruciation of their and the community's losses, this art attempted to heal some of the wounds in gay hearts and minds inflicted by both the disease and society's disdain for gay people. In a foreword to the published version of *The Normal Heart,* Joseph Papp, the play's first producer, expressed what Kramer and other gay artists were attempting to portray in their work. Papp wrote, "[T]he element that gives this powerful political play its essence, is love—love holding firm under fire, put to the ultimate test, facing and overcoming our greatest fear: death."[87]

Gay people's love and loss manifested themselves in other ways, too. In 1996, Congress designated a fifteen-acre wooded dell in San Francisco's Golden Gate Park to be the site of a memorial to those who have been lost to AIDS in this country. The concept of the AIDS Memorial Grove originated in 1989 with a group of San Francisco landscape architects who were bereft at the loss of a colleague to

AIDS. Word spread, and attorneys, botanists, designers, fundraisers, public planners, and other volunteers joined together to make the grove a reality. Kerry Enright, director of the nonprofit organization running the grove, said, "The designation of the AIDS Memorial Grove as a national landmark will not only help to raise awareness of the enormous national toll which the AIDS crisis has exacted, but it will also inform people that there is a dedicated place in the public landscape that answers a legitimate, desperate need." Even before its completion, thousands of visitors from around the world were visiting the site to grieve openly without embarrassment. Said Enright, "This is not just a place for mourning; it is a living and breathing space where people can experience the pathos of AIDS."[88]

The air was heavy with the pathos of AIDS as more than 650,000 people gathered in Washington, D.C., on October 11, 1987, for the second March on Washington for Lesbian and Gay Rights. The march was led by people with AIDS, some in wheelchairs pushed by their friends. Displayed for the first time near the post-march rallying area on the Capitol Mall was the NAMES Project's AIDS Memorial Quilt. The quilt had been laid out in a solemn ceremony at dawn, its 1,920 panels covering the equivalent of two football fields.[89] Those panels represented a fraction of the 24,698 Americans who had died of AIDS by then. People in the cities most affected by the epidemic to that point—New York, Los Angeles, and San Francisco—had sent panels to the NAMES Project's San Francisco workshop in memory of their loved ones. Most of the panels were sewed with the names of young gay men.[90]

Many of those at the march saw the quilt as a stark reminder of why they were in Washington to protest. Like the motto of the people with AIDS who carried the banner in 1983, the hundreds of thousands gathered on the Mall near the quilt joined lesbian folk singer Holly Near in the old civil rights anthem, "We are a gentle, angry people who are fighting for our lives." The timing of the quilt's premiere at the march—as the presidential campaigns were getting seriously underway—was deliberate, and its presence provided a powerful symbol of the gay community's political struggle for equal rights and of the casualties of the simultaneous struggle for sexual liberation. The day of the march and the quilt's display was NAMES

Project founder Cleve Jones's thirty-third birthday. To this day October 11 is designated "National Coming Out Day," when gay people are urged to identify themselves as such to others.

Jones recalled in an interview in San Francisco, not far from the places that inspired him, why he thought the quilt would provide an image that resonates with the American people. Jones had had to reschedule our meeting because he himself was now living with AIDS and the unpredictability of his health from one day to the next made planning difficult. He told me that he got the idea for a quilt when he and others were putting up posters for the annual candlelight march for Harvey Milk. "The *Chronicle* had a headline saying that a thousand San Franciscans had died," he recalled. "I was talking to my friend Joseph saying those thousand, they were all right here: Almost every one of that thousand had died within ten blocks of where we were standing. But you couldn't see that, couldn't walk down the street and see death everywhere."

Jones wanted something that would provide a visual image of the toll by showing the lives behind the statistics. During the candlelight march, he asked everyone to carry placards with the name of one person who had died. Using ladders he hid in the shrubbery, Jones and his friends taped the placards on the front of the federal building. "As I was looking at the patchwork of names on the wall," said Jones, "I said to myself it looks like a quilt." The word evoked warm memories for him because his great-grandmother had sewed a series of quilts to pass on to her grandchildren. An idea was born. Jones recalls thinking, "This is such a warm, comforting, middle-class, middle-American symbol. Every family has a quilt; it makes them think of their grandmothers. That's what we need: We need all these American grandmothers to want us to live, to be willing to say that our lives are worth defending."[91]

Besides its obvious link to the gay rights struggle, the quilt is one of the nation's most extraordinary examples of public mourning art. It is often compared and contrasted with the Vietnam War Memorial in Washington, D.C., because it represents a collective memorial for many individuals, and because of the way it draws people to publicly share their grief with others who also have lost loved ones. In America's death-denying culture, public mourning is traditionally discouraged. We are, after all, a forward-looking nation that brooks few exceptions to our view of Americans as an obsessively optimistic people. The quilt challenges the taboo of openly mourning our dead, thereby acknowledging the reality of death in life.

As a longtime political activist, Cleve Jones was clearly aware of the quilt's power. He describes it with such words as "soft," "gentle," and "subversive." As he puts it, "It's not ACT UP screaming in the street." He points out that the quilt has provided him and other gay people the opportunity to bring a message of compassion and even HIV prevention to places, such as high schools, that likely wouldn't otherwise be open to them. "When I go to a high school," said Jones, "I'm welcomed by the teacher, usually the principal is there. They treat me with great respect, great deference, and I speak well to these kids. I know in every class I go to there are four or five kids in that room who are going to grow up and find out they're gay. And how much of a difference it would have made in my life if when I was in tenth grade some nice-looking, well-spoken man came and talked."[92]

Despite the access that the quilt opened into the hearts of "middle America," some gay activists complained that the quilt's political potential hadn't been sufficiently exploited. Urvashi Vaid, for example, says the NAMES Project "didn't do enough to politicize people." It wasn't enough for people to attend a NAMES Project event. "Every one of them should have been asked to lobby," said Vaid. "Every one of them should have been asked to write letters. The project could have acted as a funnel to direct them—into AIDS Action Council or any of the other political organizations. But it didn't do that."[93]

Despite criticism that the quilt hasn't been political enough, it has by itself arguably done more to increase awareness of the human toll of the epidemic—and of the humanity of those it memorializes—than all the nation's gay political organizations combined. For example, in 1994 alone, forty NAMES Project chapters around the United States sponsored nearly eight hundred displays of sections of the quilt, viewed by an estimated eight hundred thousand people, according to Anthony Turney, who was then the NAMES Project Foundation director.[94] When the quilt was displayed in its entirety for the fifth time in Washington, in 1996, an estimated 750,000 people viewed it over the same days in October on which it was first displayed in 1987.

As with its premiere, the timing of the quilt's 1996 display was deliberate. As Mike Smith, a cofounder of the NAMES Project Foundation who directed the display, put it beforehand, "Several weeks before critical U.S. elections, when the spotlight is on the president and elected members of Congress, we will display the entire AIDS Memorial Quilt in Washington—to ensure that AIDS and its awful costs are given urgency on the American and international agendas."[95] In 1989, President George Bush declined an invitation from the NAMES Project to view the quilt, though he presumably saw it as he flew overhead in a helicopter on his way somewhere else. The Reagans also had declined an invitation to see the quilt in 1988.[96]

In 1996, President and Mrs. Clinton visited the quilt, marking the first time a president had done so despite the quilt's proximity to the White House. During the Clintons' visit, Cleve Jones said that someone in the crowd "startled" the first couple when he called out, "Thank you for being the first president to visit the Quilt!" Both Clintons looked at Jones and said, "Surely this can't be true." He assured them it was indeed the case. Said Jones, "I'd have to say it was the greatest moment of my life." It was also Jones's forty-second birthday.[97]

The quilt has grown exponentially from the forty panels—including Cleve Jones's original panel for his friend Marvin Feldman—that had been collected by the time of its first display during San Francisco's annual Lesbian and Gay Freedom Day Parade on June 28, 1987. In 1996 the quilt consisted of some forty-five thousand panels and covered twenty-five acres on the Mall. Despite its vastness, the quilt still represented only about one in eight Americans who had died from AIDS at that point.

However the politics of mourning are defined, it's clear that the quilt has had a tremendous impact on the way many Americans think about AIDS and, quite possibly, about gay people as well. Whether the NAMES Project alone could mobilize legions of bereaved Americans into a militant force is a dubious proposition. But perhaps the quilt's political achievement—like the gay community's terrific losses themselves—is best measured against the broad backdrop of human life, death, and how each is regarded with respect to the other. Rather than being merely a "political instrument," observes Richard Mohr, the quilt "both expresses and creates sacred values."[98] Pragmatic activists who insist that mourning is worthless unless it turns to militancy, miss an important point about the quilt and its lessons for human life. As Mohr puts it, elegy-making and mourning are worthy in themselves because they remind us of the reasons why, "in a world where suffering regularly dwarfs well-being, life is worth living in the first place."[99]

Even if the quilt were merely a tremendous, silent elegy, its power and effect would be undiminished. As it is, however, activists who downplay the quilt's political power overlook the fact that simply mourning the deaths of gay men is a political statement in that it affirms the value of their lives as equal to those of any other human being. In too many quarters, this remains a radical notion indeed.

By adapting a traditional, even archetypal, American folk art to publicly mourn and celebrate the lives of those who have died in the epidemic, the gay people who created the AIDS Memorial Quilt did more than their share for the gay civil rights movement by showing America the pain, dignity, and humor with which its gay citizens carried the weight of their knowledge of mortality. By living as people who have been unalterably changed by their sorrows and by a new awareness of their strength, gay people—survivors—bear daily witness to the transformative power of love and loss. That witness is every bit as "political" as any march and as powerful a testimony as there is of the struggle of gay people for an equal place in the nation where they also live, love, die, and are mourned.

VICTORY DEFERRED

Once the faintest stirring of hope became possible,
the dominion of the plague was ended.

ALBERT CAMUS, *THE PLAGUE*

The advent of new and stronger treatment for HIV brought renewed and strengthened hope that AIDS might yet become a manageable illness, its horrors a receding memory. But hope also has a price, and the exorbitant price and complex regimens of the new drugs rendered the idea of "living with HIV" for too many people as chimerical as it had ever been. Nevertheless, the ability of many others with HIV to benefit from new treatments meant not only profound changes for them personally, but also for the AIDS organizations that were created to help people who couldn't fully help themselves. The challenge remained to integrate HIV care into mainstream health care and social service organizations—and to ensure that all gay people receive appropriately sensitive care whatever their health needs. AIDS and gay people advocating on behalf of its victims pointed out the flaws in the American health care system, and their legacy included a system far more open to the needs and demands of its "consumers."

But even gay people too often followed the American way of neglecting things until they fall apart, focused as they were on those whose bodies were broken by AIDS and overlooking the many more who were healthy as yet but still facing the risk of HIV infection. As a new generation of prevention educators equipped gay men with information to make their own sexual and other health choices, homophobia still threatened to undermine even the best-designed prevention efforts. Community institutions were created as bulwarks against homophobia and as welcoming refuges for any and all. Even those institutions grappled with the challenge now facing gay America: how to remember the past, live fully in the present, and look to a future that may or may not be free of AIDS.

Lawrence K. Altman, the *New York Times* medical writer who first described AIDS to the newspaper's readers twelve years earlier, wrote in June 1993, "It is one of the bleakest moments in the fight against the disease since AIDS was first recognized as a new disease in 1981."[1] After the international AIDS conference in Berlin that month, Altman had observed that "only an eternal optimist" could believe that new drugs would be available anytime soon to save the lives of the fourteen million people worldwide then believed to be infected with the virus that causes AIDS.[2] People with HIV and their doctors alike were discouraged in 1993 by the findings on AZT reported at the Berlin conference from the European Concorde study, which showed that the first drug approved in the U.S. to treat HIV eventually lost its effectiveness when used as a "mono-therapy."

The goal of making HIV the chronic, manageable disease that scientists long had aimed to make it seemed as remote as ever. Casting about for new possibilities, researchers speculated that perhaps combining AZT with the more recently approved drugs ddI or ddC might improve the outlook. In fact, as early as 1985, at the first international conference on AIDS, researchers had discussed the possibility of using combinations of drugs that would address several aspects of immune breakdown at once.[3] Combination therapies already were being used effectively in treating other diseases, such as tuberculosis and childhood leukemia. Since there finally were in 1993 three approved drugs for HIV, it seemed to make sense to try them together.

Cut forward two years, and the beginnings of a very different picture began to emerge. In January 1995, the World Health Organization reported that there had now been more than one million AIDS cases worldwide—70 percent in Africa, only 9 percent in the U.S., and very likely four and a half times less than the actual number because of underreporting. The same month, David Ho, director of the Aaron Diamond AIDS Research Center in New York, and George M. Shaw of the University of Alabama in Birmingham, reported one of the most important research findings about HIV to that point. Rather than lying dormant for an indeterminate time until starting its virulent campaign of destruction, as scientists had believed for years, HIV was active from the time it infected someone. Ho and Shaw reported that, in fact, upwards of one billion new viruses are produced a day. A healthy immune system each day generates about that many CD4 cells, the main targets of HIV. For a time, the immune system keeps the virus in check; gradually, however, HIV gains the upper hand and CD4 production can't keep pace with the virus's reproduction, until the virus finally vanquishes the immune system altogether. Ho pointed out that it was now evident that the goal of drug therapy should be to inhibit the virus's ability to reproduce.[4]

By the end of 1995, the Food and Drug Administration (FDA) had approved 3TC, another drug in the same family as AZT, to be used in combination with AZT. In early December, the agency approved saquinavir, the first of a new class of drugs called protease inhibitors. While the earlier drugs such as AZT and 3TC, called nucleoside analogues (the "nukes"), interfered with the gene-replication cycle of HIV, the protease inhibitors blocked an enzyme used by the virus at a later stage of its reproduction. "This is some of the most hopeful news in years for people living with AIDS," said Donna E. Shalala, secretary of Health and Human Services.[5] The FDA demonstrated that it had learned its lesson about accelerated approval, taught by AIDS activists, approving saquinavir in record time. The agency broke its own record only three months later, on March 1, 1996, approving a second protease inhibitor, ritonavir, only seventy-two days after its manufacturer applied for approval. Two weeks later, the FDA approved yet a third protease inhibitor, indinavir, the most effective of the three new drugs. FDA Commissioner David A. Kessler was quoted as saying, "We now have some big guns in AIDS treatment."[6]

Two important innovations came to prominence in 1996: the use of viral-load testing to measure the amount of virus circulating in an individual's bloodstream and combinations of protease inhibitors with the older class of "nuke" drugs. Viral-load testing allowed doctors to tailor treatment individually to the needs of each patient. The drug combinations produced such dramatic results that even veteran scientists spoke of its being an unprecedented turning point in the treatment of HIV. Together, these two new "weapons" made 1996 a year of great moment in the history of the AIDS epidemic.

When scientists gathered in Vancouver in July for the Eleventh International Conference on AIDS, the air was electric with excitement and anticipation about the findings on combination therapies to be reported during the meeting. "By trumpeting the gains in glowing terms in advance of the meeting," noted Lawrence Altman in the *New York Times,* "a number of leaders in AIDS research and drug companies have transformed the pessimistic mood that has prevailed at the last several international meetings to one of exuberance."[7] Triple-combination drug "cocktails" were the talk of the day as researchers excitedly discussed how they had successfully reduced the amount of HIV in many infected individuals to undetectable levels, with corresponding increases in CD4 counts that would seem to indicate a rebounding immune system.

"For the first time since the early days of the epidemic," the *New York Times* editorialized after the international meeting, "scientists seem actually to be gaining ground in treating a viral menace that has been largely incurable and almost invariably fatal." The newspaper, however, noted several caveats that had been raised about the new protease inhibitors and drug combinations, including: possible severe side effects such as kidney stones and nausea; the difficulty of taking more than fifteen pills a day, some with food and others on an empty stomach; the possibility that HIV would develop resistance to the drugs if the regimen wasn't followed precisely; and the exorbitant cost of the drugs themselves. Add to the list the fact that the drugs were not working for everyone, or worked for a while and then stopped, and the relatively short period of time in which the combinations had been studied. "But even after all the caveats," continued the *Times,* "it is hard to minimize the dramatic shift in thinking that has occurred." Of course, the newspaper noted, the drugs would do no good at all if one didn't know his HIV antibody status. More than ever before, antibody testing was an essential first step toward getting treatment if one was infected.[8]

Going several steps beyond the exciting possibility of managing HIV infection, scientists speculated—and news headlines prompted some, apparently, to take the speculation as fact—as to whether the drug combinations might actually eradicate HIV from the body. For the first time in the epidemic, scientists and activists alike allowed themselves to utter the word "cure," savoring its monosyllabic elegance even as they asked a question whose implications were chilling: What if the virus continues to hide, reproduce, and develop resistance somewhere in the body where current tests can't detect it? Writing in the *New Republic* shortly after the Vancouver meeting, noted AIDS researcher Jerome Groopman said it was too early to call the inroads made against HIV a cure. But, he added, the three-drug combinations had "cause[d] the microbe to stumble severely." Even if a cure was not yet at hand, Groopman concluded, "the question has become 'when' rather than 'if.' "[9]

In early November 1996, two of Groopman's patients who were having exciting results from the drug cocktails used their access to the news media to describe their personal experiences with the new drug combinations, raising hope and stirring controversy about what many viewed as optimism that didn't jibe with the hard facts of life for most of the world's HIV-infected people. In a front page article in the *Wall Street Journal,* the newspaper's own page 1 editor, David Sanford, described his back-from-the-brink experience made possible by protease inhibitors. "The year 1996 is when everything changed, and very quickly, for people with AIDS," wrote Sanford. "I've outlived friends and peers, and now I find myself in the unusual position of telling people how I've survived this scourge, something I never thought would happen." With his CD4 count rising and viral load continuing to fall, Sanford had found renewed optimism for the future. "I am planning to one day retire with my partner of twenty-eight years, who is HIV-negative," he wrote.[10]

Two days after the publication of Sanford's article, a cover story in the *New York Times Magazine* by former *New Republic* editor Andrew Sullivan boldly described his vision of what happens "when AIDS ends." Sullivan acknowledged the caveats raised about the drug combinations, then hastily dispatched them to describe the experience of having faced mortality and lived to tell about it. Because of the new drugs, and others in the development pipeline, wrote Sullivan, "a diagnosis of HIV infection is not just different in degree today than, say, five years ago. It is different in kind. It no longer signifies death. It merely signifies illness."[11] Unfortunately, Sullivan's article focused almost exclusively on people like himself: white, middle-class gay American men with private health insurance and the best medical care available. The announcement that the "end" of AIDS was at hand would certainly be a surprise to the overwhelming majority of the twenty-three million people infected with HIV worldwide at the time, most of them poor, uninsured, and fortunate merely to have access to a rudimentary drug like AZT.[12]

Sullivan was duly chastised in the news media for what credible scientists and activists agreed was, at best, a premature declaration of the end of the epidemic. "We might be at the beginning of the beginning of the end," wrote AIDS reporter Mark Schoofs in an opinion article in the *Washington Post*, "but that depends on our resolve. If we let hope lapse into triumphalism, then we might well squander the promise of the new medicines and perhaps create an even more intractable epidemic." Schoofs noted that many researchers believed the new medical regimens would have only a limited benefit. Even if the new drugs could cure people, he cautioned, "it is simply folly to talk about the end of AIDS" because of the continued absence of an effective vaccine and the risk that HIV will develop resistance to the new drugs.[13]

The excitement continued to mount nonetheless, even as phrases like "cautious optimism" became the preferred way to couch one's hopes for the new drug combinations. New York City officials made a startling announcement in January 1997: For the first time since the recognition of the AIDS epidemic in 1981, deaths in the city from the disease had dropped sharply in 1996. Dr. Mary Ann Chiasson, the city's Assistant Commissioner for Disease Intervention Research, said the number of people who died from AIDS in New York fell 30 percent, to 4,944 in 1996, from 7,046 in 1995. Chiasson attributed the drop to the increased use of the new drugs (noting, however, that the protease inhibitors were so new that they were unlikely to have contributed significantly to the decline in 1996) and the increased availability of federal funding to pay for more and better AIDS care.[14]

As more exciting reports of treatment successes emerged in 1997, AIDS researchers and activists continued to caution against premature declarations of victory. "These new treatments are like hope with an asterisk," said Los Angeles AIDS doctor R. Scott Hitt, chairman of the Presidential Advisory Council on HIV/AIDS.[15] Besides the caveats already noted, the "asterisk" might well be the fact that not everyone with HIV would have access to the new drugs. The AIDS drug-assistance programs in twenty-eight states didn't yet cover protease inhibitors. Other states faced a flood of requests for the drugs that threatened to push them into a funding crisis. Some states, including Indiana and Missouri, went so far as to organize lotteries to determine which patients would get the treatments. As New York treatment activist Bill Bahlman put it, "We don't know what the future will bring. There's great potential there, and we already have tremendous results. The thing is to make sure this isn't just a couple-year lapse in the sickness and dying. The future scares me as much as it presents great opportunity."[16]

Moisés Agosto, director of research and treatment advocacy for the National Minority AIDS Council, tempered his excitement as he described his own experience with combination treatments. "Cautious optimism" is a hard but realistic outlook when things are looking so good after you've had a brush with your own mortality that gives you a personal kindredness with the biblical tale of Lazarus. In fact, activists were calling experiences like Agosto's the "Lazarus Syndrome." When Agosto started on protease inhibitors, his CD4 cells were in the twenties, and had been under fifty for three years. He was starting to get sick and his parents came to be with him after he'd lost a lot of weight, had microsporidium, shingles, drug-resistant thrush, and esophagitis. "It was a scary moment because I had no other options for treatment," said Agosto. Then came the protease inhibitors. "Now," he said, "my last T-cell count was two hundred eighty-six—from in the twenties. And it changed my health. It was remarkable. I got weight back. I'm making plans for the future."

Still, Agosto cautioned, realism is paramount. "I'm still afraid of what could happen," he told me. "If my viral load starts going up, I'm going to freak out. But I had two hundred eighty-six T-cells four or five years ago. Who knows, if I can have that stabilize maybe four or five more years, until there are another few drugs. . . ." His voice trailed off. Then he concluded, "Buying time—that's the way I personally see it."[17]

Buying time was everyone's goal; paying for the drugs was another story. Calling protease inhibitors the "rich man's drug," *Out* magazine noted that the cost of combination therapy that includes protease inhibitors and other antivirals can range up to $14,000 a year, excluding the costs of drugs to prevent opportunistic infections and expensive services such as viral-load tests, which typically cost about $200.[18] Describing what he called a "good news/bad news AIDS joke" in the *New York Times Magazine,* Larry Kramer noted, "For the first time an awful lot of people who thought they were dying are saying, 'Maybe we'll live through this plague after all.' And an awful lot of people should be thinking, 'If I can afford it.' "[19]

As it had been throughout the AIDS epidemic, access to information about the new treatments was still as potentially important as the treatments themselves. As *POZ* magazine publisher Sean Strub told me, "From the first days of the epidemic, access to information has been equivalent to survival."[20] But poor people of color, among whom HIV continued to spread, typically haven't had access to the same informational networks as privately insured, well-connected middle-class gay men. "Patients and doctors need to understand how to utilize these drugs," said Agosto, "because if you don't use them properly, if you're not following the rules, you're sabotaging your own health."[21] And risking your life. Lawrence Altman pointed out in the *New York Times* that many people fail to complete even the simplest course of antibiotics for common infections. "In AIDS," he wrote, "skipping just a few doses can be fatal because it can allow drug-resistant strains of HIV to take over."[22]

Unfortunately, even the efforts of advocates like Agosto and the National Minority AIDS Council to educate people of color about the new treatments faced more obstacles than just the cost. For many African-Americans, the shadow of Tuskegee hung over anything to do with medicine. Many refused the promising treatments for fear that they would once again become unwitting guinea pigs. Stephen B. Thomas, director of the Institute of Minority Health Research at Emory University, said, "It doesn't matter what breakthroughs we have. If the community doesn't accept it, it might as well not exist."[23] Even in California, where a generous drug assistance program enabled anyone who needed the drugs to get them, distrust of the medical system and the medicines themselves, coupled with a persistent stigma attached to HIV and the behaviors through which most people contract it, were making minorities miss out on the "revolution" in AIDS drugs.[24]

Attitudes in the hard-hit black community were unlikely to change any time soon towards either AIDS or medicine. Nearly two full decades into the epidemic, and with an estimated one in fifty black men, and one in 160 black women, infected with HIV—and accounting for 43 percent of all U.S. AIDS cases, despite being only 12 percent of the population—leaders of the black community still ignored the reality of AIDS. "Eyes shut, black America is being ravaged by AIDS," said the *New York Times* in a page-1 article.[25] At a Harvard AIDS Institute forum on the impact of AIDS among African-Americans, in March 1998, Henry Louis Gates, Jr., director of Harvard's W. E. B. DuBois Institute for Afro-American Research, said, "We didn't get any major black leaders to come to this. These guys don't want to touch this with a ten-foot pole." He added, "It's disgusting to me."[26] In May, the Congressional Black Caucus called for the federal government to declare a state of emergency because of the rapid spread of HIV among minority communities in the U.S., a symbolic move since there were no emergency funds available beyond the annual $3 billion the government was already spending on AIDS.[27] One had to wonder: Why the sudden concern? Could it have had anything to do with the public criticism of the black leadership's apathy by a black leader of Gates's stature?

Things were no better among Hispanics. Accounting for more than one in five American AIDS cases—109,252 cases as of June 1997—it was only in May 1998 that a national coalition of Latino leaders met to draft a plan to fight AIDS among their people. Ingrid Duran, director of the Washington office of the National Association of Latino Elected and Appointed Officials, said, "AIDS really isn't an issue that NALEO has given much attention to. . . . It's been seen as a gay and lesbian issue—not a Latino issue." Duran said that the 5,400-member NALEO would lead efforts to sponsor an AIDS education meeting for the twenty-member Congressional Hispanic Caucus.[28]

Despite the same old denial in the nation's minority communities even as their own people were devastated by AIDS, ever-optimistic Americans proclaimed a "new era" in the AIDS epidemic.

Indeed, the continuing drop in AIDS deaths in this country was astounding. National figures showed that for the first six months of 1997 alone, AIDS deaths in the country had declined 44 percent. News headlines continued to proclaim the good news: "AIDS Deaths Drop 48 percent in New York." "California AIDS Deaths Plummet 60 percent." "No Obits," proclaimed San Francisco's *Bay Area Reporter* in August 1998. For the first time in more than seventeen years, the gay weekly contained no AIDS-related obituaries. The full-time reporter whose job was to edit the obituaries had left two months earlier because there was so little to do.[29]

Yet other news stories revealed just how premature the victory celebrations really were. As many as half of those who had been "revived" by the drug combinations were failing.[30] A survey by GMHC found that nearly three-quarters of its clients taking protease inhibitors had missed a dose in the previous three months—one in ten of them missed a dose on the very day they participated in the study.[31] A telephone survey of 655 people revealed that 43 percent of them had not adhered to their drug treatment regimen.[32] As if the failure rates and nonadherence weren't alarming enough, an estimated ten to twelve million new cases of sexually transmitted infections—mostly spread in the same ways as HIV—were being reported each year to the Centers for Disease Control.[33] Throughout the world, the United Nations estimated there were now 16,000 new HIV infections each day.[34]

Deaths attributed to "complications associated with AIDS" would, unfortunately, continue to appear in obituaries into the foreseeable future.

*

For the time being, the implications of being able to live reasonably well with HIV infection reverberated beyond the many individuals for whom the drug cocktails were having salubrious effects. By early 1997, viatical settlement companies—whose business it is to wager on the imminent demise of people with life-threatening illness by buying their life insurance policies—were in a state of panic because of so many fewer clients. Peter Freiberg reported in the *Washington Blade*, "Some firms folded, some are no longer purchasing policies from people with AIDS, and many are offering significantly less money for policies than previously." But the industry's travails were in inverse proportion to the hope raised by the new drug treatments. Kiyoshi Kuromiya, director of Critical Path AIDS Project, an electronic treatment information network, said that while people with AIDS "don't have as much of an asset" in selling their life insurance policy, they had something far better. "They have a future," he said, adding, "I'd rather have that. I'd rather have a reason to live."[35]

With the advances in treatment and new hope, AIDS service organizations, long used to assisting clients mainly during the more advanced stages of AIDS, now faced the challenge of retooling their services to accommodate those who were more healthy than sick, and looking forward to longer lives rather than facing certain death. As Sandra Thurman, a former director of AID Atlanta appointed by President Clinton in 1997 as his third AIDS "czar," put it, "We're in an incredibly pivotal time in the epidemic where we are looking at how to help people live rather than how to help them die. It's a huge shift logistically as well as psychologically."[36]

Instead of helping clients deal with declining health, AIDS service providers were now helping at least some of them find jobs. In 1998, the city of Boston launched a "Reentering the Job Market" initiative to help people with HIV who were doing well with the drug "cocktails" go back to work.[37] And in Chicago, Howard Brown Health Center and Test Positive Aware Network in 1998 formed programs to offer clients career guidance, interview skills, job skills, and legal advice on privacy rights and health care benefits.[38]

The "new era" in the epidemic brought a number of challenges to AIDS service organizations. Now that people were living better and longer, the giving public saw less need to donate money to fund AIDS services. As a result, Daniel Zingale, director of AIDS Action Council, said that at least half the council's 2,400 member organizations had cut their budgets in 1997. With fewer AIDS deaths, the NAMES Project was one of the hardest-hit groups, slashing its $5 million budget by 30 percent. In Boston, revenue from the 1997 AIDS Walk dropped $400,000, forcing AIDS Action Committee to reduce its $10 million budget. AIDS Project Los Angeles's 1997 dance-a-thon brought in $250,000 less than in 1996. After GMHC launched a campaign around the theme "Keep on walking, we're not there yet," more people than ever participated in the 1997 New York AIDS Walk, but they raised $400,000 less than in the previous year. New York's 1998 walk raised $800,000 less than in 1997. By early 1998, the world's oldest AIDS organization was described as "beleaguered," as dwindling donations forced it to cut its budget from $30 million to $25.5 million and to eliminate some of its 260 staff positions.[39]

Expanding optimism and shrinking donations forced some AIDS service organizations to consolidate operations, explore alternative fundraising techniques, and provide accountability in a way they hadn't done since the CARE act's hundreds of millions had fertilized so many thousands of seedling groups throughout the country. The AIDS Resource Center of Wisconsin, for example, merged with five smaller regional organizations and increased its overall budget from $7 million to $8.5 million. Director Doug Nelson said, "There is not any question it was time for us to make sure we were the most cost-effective in our operations."[40] And in neighboring Minnesota, Lorraine Teel, director of the Minnesota AIDS Project, assured contributors that, despite "isolated naysayers" who criticized the AIDS industry, her agency's total overhead costs were less than 18 percent. "We are good stewards of donated funds," she said, "and we are able to maximize the donor's dollar."[41]

There was more talk of "mainstreaming" AIDS services as the epidemic increased among poor people of color. AIDS Action Council's Zingale said that the organizations formed by white gay people early in the epidemic have both an opportunity and an obligation to share their experience with minority communities in particular.[42] Besides giving up what Gil Gerald calls the gay community's "sentimental attachment" to the organizations they created, "mainstreaming" would likely alter AIDS "exceptionalism"—the special "set aside" of funding in the Ryan White CARE Act and treatment of HIV as unique among Americans' medical needs. Even in the early nineties, the National Academy of Sciences noted that as AIDS affected fewer white gay men and more poor, politically disenfranchised people, the exceptions that gay advocates gained for AIDS had already begun to wane.[43]

For early leading AIDS advocates in Washington, though, carving out exceptions for AIDS was never the long-range goal, even if that is precisely what the government did in the Ryan White CARE Act. Former AIDS Action Council director Jean McGuire said, "We evolved in resistance to and in the face of public neglect. But we'll never be able to keep up with the momentum of the epidemic." She added that integrating AIDS services in mainstream organizations was always the ultimate goal.[44] McGuire's former colleague Tom Sheridan concurred. "Building a new mousetrap just for the AIDS epidemic," he said, "was not sustainable for the long term from political or financial perspectives. There shouldn't be any clinic in America that isn't doing HIV and AIDS-related services."[45]

At the 1995 Seventh National AIDS Update Conference, in San Francisco, Mervyn Silverman said in a panel discussion on specialized versus integrated HIV medical care, "We have to mainstream the AIDS patient because, one, there are not enough HIV 'specialists' to care for all of them; two, everyone needs to understand how AIDS relates to their specialty; and three, setting AIDS apart makes it a target."[46] Silverman elaborated in a follow-up interview, "It needs to be mainstreamed because of homophobia, people trying to compartmentalize it and not see it as a problem for them. We can't continue to have an AIDS unit in a hospital—every physician needs to care about it. At the same time, we can't normalize it like 'Cancer Month' and then forget it."[47]

Of course mainstreamed HIV care would mean that gay men with HIV are cared for by health care providers who aren't necessarily gay themselves. This raises the question as to whether we weren't risking going "back to the future," returning to the situation at the start of the epidemic when gay people formed their own parallel health care and social service systems because they didn't receive sensitive care by mainstream providers. Would gay men with HIV—regardless of their race—receive appropriately sensitive care? What role could AIDS-specific organizations continue to play in their care?

These questions were answered in Chicago in the formation of a unique collaboration between Howard Brown Health Center and nearby Illinois Masonic Hospital. To provide HIV clients with a "continuum of care" that includes a full range of medical and hospital services, the gay clinic and the hospital agreed to what amounted to a mutually beneficial affiliation. The health center offered the hospital access to HIV and other gay patients, and the hospital guaranteed to provide gay-friendly services. Howard Brown executive director Eileen Dirkin attributed the hospital's interest in the arrangement to an article about gay and lesbian health care in *Modern Healthcare,* which portrayed the gay community as an untapped and potentially lucrative market for mainstream health care providers. Besides the potential profit, Dirkin said the hospital was interested in being perceived as a "good neighbor" by creating a welcoming environment for the diverse people who live in the Lakeview area.[48]

Besides improving and increasing its HIV health services, Howard Brown's board president Frank Pieri noted that the arrangement allowed the agency to expand its range of services to address the many other health concerns gay people have besides HIV. "There are more and more men who are getting older now," he said, "who have been essentially 'out' since their early twenties, for most of their lives. As they get older, and as they have other health concerns, I think they are going to demand services that are gay-friendly." He pointed out that gay men in their forties and fifties have the same health risks and concerns—such as prostate cancer and heart attacks—as their heterosexual counterparts. Yet, he added, "All of these issues have not been looked at because we have been so overwhelmed by AIDS, so preoccupied. It really has caused us to be so narrow-focused because it has been so overwhelming." But other health concerns would have to be addressed, because of course death is the final issue in every life. As Pieri put it, "It'll be interesting to see when people start losing lovers in twenty or twenty-five years to a heart attack if that's going to be acknowledged as being as much of a loss as a lover lost to AIDS at forty. Is one loss perceived as more tragic than another?"[49]

Or, to rephrase the question, is one serious health problem more important than another if each is disruptive, even threatening, to its respective sufferer's life? Should a gay man with a heart problem get a different level of care than another gay man who has HIV? Should a lesbian have to settle for possibly insensitive care by a mainstream provider because the gay health clinic is so overwhelmingly focused on HIV care? In society at large, the question is whether anyone, no matter what their diagnosis, should receive less than the level of services carved out specifically for people with AIDS. Ken Mayer, the infectious disease doctor at Boston's Fenway Community Health Center, says, "There has to be more to life than AIDS."

Clearly, AIDS brought in resources to help build the expertise and capacity of the gay health clinics. But, Mayer noted, "If you don't take into account the fact that there are next generations, there are survivors, and a community grieving," you lose sight of the need for ancillary services, such as mental health services, as well as the reality of most gay people's lives. Given the range of health needs beyond HIV that are as varied as the people who have them, Mayer told me, "It becomes ludicrous to build all these programs for the community you serve around this one disease. This is *one* disease that has an impact, and people have complex lives."[50]

It wasn't only because HIV was so prevalent among gay men that it overshadowed other gay health services. Funding, both from the federal government and private sources, was far more abundant for HIV services than for other gay or lesbian health needs. At the same time, the fact was that fundraisers spent most of their time raising AIDS dollars because the issue was visible and the money there for the asking. For example, of the $12.3 million spent by Washington, D.C.'s Whitman-Walker Clinic on programs in fiscal 1995, only $791,788—about 6.4 percent—went for non-HIV programs including lesbian, mental health, and alcoholism services. Ninety-eight percent of the clinic's $8.4 million in government grants, United Way, Combined Federal Campaign, and donations from clients was designated for AIDS services. Whitman-Walker's medical director, Peter Hawley, said, "AIDS is so overwhelming, consuming, and visible that I think sometimes we lose sight, even those of us who work here, of all the gay and lesbian-specific things we'd like to do." But the clinic's acting director of development estimated that less than 10 percent of his department's time was spent on non-AIDS fundraising.[51] This begged the question: Was there so little money for non-AIDS gay and lesbian health programs because it was unavailable—or because Whitman-Walker fundraisers spent so little time trying to generate it?

There certainly seemed to be a greater interest in broader gay and lesbian health issues in other quarters. Christopher J. Portelli, executive director of the National Lesbian and Gay Health Association (NLGHA) at the time of our interview, said that gay health clinics and other health care providers that constitute the association's membership were in fact recognizing that while HIV would be with us for the foreseeable future, they must also address other health concerns of gay men and lesbians. "We're soon going to see a new mission of these lesbian and gay health clinics," he said, "as we begin to deal with the fact that HIV and AIDS are not going to go away, and that we need to take care of our health needs and the problems we have with access to health services, and to become model institutions, if you will, of services to our community of an entire panoply of primary care needs, not just HIV/AIDS-related services."[52]

The American Medical Association itself took a stronger interest in the health needs of gay people. In a 1996 report, the AMA urged physicians to make a greater effort to "recognize" when a patient is gay. The AMA's Council on Scientific Affairs noted that as few as 11 percent of primary care physicians routinely take a sexual history from their new adult patients. Without the information provided by a frank and nonjudgmental sexual history, the AMA noted, doctors often failed to "screen, diagnose, or treat important medical problems," including HIV and other sexual diseases.[53] Joe O'Neill, the principal author of the AMA's new policy on gay and lesbian patients, noted that although there are few physiological differences between gay people and heterosexuals (there are different manifestations of sexually transmitted diseases, and different risks for certain cancers among lesbians) "ultimately the most important issues are around access to care, and on the psychiatric or psychological end." The greatest change in the AMA's policy, he said, was in "not medicalizing or pathologizing the homosexual patient."[54]

Two and a half decades after gay people convinced the medical establishment to view them as "normal," the nation's leading medical organization finally acknowledged that physicians need to educate themselves about the health needs of their gay and lesbian patients.

Chris Portelli sees the shift in the AMA's position as the result of a "second wave" among health care providers serving gay people, stemming from the recognition that "AIDS isn't an isolated and single problem, but rather it's connected to our whole body, our whole self, and how we approach life." Besides AIDS, though, he said it also is due to a growing number of gay and lesbian health care workers "coming out," and an increased number of gay health programs throughout the country. He also noted that one of the most crucial factors in raising the gay community's awareness of broader health issues was a political one.

The election in 1992 of Bill Clinton, after his overtures to the gay community during the campaign and his promise to reform the nation's health care and insurance system, raised the hopes of gay and lesbian health care professionals that at last the health needs of gay people would be taken seriously in a reformulation of the system many Americans found so lacking. Portelli said there was much excitement that finally the government "would begin to listen to the story about how, in the midst of government neglect, the community learned to mobilize and take care of itself." He added, "We all hoped, upon hearing that story, the government then would fling open its coffers and help us go the next step, which would be to shore-up that self-care and all of those nonprofit health centers that, at that point, were surviving on private donations and very little government assistance."[55]

But then, as Portelli put it, the great national discussion about health care reform in 1993 "went nowhere." Those with vested interests—mainly the insurance industry—pumped millions of dollars into a campaign aimed at maintaining the status quo. Just as suddenly as Bill Clinton the candidate had proclaimed health care the nation's number one concern, Clinton the president let this concern be pushed back out of sight and out of mind—though it was very much on the minds of the forty-one million uninsured Americans and the millions more who had been herded into managed care plans and HMOs whose business it is to make profits by spending as little as possible for actual health care.[56] For people with HIV, as for anyone affected by chronic or life-threatening illness—especially those who are poor—health care and insurance continued to be priorities of the first order, even if they were no longer a national priority.

Though there have been significant improvements in the level and variety of AIDS-specific services available under the Ryan White CARE Act, the epidemic highlighted the flaws in the nation's health and insurance systems. Early in the epidemic, Ginny Apuzzo warned at a congressional hearing, "This disease, left unchecked, will bring down health care in America." Even though it didn't exactly bring it down, AIDS did raise important questions about the nation's health care system and its ability and willingness to respond to a public health catastrophe. Apuzzo, now the highest-ranking openly gay staff member in the Clinton White House, says, "The epidemic certainly confronted this country—the richest, most advanced country in the world—with the fact that it was not prepared to deal with a public health emergency." While she believes the federal government ignored AIDS as long as possible because of those it was affecting, Apuzzo, like other politically astute advocates, sees the situation in broader terms. "I believe that AIDS is every single crisis this society has looked at and ignored historically," she said. "I believe it's sexist. I believe it's racist. I believe it's homophobic. I believe that the face of AIDS is homelessness and drug addiction. It's all the things politicians have said they want to address and never touch."[57]

Tim Westmoreland, who organized the early congressional hearings on AIDS, says the main flaw in the health care system that AIDS highlights is its emphasis on acute illness rather than early intervention and prevention. "We have a health care system whose financing schemes are focused on taking care of people in their last stages of death and dying," he told me. Even AIDS advocates and service providers focused mainly on caring for people who were already infected with HIV, particularly in the later stages of the disease. But whether it's the federal government, insurance companies, or AIDS advocates, Westmoreland said, "It's not an accident that this occurs in a nation where we don't fix our bridges until they fall down on the highway. It's a national thing, not just in health, it's in everything that we don't do something until it's a crisis."[58]

Former AIDS Action Council director Dan Bross told me that the organization seemed to face an uphill battle in getting AIDS service organizations to understand the relevance of their work to broader discussions of health care. "It's difficult to get ASOs to see their interest in legislation and policy discussions that don't have 'AIDS' specifically on them," he said.[59] But building strategic alliances with non-AIDS organizations would be essential to ensuring that HIV services continued to receive attention and funding. In the larger scheme of things, notes Jean McGuire, the most important issue behind discussions of reforming any of the components of the nation's health and social welfare systems was something as intractable as it is ignored. "The truth," she said, "is that if our systems really want to learn from what happened in AIDS, they have to take up poverty, and I don't see that happening. After we saw such a defeat with health care reform, I think one thing that will have to happen is things will have to get much worse before there's a will to change them."[60]

Prompted by the broader issues that AIDS has raised about America's health care system, the Robert Wood Johnson Foundation by the mid-nineties had resumed its pre-AIDS focus on broad, systemic health issues rather than focusing specifically on single diseases such as AIDS. The foundation that led both the nation's private philanthropies and the federal government to fund AIDS services recognized that AIDS is in many ways a case study of the larger issues in the health care system in general, including access to care, the drug approval process, antidiscrimination protection for people with chronic illness or disabilities, and the linkage of health insurance to employment. RWJ's Paul Jellinek explained, "We began to realize that in every case we were running up against the same systemic problems. While you might be able to get a Ryan White CARE Act—by definition an 'emergency,' an exception to the rule—there were no real changes to Medicaid, for instance, and you still had to wait two years for home and community services." Jellinek said RWJ is now advocating for the kinds of policy changes that benefit people with all kinds of health challenges. He pointed to the Americans with Disabilities Act as an example of reform that, for RWJ, "represents a higher level of change" because it benefits people with a variety of disabilities rather than any one group.[61]

Cliff Morrison recalls that when he traveled throughout the country to work with local communities as part of RWJ's AIDS program in the late eighties, "People would say AIDS would be the straw that broke the camel's back." More than anything, he said, the AIDS epidemic "highlighted the cracks and flaws in the system." True as this was, people like Morrison found ways to fill some of the cracks and minimize the flaws. When Morrison created the AIDS unit at San Francisco General Hospital, in 1983, the unit's client-centered approach was viewed as a radical departure from the usual physician-centered approach to health care. But, says Morrison, "I kept saying to people I think this can be a model for other things in the institution, doing what we do for these patients for *all* patients. People were asking whether I was coddling this particular group of patients, bending over backwards. I said no, attitudes in health care had to change."[62]

If their long-term viability was in question, the AIDS service organizations formed by gay people certainly provided at least partial and impressive solutions for the short term. As AIDS fundraising pioneer Michael Seltzer puts it, "We showed some of the solutions of the health crisis in America through the organizations we put in place that were community-based, volunteer-driven, and provided low-cost health-care-related services that kept people out of expensive hospitals. That's something we as lesbian and gay people can be proud of. Our agencies are models for better health care delivery for this country." What's more, notes Seltzer, AIDS advocacy provided a model for people with other kinds of diseases and health concerns. "Now you have people with breast cancer using ACT UP tactics," he said, "because we demonstrated that people have to take control of health care."[63]

As both a onetime target of ACT UP and the federal government's top AIDS scientist, Tony Fauci says that gay people certainly were effective advocates and left a powerful legacy for others. Although there had been some degree of consumer activism in health care before AIDS, Fauci said, "I think the gay community has brought that to its now prototypical art form for a number of reasons. It's dangerous to generalize, but fundamentally the gay community that's evolved is a very competent, highly intelligent, well-placed, experienced, politically adept group. So when you get a group like that whose lives are on the line, and they decide they want to become consumer activists, they become one hell of a consumer activist!" Whereas advocates for other diseases typically are heterogeneous— "You've got old people, young people, people who are at various socioeconomic levels," said Fauci—the majority of those advocating on behalf of AIDS benefited from belonging to the gay community. "You put the gay community together," he said, "and you have a very highly polished, educated, well-placed group that, as a group, has been more effective than many other consumer 'groups' were."[64]

As effective as this community has been, though, heightening consumer awareness of health care issues has been merely a by-product of gay people's efforts to bring attention to AIDS and the flaws it revealed in the health care system. For gay men and lesbians, the more fundamental issue has consistently been that of fairness and equality for all citizens in the far bigger enterprise known as the United States of America. As former GMHC director Tim Sweeney puts it, "We are working toward a transformation so that, hopefully, next time there won't be such social bias when it comes to a disease."[65]

But the social bias against gay people, and political bias against disturbing the status quo, continue to prevent the kinds of reforms that would make AIDS, and any other health emergency that might come along, a top priority as well as a situation that can be managed effectively by a well-designed and equitable health care delivery system. Paul Boneberg, who now works on international AIDS issues, likens the role of gay people in the AIDS epidemic to that of the "canary in the coal mine" used by miners to test the safety of the air in a newly opened shaft. If the canary dies, the miners leave and try a different approach. He explained, "We're like the canary saying, 'Hey, trouble! There's a problem here.' We're saying it when one canary dies, and they keep going. Then another canary dies. And that's exactly what's happening to our people. They get sick, and the last thing the canary says is, 'Be careful, take care of yourself, it's really bad.' And nobody wants to listen to the canary." For whatever reason—though it's almost always money and politics—Boneberg added, "Those miners want to move forward to the point that they don't care that the canaries are all dying, or what's being said."[66]

How many more "canaries"—gay men, poor people of color, those considered "expendable"—would have to die before the United States finally found the political will to try to save them? What would it take before the nation's leaders did something that truly mattered in the fight against AIDS and other life-threatening illnesses, such as funding realistic and useful prevention efforts? Or creating a health care system in which people with a life-threatening illness don't have to worry about losing their health insurance when they become too sick to work? Or demanding fair pricing of drug treatments and providing funding support so that no one who needs them will have to go without them? Would all the "miners" have to be affected in a more personal way?

*

Lost in the excitement over the new combination treatments for HIV was the fact that "men who have sex with men" continued to account for the largest proportion of new HIV infections in the country,[67] and that there continued to be a lack at the national level of any real emphasis on prevention strategies that work. Even in the gay community, there has been a resounding lack of passion for prevention, despite the fact that vastly more gay men are at risk for HIV infection than those already infected. In a 1996 article in the *Washington Blade*, Tom Coates, director of the AIDS Research Institute and the Center for AIDS Prevention Studies at the University of California–San Francisco, and Mike Shriver, now the policy director for the National Association of People with AIDS, noted that gay men had done well in arguing for the "right" to HIV treatment. But, they asked, "What about the right to be protected from HIV in the first place?" The new treatments are exciting and should be pursued wholeheartedly, said the HIV-positive authors, adding, "Blindly running after the promise of a cure, regardless of tantalizing hope, is never to be an excuse for abandoning HIV prevention."[68]

As viral loads declined with the use of protease inhibitors and drug "cocktails," so did the practice of safe sex, at least for some men. Almost as soon as it was revealed that the amount of HIV in the body could be suppressed to undetectable levels in some people, the question arose as to whether it was now safe to have unprotected intercourse—assuming that a low viral load meant a low chance of transmitting HIV (notably, this was only an assumption).[69] Michael T. Isbell, associate director of GMHC, said, "The very hopeful developments around the protease inhibitors may make our jobs as educators even more difficult." Besides the premature "all clear" some inferred from the promising effects of the new treatments, the new challenge to prevention educators was in part the result, oddly enough, of the educators' own success in giving hope to HIV-positive people. Ben Schatz notes, "The HIV service sector has been saying, 'You can have a full, vibrant life and be HIV positive.' The more people believe this to be true, the less likely they are to believe that contracting HIV is the worst thing that can happen to them."[70]

Others also challenged the message about living and "thriving" with HIV. If it's such a seemingly benign condition, they asked, why bother trying to avoid contracting HIV? "We talked about 'living with HIV' or 'living with AIDS,' " says psychologist Walt Odets. "If these men are thriving with AIDS, what's so important about my not having HIV? Saying these men are thriving with AIDS, but it would be better if you thrived without it, got awkward." To avoid the awkwardness, prevention messages tended not to distinguish between HIV-positive men and those who were uninfected. Formulated before the HIV antibody test made it possible to know who is and isn't infected, the messages blurred the lines so as not to make those with HIV feel "left out" by aiming to keep HIV-negative men uninfected. But, said Odets, "We're not going to keep men negative by saying you're going to have to live with the same limitations that HIV-infected people live with because that's the only socially acceptable way."[71]

Odets argues that HIV-negative men were for too long "abandoned" because of the necessity to care for those with HIV and AIDS. But the epidemic affected HIV-negative men profoundly, he said, even if they were not infected. If we are serious about preventing new infections, prevention education must accept that people are going to make individual choices based on their own and their partner's HIV antibody status, their understanding of the information available to them, and their personal values. Odets contends that prevention aimed at uninfected men—primary prevention, as opposed to secondary prevention, which targets the already-infected—must acknowledge the psychological realities of being a gay man at a time when AIDS has been so closely identified with gay men that many use the terms "AIDS community" and "gay community" as though they are synonymous.

To illustrate the point, Odets recalled a focus group conducted in San Francisco to investigate the psychological issues with which gay men are dealing. After an HIV-positive man complained about uninfected men "whimpering all the time about survivor guilt," Odets said an HIV-negative man pointed out that, although he didn't have HIV, he did have ten or eleven dead friends and a dead lover. "I don't know what you want to call that," Odets recalls the man saying. "But I feel like I've got a problem, too."[72] Odets likens uninfected men to a family's "good child," presumed not to have any needs by parents who are preoccupied with other problems, possibly another child who is sick or needy. But, he contends, anxiety, depres-

sion, loneliness, and homophobia—now even more insidious because of a common association in the minds of many, including some
gay men, of homosexuality with a lethal disease—are serious needs
that must be attended to if gay men are to remain uninfected and
survive the epidemic.

Tom Coates says prevention efforts must become more sophisticated, incorporating what is known about motivation and behavior
from the behavioral sciences, and including a variety of approaches.
"As the epidemic evolves," he told me, "the reasons people have unsafe sex also change over time. What we don't understand is what's
going to motivate people to stay safe in the long haul. The only way
we can do that is by constantly keeping our ear to the ground, talking
to people."[73]

As important as listening to people's concerns, though, Coates
says accountability in the community and individual responsibility
are two key determinants of whether the gay community will continue to reduce, if not eliminate entirely, new HIV infections among
gay men. Whatever one's personal view of sex clubs, for example,
Coates said it is incumbent upon the community to discuss their
pluses and minuses. Speaking during our interview of the Crew Club
in Washington, D.C., Coates said, "Maybe as a community we need
to get a grip, be controversial, challenge one another. Should this
bathhouse on Fourteenth Street be open? Is it a very good thing for
this community?" On a personal level, he noted, the community
hasn't told gay men to find out, first of all, whether they are positive
or negative, and, if positive, to care enough for other people, their
brothers, not to want to infect them. On the other hand, fear of
alienating those who are infected has kept the community from telling the uninfected their lives will be better by staying uninfected. "I
think we fear our community is too fragile to withstand that kind
of division," said Coates. "But if we're a strong community, we ought
to be able to tolerate that kind of diversity."[74]

The matter of either personal or communal responsibility has
not been popular in a community that prizes sexual "freedom." Many
men believe it to be the responsibility of the passive partner in anal
intercourse, if he is HIV-negative, to insist his partner use a condom.
For example, nearly a third of the men in one study who knew they
were HIV-infected at the time they engaged in unprotected anal in-

tercourse reported thinking, "I may be infected already, but if this guy is willing to fuck without a condom that's his affair. I'm not responsible for him." At the same time, almost one in five uninfected men reported thinking, "If this guy was really infected, he'd be a lot more careful about taking a risk than he's being now. The fact that he's willing to fuck without a condom means he can't be infected."[75] Strangely, the views of both negative and positive men echoed the heterosexual male chauvinism that sees the woman as responsible for birth control—only in this case, with two men involved, each assumes the other should be the responsible one, though the stakes are considerably higher than an unwanted pregnancy.

Among those who challenged the "political correctness" that was loath to insist upon responsibility by the HIV-positive partner was a gay man with AIDS who admitted to episodes in his own sexual history of not informing his partners that he was infected. Washington, D.C., AIDS activist Greg Scott said, "None of us, when we go for testing and counseling, are truly told that we're supposed to be responsible—that we, as HIV-positive people, have an enormous, grave responsibility in this. A lot of the politics of it have been about a fear of stigmatizing positive people. It's an attempt to equalize all people in this fight, but it's a lie, because those of us who are infected have very different responsibilities than those who are not infected."[76]

Of course personal responsibility implies individual choice, which means that some people will make different choices than others, based on the same information and their own values. If they are to be held accountable for their choices, those choices also must be respected, even though they may differ from the choices that prevention educators might like them to make. As Eric Rofes puts it, "Equating education with prevention and giving lip-service to individual agency in sexual matters is the core contradiction of safe sex campaigns." He added, "Education under democracy aims for people to govern themselves, invent their own lives, and accept responsibility for their actions."[77]

In recognition of the individual choices and differences in gay men's sexual practices, the terms "harm reduction" and "negotiated safety" came up regularly in the nineties in discussions about reshaping HIV prevention for the foreseeable, AIDS-haunted future. Simply described, harm reduction, an approach long used in the treatment of substance abuse, aims to reduce the negative effects of harmful behavior. If a man is going to engage in unprotected sex, for example, the potential harm (HIV infection) could be reduced substantially by having less risky unprotected oral, rather than extremely high-risk unprotected anal, sex. Sexual partners with the same serostatus are said to negotiate safety when they agree not to use condoms during intercourse, since for two uninfected men, HIV is not present, and for two positive men it is already there so neither risks becoming infected. One Australian study found that in fact negotiated safety was widely used by gay men, particularly among couples in which both partners were seronegative.[78]

In 1995, Boston's AIDS Action Committee launched an HIV prevention campaign for gay men that respected their right to choose their sexual practices, and helped inform their choices by providing frank information about the differences in possible risk between oral and anal sex. The campaign was innovative, even radical, in that it acknowledged the realities and ambiguities of gay men's lives in the ongoing epidemic, rather than the kind of black and white, all-or-nothing approach that prevention educators had used for years. In a series of ten small posters, targeted to gay men of different ages and races, and placed in the men's rooms of gay bars, AIDS Action Committee offered messages such as, "Oral Sex *Is* Safer Sex. . . . Oral sex is much less risky than anal sex. Unprotected anal sex is responsible for almost all HIV transmission between gay men. If we all agree to use condoms when we have anal sex, we could end this epidemic." The risk reduction campaign, aimed at both infected and uninfected men, emphasized the importance of remaining HIV-negative, using images of both negative and positive men to convey the message. One poster pictured a man, probably in his late twenties, who says, "Honestly, I wish I were negative again. . . . If you are negative—stay that way."

Although oral sex has been one of the "gray" areas of sexual behavior—low-risk but not zero-risk, as the Gay and Lesbian Medical Association deemed it in 1996—some doctors and AIDS educators resisted saying so frankly lest gay men do with impunity what virtually all of them had been doing anyway throughout the epidemic: having oral sex without condoms.[79] AIDS Action Committee director Larry Kessler said that those who saw the campaign as controversial missed the point. "Some people think we're pushing oral sex," he said, "and miss the risk reduction nature of it all."[80]

In addition to the poster campaign aimed at reducing "harm," AIDS Action Committee aired a thirty-second public service ad on local television stations, intended to increase the self-esteem of gay men. Brian Byrnes, director of AIDS Action Committee's gay male education program, said, "It is often difficult for us to convince gay men at risk of HIV infection to care for themselves and their sexual partners when the messages they receive about themselves are so negative." The agency borrowed the ad from Seattle's Northwest AIDS Foundation, which created it in response to public health studies indicating that a gay man's reducing his risk for HIV infection is directly correlated to his self-esteem and sense of self-worth. The ad aimed to break down negative stereotypes of gay men, and concluded with the message, "Ending AIDS begins with pride."[81]

Like growing numbers of gay health professionals, Dana Van Gorder, coordinator for lesbian and gay health services in the San Francisco Department of Public Health, believes that issues of well-being should take precedence over technical information about HIV. He explained, "Gay men had major psychological issues before the epidemic came along, and the epidemic made it worse. So many gay men feel they live in isolation, and that they've lost their biological families *and* support networks."[82] Stacked against the pain of living, the risk of HIV infection—particularly at a time when new treatments are so promising—may seem for some a reasonable price to pay for a bit of intimacy with another person. But, Van Gorder argues, if prevention education is going to work it must first help gay men to value and protect themselves in order to live and be well for a brighter, hopefully AIDS-free, future.

In a series of articles for the *San Francisco Sentinel*, Van Gorder described how HIV prevention for gay men has become far more than a medical issue. "HIV prevention should no longer be thought of simply as the effort to keep gay and bisexual men free from HIV," he wrote, "but as a movement to help them grow old, valued, and fulfilled." The first step, he noted, "is an uncensored, community-wide discussion about all of the factors that challenge our ability to remain uninfected."[83] Underscoring the interrelationship between gay men's personal choices and their relationship to the community,

Van Gorder told me, "Somehow the community has lost sight of the notion that it needs to provide for its future and for its survival. Some people have to be willing to stand up and say, fine, you get to make your choices—yet we also need to encourage you to make sure you make a good choice, an informed choice, and that you make the choice within an environment in which you are comfortable that you have come to the right conclusion."[84]

In the earliest days of the epidemic, Donald Krintzman, the first person with AIDS ever to be interviewed in the press, recognized that the key to dealing with the AIDS epidemic just then beginning to break out among gay men was going to be the gay community's ability to pull together and keep everyone focused on a future free of AIDS. "If we embrace the community concept," said Krintzman, "if we can engage our collective intelligence, courage and maturity, our emphasis will be on the overcoming rather than on the suffering of this disease."[85] Only two years later, *Washington Blade* editor Steve Martz observed that the term "gay community" had already taken on new meaning because of the way gay people had responded to AIDS. Wrote Martz, "One can tell where a true sense of community exists by the way its members treat the weakest among them and, by that yardstick, the compassion that gays are showing to those afflicted with AIDS is a wonderful sign of strength."[86]

From a historian's point of view, John D'Emilio observes, "For better or worse, the AIDS epidemic has helped to foster, at least among some of us, a sense of community in its fullness that we might not have felt before." He added that the widespread experience of sickness and death among gay men has "created an emotional level of connection that extends further for more people." The greatest challenge to gay individuals and the community as a whole, said D'Emilio, continues to be homophobia—which gay people still too often turn in upon themselves. "The fact that gay men are still seroconverting tells us something about the complexity of what sexuality is all about," he said, "but also how we've underestimated the power and depth and insidiousness of homophobia. If our lives were easier, without the effects of our oppression and the ways we've internalized it, safer sex would be a lot easier to be integrated into our lives because the desire for sexual passion and intimacy and connection would not have this added layer of desperate meaning attached to it that the oppression creates."[87]

Another challenge to the community's ability to help gay men imagine healthy and long lives is, paradoxically, its very willingness to do its own prevention campaigns, care for those with the disease, and push for political attention and public financial resources to underwrite the costs of prevention and care. Laudable and necessary as these efforts are, they have had the unwanted effect of linking gay people with the epidemic in a way that has made it difficult for many, gay and nongay alike, to separate gay identity from AIDS. Even the cultural outpouring inspired by AIDS has resulted in once again linking homosexuality to a medical diagnosis—precisely what gay people, like Larry Mass, feared early in the epidemic.

The art created by gay people in the AIDS years unwittingly conveyed a sense that AIDS was their only concern. Not only was this grossly reductionist, it was harmful to the broader efforts of the gay civil rights movement to show gay people as multifaceted human beings—just like heterosexuals. Gay writer and GMHC cofounder Edmund White, living with HIV himself, disputed the view that AIDS is, as some argued, the only "legitimate" subject for gay writers and artists. Said White, "Gays, even in their own eyes, get reduced to a single issue, which is after all a medical one. There is a kind of 'remedicalization' of homosexuality going on, which I find very dangerous."[88]

Since the early seventies, the community has sought to counter the negative, even pathological, images of homosexuals by nongay people and gay people themselves who may be uncomfortable with their own sexual orientation. One way it has done so is in the creation of community institutions, places where people can share their lives with others like themselves and feel at home. For a community now suffering the twin plagues of homophobia and HIV, community institutions offer safety and solace. As Ginny Apuzzo put it, "We need institutions where people can bring the grief and the pain and the despair and find a way to relieve it."[89]

One community institution that predated AIDS adapted to the community's needs in the epidemic and now looks to a future beyond it. This is the Gay and Lesbian Community Services Center in Los Angeles, the largest gay community organization anywhere. The center has played a pivotal role in nurturing gay people through the epidemic and is, according to its director Lorri L. Jean, helping them to imagine a healthy, even happy, future in spite of—and hopefully beyond—AIDS. "We live in a society that tells us from the day we're born that there's something wrong with gay and lesbian people," said Jean, "and many buy it." At the heart of the center's programs, she said, is an effort to build self-esteem. She explained, "We try to show people that you can be gay or lesbian and 'out,' and you can lead happy and productive lives, that your future is not just one of sadness and discrimination and bigotry, but that we do have some power over changing our lives. Part of that is about hope. We try in all our programs to promote hope and self-esteem because if you feel good about yourself, even if you have HIV or AIDS, you [will believe that you] are unique and worth preserving."[90]

The important work of gay community institutions like the center notwithstanding, many gay men have looked outside the community itself for a sense of connection and support that transcends sexual orientation. For Dana Van Gorder, it was a matter of interacting with heterosexual friends who, because they didn't live in the war zone he did, where so many young men have died, could remind him that life is for the living. "I had to look outside the community for support and to gain perspective," he told me. "When I talk to my straight friends in Los Palos, and they say 'are you staying safe?' there's an assumption on most [gay] people's part that that's homophobic, that they're meddling in my sexuality. The point is that they don't want to see you getting sick, they love you."[91]

Others, particularly gay men of color, have found identity and support in their ties to families and communities to which they belong through race and ethnicity, religious faith, or culture. For Randy Miller, connection to the black community provides a source of strength and perspective. While many gay men, particularly white men, leave their families for places like San Francisco, Miller notes that other "paradigms" are available. One of them, chosen by many minority gay men, is to stay in one's community of origin and figure out how to live as an "out" gay person among family and childhood friends, drawing on the community's sense of shared history and response to life's vicissitudes. "As a black gay man," said Miller, "I draw on my community's sense of history about dealing with slavery and oppression for hundreds of years in this country." What this has meant, said Miller, is that although AIDS has been "a horrific thing," it doesn't rattle his sense of personal identity the way it has for many white gay men whose identities are bound up strongly in their sexual orientation. "It's a horrific thing like many horrific things I have to survive," he said.[92]

For the Reverend Carl Bean, being connected to the broader world is not only important in coping with AIDS but in life generally. "It has never attracted me to be in a Castro or West Hollywood," he said. "I like talking to the old lady in my building in L.A.—she has a nephew who is gay. She's a delight, a wonderful woman. I have a Russian couple who moved over here recently, and we talk. There's gay folk in my building, and there's Asian folk, black folk, Jewish folk, Greek folk. To me, that's humanity. Coming from a past of segregation, I don't understand wanting to create segregation. How are we ever going to love, share, bring about these things that we say our country is built on if we're afraid to know each other?"[93]

One gay institution that fosters a spirit of community among gay people doesn't have the word "gay" in its name. San Francisco's Café Flore has been drawing coffee drinkers and people watchers since 1974. NAMES Project founder Cleve Jones had been a regular for more than twenty years, and had been interviewed earlier in the day for a history of the café, when we talked about the always hopping coffee shop on the edge of the Castro district in San Francisco. Psychologist John Newmeyer described Café Flore as a community institution ideally suited to usher young gay men in particular into the gay community. He noted that comfortable, welcoming places like Café Flore are especially important when, as he and others expect, young gay men will continue to represent the leading edge of the ongoing AIDS epidemic in the United States. Newmeyer predicts that upwards of 15 percent of young gay men in San Francisco alone will ultimately be infected.[94]

Clearly prevention aimed at young gay men must be a top priority for the gay community and the nation, and community institutions must welcome and support them. But what of the not-so-young gay men who continue to be at risk for HIV infection? AIDS advocates often speak of the young men at risk, overlooking the fact that the emphasis among many gay men on the young, and youth in general, has been an important obstacle to the ability of older men to look to the future and embrace the idea of a healthy, long life. As Dana Van Gorder put it, "It is fairly clear gay men are experiencing a lot of problems 'growing up' and dealing with the transitions in their lives from sexually attractive men in their twenties, whom everybody is sort of after, to men in their thirties, forties, and early fifties, and feeling that they don't look quite as good anymore and can't quite figure out how to deal with that transition."[95]

In a 1996 *New York Times Magazine* essay called "The Wrinkle Room," author Andrew Holleran, whose despairing novel about a middle-aged gay man, *The Beauty of Men*, had just been published, lamented the passing of youth and voiced the uncertainties of being an "older" gay man in a youth-obsessed culture. "Wrinkles, of course, are not confined to gay men of a certain age," wrote Holleran. "Gay men's identity, however, is thought to be based, more than most people's, on being *un*wrinkled." He described a film star who, now old, was unrecognized as he emerged from a nightclub. He then described a gay friend who, at forty-five, was obsessed with being let into a popular night spot called Club U.S.A. "In this mindset," wrote Holleran, "the doorman at Club U.S.A. does become the Grim Reaper, and a certain estrangement ends up feeling like ostracism."[96]

Fortunately, not all older gay men concurred with Holleran's bleak assessment. In a follow-up letter to the editor, septuagenarian composer and writer Ned Rorem observed, "When Andrew Holleran, age fifty, defines gay men's identity as based, 'more than most people's on being unwrinkled,' where does that leave me, age seventy-two, and my contemporaneous gay friends? Like everyone, we sowed wild oats, but as the bloom faded, we readjusted our tempo and talents to the inevitable, and did so as individuals."[97] Many older gay men, particularly those who had suffered the losses of the AIDS years, also recognized the importance of being mentors and role models for younger men. Arnie Kantrowitz, about to turn fifty-six a week after our interview, found great satisfaction in helping young people avoid the terror of coming to grips with their homosexuality. Speaking of his own sense of isolation as a young person, he said, "What a difference it could have made for me to have contact with someone."[98]

Still other men responded to the existential issues raised by aging and loss through the time-honored means of parenting. Boston psychiatrist Marshall Forstein told me, "I come from a family that has always instilled in me how important connectedness is with the people who came before and will come after. I think where gay culture has suffered is in our unwillingness to see our connectedness over time." He explained that his own decision to adopt a child, more than a decade earlier, grew out of a desire to leave a legacy in the world. "I'm not saying parenting is the answer to the question of generativity," said Forstein, "but it's the particular route where I have addressed my issues of what I'm contributing to the world, what I leave behind, and how I find a place in the marching on of time." He added, "I think for so many years gay people lived in a world that said you are not acceptable the way you are, you are intrinsically defective. Well, with those internalized beliefs, why would you care about leaving something behind?"[99]

Torie Osborn believes there is a direct correlation between the AIDS epidemic and the seeming upswing in the number of gay men raising children, what she called a "gayby boom." Said Osborn, "There's a huge transformation of values, a huge resurgence of spirituality and of connecting to kids. If I look at my friends across the country, gay and gay-identified, the people who are coping the best with the epidemic are the ones who have kids in their lives and straight people in their lives." One example, said Osborn, was her HIV-positive male friend who decided to adopt a child. She recalled him saying, "I want to see life at the beginning. I think I will die sooner if I don't stop seeing life only at its end."[100]

Unfortunately, the efforts of gay people to enjoy the fullness of life remain limited by the homophobia of American politics that forces them to be second-class citizens. The support of same-sex marriage that people like Larry Mass called for in the earliest years of the epidemic as a means of channeling the sexual energy of gay men away from unsafe situations and into committed relationships is as ignored in the late nineties as it was in the early eighties. When President Clinton signed the so-called Defense of Marriage Act, in 1996, he claimed he did so merely to silence an "unpleasant debate" about whether gay people should have the legal right to wed and the same benefits that heterosexual couples take for granted.

If gay people thought they had somehow "proven" themselves by responding with compassion and humanity in the AIDS epidemic, they were brutally reminded all over again of their outlaw status in American society as states raced to join the federal government in denying equal rights for gay men and lesbians through measures to prevent the recognition of same-sex marriages. A Valentine's Day 1997 issue of the *Washington Blade* reported that when Mississippi two days earlier became the seventeenth state to ban legal recognition of same-sex marriages, Republican Governor Kirk Fordice proclaimed, "For too long in this freedom-loving land, cultural subversives have engaged in trench warfare on traditional American values." He added, "These radical subgroups have distorted the national agenda and defiled time-honored customs for their own selfish purposes. Today, the state of Mississippi takes a significant step to protect the foundation of a healthy society."[101]

As conservative politicians protected their fear- and hate-driven versions of a healthy society, gay people continued to create new ways to protect their lives. "Healthy people are more likely to make healthy choices," observes University of Minnesota psychologist and sex educator Simon Rosser. "Rather than beating people over the head with a technological argument about needing to use a condom, we need to face the tougher question about how to build a healthy community because in the long term it's going to be healthy people who will make a difference in the epidemic."[102] Gabriel Rotello in *Sexual Ecology* describes this as "transformative change," which, he says, involves "the integration of sexuality into the whole of life, a life that respects sex but does not make it the central point of existence."[103]

Just as it launched nationwide trends in rock music and gourmet-coffee drinking, Seattle in the mid-nineties pioneered a new, integrated approach to prevention education for gay men that promised to revolutionize the field and revitalize the gay community by viewing prevention as a subsection of gay community-building. In 1996, a Seattle group called Gay City Health Project electrified an audience at the National Lesbian and Gay Health Conference, held in Seattle, with its vision for the health and well-being of the gay community. The group's director, John Leonard, described Gay City's vision this way: "Imagine no more poignant memorial services. No more 'twenty-

something and HIV-positive' support groups. No more AIDS protests, no more AIDS fundraisers. And no more fucking red ribbons.
Imagine a future of equality, diversity, community. Imagine a time
when gay men count gray hairs, not T-cells. Imagine a world where
we're raised to love ourselves as healthy, whole, and beautiful. Imagine a place where holding hands is not an act of courage. And having
sex is not against the law. Imagine no more fear, no more grief.
Imagine no more new HIV infections."[104]

From its beginning as a county health-department task force exploring prevention options for gay men, Leonard said, "Gay City
wasn't just about something bad that we wanted to prevent, but
about something really good that we wanted to create." The group's
mission, he explained, is "building community, promoting communication, and nurturing a culture where gay men see their lives as
worth living." Drawing on well-established educational models, the
group created its programs in response to what they heard from
gay men. Said Leonard, "We were told to build community, build
connections among gay men, build a greater sense of responsibility among men for each other, and help men feel better about being gay."

In January 1994, Gay City held the first of a series of extremely
well attended forums, "Why Are Fags Still Fucking Without Condoms?" Three hundred people attended. I asked Leonard how people
reacted in the forum when men spoke up about their unsafe sexual
experiences, a taboo subject among gay men who looked at prevention educators as authority figures. "I remember a collective sigh of
relief that finally somebody was saying it," he said. "I don't think
anybody was shocked because I think on some level we knew that
we weren't being good little boys all the time, but it wasn't okay to
talk about and people did and do feel a lot of stigma admitting that,
especially if they're HIV-positive."

Hundreds more have showed up at subsequent Gay City forums,
each one dedicated to timely issues such as dating, oral sex, coming-
out, relationships between HIV-positive and HIV-negative men,
drug and alcohol use, and other topics of interest to gay people that
don't, at first blush, look like HIV prevention. More than seven hundred participated in a May 1996 forum on "charting our futures"
featuring lesbian activist Urvashi Vaid. A forum on gay history the

following month grew out of one young gay man's standing up in an earlier program and saying, "I don't know who Judy Garland was. Talk to me about pre-Stonewall. It would help me feel better about the gay community and other gay men to know a little about where I came from."

As Leonard explained, "We talk about how you need more than just condoms and practice putting them on a banana to practice [safer sex] over the long run. You need to address broader social issues, and those have to do with self-esteem and feeling a part of a community that you feel connected to." He said that gay men in Seattle have responded very positively to Gay City's positive vision. "In the surveys we do," he told me, "people report that coming to forums, even if not directly about HIV prevention, has an impact on them that makes them leave the forums feeling more pride and connection to the gay community, and feeling greater motivation to practice safer sex and take care of their health."[105]

In 1998, similar programs were launched at the nation's two oldest AIDS organizations, GMHC and the San Francisco AIDS Foundation. In a series of small workshops, GMHC's new "Beyond 2000" program encouraged gay men to examine and discuss how their own sexual behavior fit in with their ideas about masculinity, sex, and drug and alcohol use. The AIDS Foundation's new program, "Gay Life," was intended to create a sense of community and build self-esteem. Rene Durazzo, the foundation's deputy director of programs, said, "Gay Life was constructed in appreciation for the fact that men's whole lives impact their sexual decision-making." Based on a study by the University of California–San Francisco, and funded equally by the city and the foundation, the new program featured a major publicity campaign, forums, social events, one-on-one and couples counseling, and a "Black Brothers Esteem" group for African-American gay and bisexual men. Like Seattle's Gay City, the foundation's program included a series on gay culture and community history. More than anything, it recognized and affirmed the individual decisions gay men had been making throughout the epidemic. Said Durazzo, "It was important for us to step back and refocus and resituate ourselves in relationship to those decisions, to be less health educators and more facilitators and supporters of men finding safe places to self-reflect and sort through the decisions they want to make."[106]

The reinvention of HIV prevention not only marked an adjustment to the fact that gay men would continue to be affected profoundly, but it signaled a maturing, sophisticated community that was once again creating its own ways to survive and thrive even amidst the ongoing assaults of HIV and homophobia. Helping to make gay men aware of their history and invested in their community, and increasing their understanding of the political implications of their personal behavior, could only serve to strengthen the gay civil rights movement. At the same time, reinforcing the pride and self-esteem of individual gay men offered them the support they needed if they were to greet their "future worth living for" with open arms, strong hearts, and the desire to savor life's sweetest pleasures after knowing too well and for too long its bitterest realities.

*

"People with AIDS are dying!" shouted the heckler from the 1,500-member black-tied, evening-gowned audience at the Grand Hyatt Hotel in Washington, D.C. "Sit down!" yelled others in the audience. They weren't yelling at the speaker on stage but at the gay man among them who'd had the temerity to shout his rage. Was it Larry Kramer heckling Ronald Reagan's first speech on AIDS in 1987? Hardly. This was an orgy of mutual admiration. "We love you, Bill!" erupted repeatedly from the crowd who'd paid hundreds to see and hear Bill Clinton become the first sitting president ever to address a gay rights group when he spoke on Saturday night, November 8, 1997, at a $300,000 Human Rights Campaign fundraising dinner. Clinton once again warmed gay hearts—as he'd done in his first campaign, if rarely afterward—by quoting his predecessor Harry Truman's speech to the NAACP fifty years earlier, vowing equality for all Americans. "And when I say all Americans," Truman said, "I mean all Americans." Clinton added, "Well, my friends, all Americans still means *all* Americans."

With his trademark political panache, Clinton addressed—and dismissed—his heckler. "People with AIDS *are* dying," he said. "But since I've become president, we're spending ten times as much per fatality on people with AIDS as people with breast cancer or prostate cancer. And the drugs are being approved more quickly. And a lot of people are living normal lives. We just have to keep working on it." The audience gave him one of many standing ovations.[107]

Applause was the furthest thing from the minds of the Presidential Advisory Council on HIV/AIDS a month later when it issued a "progress report" that harshly condemned the Clinton administration's efforts on AIDS. After beginning by saying that, yes, Clinton had been the first president "to take serious action to address the AIDS crisis," the thirty-member council said the administration "has sometimes failed to exhibit the courage and political will needed to pursue public health strategies that are politically difficult but that have been shown to save lives." In particular, said the group, federal prevention efforts were still ignoring recommendations to provide "frank, explicit, culturally relevant HIV prevention information to those at risk for sexual transmission." Like the Reagan and Bush administrations, the council said the Clinton administration "has failed to lay out a coherent strategic plan of action." The report noted that upcoming measures of the administration's commitment on AIDS would include its proposed AIDS budget for 1999 and its actions on needle exchange as a prevention measure for the ever-growing number of injection drug users at risk for HIV infection.[108]

The president's proposed 1999 budget indeed offered increased funding for AIDS programs, a total of $3.9 billion for AIDS research and services—a $314 million increase over 1998. Of that amount, $1.3 billion would go for Ryan White CARE Act services, a 14 percent increase. Another $385.5 million, a 35 percent increase, would be allocated for the AIDS Drug Assistance Program. The federal AIDS housing program would increase 10 percent, from $204 million to $225 million. And the National Institutes of Health would receive an additional $124 million for AIDS research, bringing its share of the AIDS budget to $1.731 billion. As for HIV prevention, Clinton proposed to increase the CDC's HIV prevention budget by $5 million, for a total of $637 million. In actual fact, the increase wasn't even for AIDS prevention per se but for a special program aimed at curtailing inequities in health care for minority communities. Nevertheless, Clinton's AIDS policy advisor, AIDS "czar" Sandra Thurman said, "This is a statement by the president that his resolve to ending this terrible epidemic remains firm."[109]

The firmness of the president's resolve was called seriously into question only two months later when Clinton stunned Thurman, his secretary of Health and Human Services, his own HIV/AIDS council, AIDS advocates, and scientists alike when he unexpectedly announced on April 20 that, despite scientific evidence that needle-exchange programs help to curb the spread of HIV among drug users, federal funding could not be used to support such programs. Although Health and Human Services Secretary Donna E. Shalala, like most of the administration's senior health officials, had argued that funding needle-exchange programs made sense, Clinton's political heart went with Barry R. McCaffrey, the retired general who heads the Office of National Drug Control Policy. McCaffrey persuaded Clinton that funding needle-exchange programs would open the administration to criticism that it was "soft on drugs." So Clinton declared that—despite findings from the National Institutes of Health that the programs were effective in reducing the spread of HIV, and despite the endorsement of the AMA and the National Academy of Sciences—they would have to get along without the federal government's support.[110] Dr. R. Scott Hitt, chair of the president's HIV/AIDS council, said, "At best this is hypocrisy. At worst, it's a lie. And no matter what, it's immoral."[111] The *New York Times* said, "Instead of making a principled decision, President Clinton is fecklessly trying to appease conservatives with a policy that will cost thousands of lives."[112]

Some things never really seem to change in America, no matter which politician occupies the Oval Office. Ironically, just a year before Clinton had challenged the American scientific community to make an AIDS vaccine its "first great triumph of the twenty-first century."[113] As it had done since Reagan was president, though, politics once again trumped science when it came to preventing the further spread of HIV, if it meant upsetting conservative moralists.

As federal HIV prevention efforts remained captive to politics, and gay politicos patted one another on the back for landing the president at their exclusive dinner, ordinary gay people were as hated and persecuted as ever. The number of gay men and lesbians discharged from the military was higher than ever under Clinton's

"Don't ask, don't tell" policy, which the president had intended to allow gay members to serve so long as they "kept quiet" about their sexual orientation.[114] Nineteen states still had laws against sodomy, selectively enforced against gay men.[115] A study of high school students found that more than one-third of gay teens had attempted suicide; more than a quarter of them had "missed school because of fear for their safety" in the previous thirty days.[116]

Another study found that while middle-class Americans prided themselves on their nonjudgmentalism, they didn't hesitate to call gay people "sick," "perverted," and "mentally ill." An August 1998 *Newsweek* poll found that while most nongay Americans say gay people deserve equal rights in housing and jobs (83 percent and 75 percent), 54 percent believe homosexuality is a "sin."[117]

As the president of the United States answered questions from a grand jury about his own sexual behavior, the radical right exploited Americans' ambivalence about homosexuality to inject their particular brand of poison into the national debate. Never ones to miss a chance to show that behind their so-called "Christian love" was a frightening, even fascistic, level of fear-driven hate, a coalition of conservative groups—including the Christian Coalition and the Family Research Council—launched a high-profile campaign in the summer of 1998 aimed at portraying gay people as sick patients who could be "healed" through prayer and counseling. Hoping to pressure Republicans to toe their line as the November elections approached, the group sponsored newspaper ads quoting none other than the Senate majority leader, Trent Lott (R-Mississippi), who in June had likened gay people to alcoholics and kleptomaniacs.[118]

Across the country, the *Washington Blade* reported, "Gays are on the defense in matters of marriage and family issues, and on the offense in trying to secure basic protections against discrimination and violence." Despite a drop in serious crimes across the country, reported incidents of hate crimes based on sexual orientation actually rose 8 percent from 1996 to 1997, according to the FBI.[119]

In the rarefied air of the Human Rights Campaign's offices, things didn't seem that bleak. Heady from a sense of "power" from their evening with the president, HRC announced in early 1998 that, together with the Metropolitan Community Churches, they would sponsor a fourth national gay civil rights march on Washington in the spring of 2000. Shirking the consensus-building among gay community organizations that had gone into planning the three previous national marches, the "Millennium March on Washington for Equal Rights" was viewed by many national gay and lesbian activists as a power grab by HRC director Elizabeth Birch, a ploy to increase HRC's membership toward Birch's stated goal of one million members by 2000. Words like "self-aggrandizing" were used as often as "effective" in describing Birch, and her own words at times seemed to betray her—as in a 1998 profile in *Out*, which quoted her as saying, "Imagine what you would have done if three years ago you woke up and found that someone had handed you the movement."[120] But most gay activists, who for years had lamented their lack of a charismatic individual to focus and lead the gay civil rights movement—as Martin Luther King, Jr., had done for African-Americans—weren't quite as ready to anoint Birch as she herself seemed to be. Just as AIDS service organizations did with their arguments about the "needs" of people with AIDS, Birch sometimes conflated her organization's interests with those of "all" gay people.

Robin Tyler, a lesbian comedian and events promoter hired by HRC and MCC to "produce" the Millennium March, asserted that HRC enjoyed the support of the "overwhelming majority" of gay people in the U.S. Although no one has ever produced a reliable measure of the number of gay people in this country, it seems reasonable to say there are vastly more than the two hundred thousand—mostly white, more-affluent-than-not—who made up HRC's membership at the time it announced plans for the march. Nevertheless, said Tyler, "If there's anything we've learned from the nineties it's that the majority of this movement is mainstream. You can't deny this and there's nothing wrong with this."[121]

Gay people were certainly brought further into the mainstream of American popular culture in the nineties, even if they were still reviled, discharged, arrested for having sex, and otherwise treated like second-class citizens in their own country. "Lesbian and gay figures are becoming commonplace in mainstream media," wrote gay reporter David W. Dunlap in a 1996 *New York Times* article. "And established institutions are growing less timid in courting gay and lesbian audiences." Dunlap added that capitalism—the power of the almighty American dollar and the chance to tap into the alleged affluence of gay Americans—was a likely explanation for this growing interest in the gay "market."[122]

Not everyone welcomed the increasing "assimilation" of gay people. In the purplest prose and most sweeping of generalizations, Daniel Harris lamented in *The Rise and Fall of Gay Culture* that acceptance of gay people into the American mainstream meant the loss of an "ethnic" subculture as bitchy camp humor and the sense of always being an "outsider" gave way to what he saw as the bourgeois banality that characterized the mainstream. "The end of oppression," wrote Harris, "necessitates the end of the gay sensibility."[123]

Indeed, change was afoot. Even the stodgy *New York Times* had finally begun referring to homosexuals as "gay." Movie studios were producing more gay-themed movies than ever, even if they were still serving up gay stereotypes. Gay New York City police officers in 1996 marched for the first time in the city's gay pride parade, nearly three decades after the police raided the Stonewall Inn and set off the modern gay civil rights movement.[124] Arch-nemesis of the seventies Anita Bryant was now selling copies of her gospel-music cassette, "I Am What I Am" in the lobby of her Anita Bryant Theater, in Branson, Missouri. When she wrote the song, Bryant said, she had never heard Jerry Herman's song of the same name—the defiant show-stopper sung by a drag queen in the musical *La Cage aux Folles*.[125] In 1997, closeted lesbian comedian Ellen DeGeneres came out on her television show *Ellen* and the mainstream media couldn't get enough of the spectacle. The gay media that year lost a pioneering voice, the community's earliest source of information about AIDS, which had later lost all credibility by championing the most outlandish explanations of the disease, when the *New York Native* ceased publication.[126]

In 1998, gay people were still on America's mind—and even stirred Americans' hearts. When Wyoming college student Matthew Wayne Shepard was savagely beaten and left tied to a rail fence to die alone on a cold October night, front-page news headlines, outraged gay people, clergy, and even elected officials joined their voices in denouncing the violence against gay people. The *New York Times* editorialized on 17 October, the day of Shepard's funeral, "It is a murder that seems to have aroused the deepest sympathies of the nation, a case in which law, religion, love, dignity and politics all seem on the side of a dead young gay man. It is a rare moment, and politicians and preachers had better take a lesson."

In such a state of flux, perhaps it was natural that disagreement erupted once again among urban gay men about what it "means" to be gay. In arguments that harkened back to the seventies, a handful of gay academics and porn stars calling themselves "SexPanic!" claimed—like John Rechy's "sexual outlaw"—that promiscuity is the essence of gay culture. One SexPanic! member, Rutgers University English professor Michael Warner, said, "It is an absurd fantasy to expect gay men to live without a sexual culture when we have almost nothing else that brings us together."[127]

On the other side were prominent gay writers including Gabriel Rotello, Michelangelo Signorile, and Larry Kramer, demonized by SexPanic! as "neo-conservatives." In an op-ed article in the *New York Times*, Kramer wrote, "Promiscuous gay men must hear the message, 'Enough already! Haven't you learned anything from the last seventeen years?'" He added, "Fortunately, more and more gay people are beginning to realize that it's time to redefine what it means to be gay. Allowing sex-centrism to remain the sole definition of homosexuality is now coming to be seen as the greatest act of self-destruction."[128] Kramer's commonsense message was the same as it had been in *Faggots*—and he was still being reviled for it.

If Rip Van Winkle had fallen asleep in 1978, when *Faggots* was published and Kramer was vilified for daring to challenge the gay "norm" of promiscuity, and had then awakened to the arguments of SexPanic! twenty years later, he could have easily overlooked the fact that hundreds of thousands of gay men had died horrific deaths because of a sexually transmitted disease. On the eve of the AIDS epidemic, Edmund White—a forebear of SexPanic!—said that for gay men at that point there were "few ways besides sex to feel connected with one another." Without knowing how prophetic his words would be, White added that "in the future there might be surer modes for achieving a sense of community."[129]

Nothing was surer than the devastation of the AIDS epidemic.

Not only did SexPanic! flout the epidemiologic facts of AIDS, but it ignored the fact that gay men because of the epidemic now shared so much more than a priapic brotherhood of sexual rebellion insisting on a dubious "right" to promiscuity. Despite the many ways that gay people across the United States banded together to care for their own, and to preserve the memories of the community's terrors and triumphs, some continued to question the legitimacy of describing the nation's millions of gay men and lesbians as a genuine "community." But as overused a term as it has become by its application to groups of people who share even the vaguest of commonalities, gay people could indeed consider themselves a community by virtue of their sharing a profound experience and responding together to address it.

In *Habits of the Heart*, sociologist Robert N. Bellah and his colleagues observe that genuine communities are such because they share a past and look together to the future. "For this reason," note the authors, "we can speak of a real community as a 'community of memory,' one that does not forget its past." In order not to forget that past, they said, a community continually retells its story, "its constitutive narrative," offering examples of the men and women who have embodied and exemplified the meaning of the community. Besides tying us to the past by reminding us of our shared history, they said, genuine communities "turn us toward the future as communities of hope."[130]

I asked five gay leaders who played pivotal roles in the community's response to AIDS to reflect on the hard work and terrible cost of becoming a *genuine* community, a community of memory and hope. Cleve Jones said simply, "I think what we did mattered, and I think we did the right thing. Even with all the mistakes, stupidity, and suffering, I'm still proud of it."[131] Rodger McFarlane, whose personal phone line became the hotline that was the first AIDS service ever offered in the world, said, "Most people don't have a sense of their own power. They don't realize that one queen stepping outside a hospital administrator job and doing something different can make history." He added, "We made history and changed the lives of millions of people just by stepping out from our own roles."[132] Speaking of the AIDS services provided by the gay community, Paul Kawata said, "I think the infrastructure that we built as gay men while we lost what we lost was extraordinary, heroic, unfathomable—and our legacy."[133]

Ginny Apuzzo offered her own political vision in describing the political implications of the gay community's experience with AIDS.

"In this country, this movement will prevail," she said. "If we hang in there, where civil rights and human rights are concerned across the board, and go for the generic issue of oppression, then we can make a difference, and we will prevail, and we will make the country a better place. I think that we are this country's last, best hope because no other group has representatives in every corner of the oppressed world in this country. We cross every line."[134]

Gay people will continue to fill important roles in the ongoing epidemic and well beyond in the broader arena of social and cultural life, bearing witness in their words and deeds to the losses and the possibilities that constitute their experience of the AIDS epidemic. To accomplish this, a clarity of vision and certainty of purpose are the important second steps, behind the willingness to serve. "It's a war," said Reggie Williams. "It is a fucking war, and it has affected so many people's lives, taken so many precious, beautiful, talented people away from us." As painful as it has been for himself personally, living with AIDS and losing so many friends, "the reality is it *is*," said Williams. "And we've got to keep at it, we can't stop. When someone stops, someone has to pick up that sword and keep pressing on. Pick up the sword and keep fighting this battle to the bitter, fucking end, until it is out of our lives forever."[135]

Remembering the past is essential to the "future worth living for" that HIV prevention educators say gay men must imagine and work toward if they are to sustain themselves individually and the community in general. To preserve the collective memory of the epidemic and its effects, novelist Fenton Johnson says a "genuine" gay culture must emerge. Because one of the principal acts of culture is devising means of passing along wisdom, Johnson said, "It will be interesting to see whether ten years from now we have figured out ways of passing on what we have learned, or if in fact we have sunk into the general morass of materialism and consumer society and forgotten what we have learned out of this experience." Johnson noted that gay survivors of the epidemic have an opportunity and obligation to share the wisdom gained from their experience, in the hope that others may learn, too. "Fortunately, HIV is a passing phenomenon," he said. "But we have to preserve and remember what there is to learn from the passing phenomenon—just as the Jews are not engaged in the Holocaust now, but try actively to preserve its memory because of what it taught them, and what it can teach culture as a whole."[136]

Although AIDS is obviously not only a disease of gay men, preserving the painful "heritage" of the AIDS epidemic requires that the gay community claim it in a certain sense as a "gay disease," in that it has affected—and still affects disproportionately—so many gay men, even as it affects others. Ben Schatz observes that there are many in the gay community who have tried so hard to be inclusive that they're excluding gay men, which has, for example, hampered efforts to get proportionate prevention funding. He drew an analogy to the experience of the Jewish people and the Holocaust to illustrate how gay people can claim the uniqueness of their experience while respecting that of others. "Jews were not the only people who suffered in the Holocaust who need to be recognized," said Schatz. "Yet the Jewish community has never been hesitant to speak about the special situation of the Jewish community." Gay people were reluctant to make any claim that they were being treated differently, suffering in a particular way. "But," said Schatz, "the whole government response has been fashioned by homophobia. The way people view AIDS is profoundly affected by homophobia." When Schatz first raised the issue, in the late eighties, gay people—eager to "de-gay" the epidemic—resisted. But he persisted. "As long as you convey the message that we are unimportant and trivial," he told them, "you are enhancing the disease that is causing the symptoms we are suffering."[137]

Arnie Kantrowitz says that learning about the Holocaust—"carry[ing] that torch forever"—is his "way of being a Jew." He explained, "I got fascinated by human behavior in the extreme. And the concentration camps were that. For us, the epidemic was that, too." Although he doesn't subscribe to a theory that the AIDS epidemic was purposely unleashed for political purposes, like the Nazi Holocaust, Kantrowitz points out a number of parallels between the experiences of Jews during the Holocaust and those of gay men in the AIDS epidemic. "The effects on us were quite similar," he said, "being ostracized from others, in this case because they thought we were all infectious. You'd go to somebody's house and see that they were nervous seeing you drink out of a glass. Or parents pulling their kids out of school. It was a terrifying time."

When gay men were demonized by right-wing extremists and others in the mid-eighties, Kantrowitz helped to found the Gay and Lesbian Alliance Against Defamation (GLAAD) to counter the sometimes hysterical and fear-mongering portrayals of gay men in the news media. "As somebody who was so steeped in the Holocaust," he told me, "I felt tremors going on, like the same thing was about to happen. It's part of human psychology that it's very hard to hurt someone like yourself, so you have to make them a 'thing.' The Nazis went far with that, where they called trains full of people shipments 'of units.' They dehumanized them to a level where they talked about people as though they were countable stock. It was a very effective device and ready to be used again by anyone." Talk of quarantine was not taken lightly by people familiar with concentration camps. "I was terrified and so were a lot of people," Kantrowitz recalls. When GLAAD called its first meeting, five hundred people showed up. "That shows you that the mood of fear was widespread," said Kantrowitz, "not just that the epidemic would kill us but that our neighbors would run rampant, tattoo us, and isolate us."[138]

Besides the memory of terror and fear, Kantrowitz says that a powerful legacy of wisdom and hope has emerged from the devastation. In "Friends Gone with the Wind," he quotes a man named Filip Müeller, one of the inmates who emptied the gas chambers at Auschwitz, who described in the movie *Shoah* what he saw and learned from his horrific experience: "With our own eyes, we could truly fathom what it means to be a human being," said Müeller. "There they came, men, women, children, all innocent. They suddenly vanished, and the world said nothing! We felt abandoned. By the world, by humanity. But the situation taught us fully what the possibility of survival meant. For we could gauge the infinite value of human life. And we were convinced that hope lingers in man as long as he lives."[139]

It will remain a challenge to get nongay people to look at and learn from the experiences of gay men in the AIDS epidemic when heterosexuals, white American men in particular, typically have little if any understanding of the experience of being oppressed and marginalized. The profoundly human experiences of gay people in the AIDS epidemic too often have been brushed aside simply by viewing gay people as "them" and not part of "us." Fenton Johnson describes his own frustrating, embittering experience of speaking to a straight, educated, white man about his privileged place in the world, and realizing the man's complete obliviousness even as he complained of being discriminated against as a straight white man. Said Johnson, "This would be laughable if he weren't serious." Resisting the desire to either laugh or punch the man, Johnson realized his challenge was "to figure out some way to reach this person, enlightening him to the enormous grace that he has been given by virtue of his position in the universe so that he might realize how big the gift is that he has been given and how little he has done to deserve it."[140]

Lessons learned from the AIDS epidemic transcend the already artificial boundaries between homosexuals and heterosexuals, because they go to the heart of what it means to be human. But as with "coming out" as a gay person, the challenge for AIDS survivors is largely to live as witnesses to the horrors they have experienced and the changes they have wrought in individuals and the community. Bruce Patterson, the former GMHC hotline director, says, "You can't go through something like that without feeling a profound change going on inside. It's given us a perspective beyond our years."[141]

In the AIDS years, young gay men often found deeply human connections with considerably older people because of striking parallels in their experiences. In "A Woman of a Certain Age," John Preston described a Yankee matriarch in Portland, Maine, named Franny Peabody. In the twilight years of a long life, the Republican, Episcopalian shoe-factory owner was now a Democratic, Unitarian AIDS activist. Her grandson, Peter, died of AIDS early in the epidemic, and ninety-year-old Franny was determined to do everything in her power to help end for others the loneliness and social ostracism her own family experienced because of the disease. Over lunch with Preston, who hadn't told Franny of his own AIDS diagnosis, the pillar of Portland society described what she had learned from the gay men with AIDS she had known through her volunteer work on behalf of the AIDS Project of Southern Maine.

"Franny is seldom very emotional," wrote Preston. "She is, after all, a Yankee matriarch." But once, during lunch, there were tears in Franny's eyes. "My dear, it's so horrible," she said. "All *my* friends have died as well." Seeing that Preston was puzzled, Franny explained, "You see, my dear, all the people I know now are the children—sometimes the grandchildren—of the people I knew when I was young. The ones who are my own age are gone. I'm left calling sixty-year-old women 'girls,' and I sit and feel so alone some times. This is what you must be feeling." For her own part, Franny said, "At least I am no longer frightened of death."

Taking Preston's hand, she continued, "That's the one thing you young men have given me. You have shown me that one can die with dignity and with courage. I was so petrified of death, it was so frightening, but now I understand that death comes, that one can greet it with a sense of propriety. I've sat with so many men and watched life leave them. So many, and they were all so brave. You will be, too. You already are."

The two sat quietly a moment. Then Franny sat up, smiled, and said, "And now, my dear, how about a cocktail?"[142]

Like Franny Peabody, gay men in the AIDS epidemic learned to cope with the reality of death while getting on with the business of living. As a result of working with AIDS professionally and as a volunteer, and dealing on a personal level with the illness and deaths of so many friends, Bruce Patterson says, "AIDS has given me a new appreciation for life." At the "advanced age" of forty-one, Patterson said he was celebrating life by going out dancing once or twice a month. "That part of living, that joyous abandon is really something I don't take for granted anymore," he said.[143] After years of mourning, many gay men, like Patterson, rediscovered "the crazy compulsion with which we resolved all the tangled impulses of our lives— the need to dance," as Andrew Holleran put it in *Dancer from the Dance.*[144]

Boston psychologist Steven Schwartzberg likens the lives of gay men in the face of AIDS to the experience of driving past a grisly bus accident. "It looks terrible and awful," he said, "but then you remember there's dry cleaning to pick up." He added, "We need to remember that we are living with an ever-present bus accident—and we still need to pick up the dry cleaning."[145] Approaching the third decade of the epidemic, Eric Rofes says the fact of the ongoing epidemic and the need to look to a brighter future require a challenging psychological balancing act. "We need to accept the fact that AIDS has happened," he told me. "It's not about accepting that there might not be a cure in our lifetime, but it's about psychologically accepting the fact that AIDS has happened, accepting that people are dead and we're never seeing them again, accepting that we're going to be burying friends and lovers the rest of our lives, accepting the fact that our sexual lives have changed, accepting the way that in politics and the public image the linkage of homosexuality and disease and death are going to be there for many generations."[146]

When gay people come out of their closets and let nongay people know and love them for their true selves, when gay people stand up and insist without apology that their losses and heroism in the AIDS epidemic be counted—as they should be—among the greatest of human tribulations and accomplishments, and when nongay people finally acknowledge the full and shared humanity of gay people, the true magnitude of the AIDS epidemic in this country will be understood.

At an ACT UP rally in Albany, New York, on May 7, 1988, film historian Vito Russo, who died from AIDS in 1990, put it like this: "Remember that some day the AIDS crisis will be over. And when that day has come and gone there will be people alive on this earth: gay people and straight people, black people and white people, men and women—who will hear the story that once there was a terrible disease, and that a brave group of people stood up and fought and in some cases died so that others might live and be free. I'm proud to be out here today with the people I love, and see the faces of those heroes who are fighting this war, and to be a part of that fight."[147]

Until the day when the deferral of victory over AIDS finally yields to a victory celebration of the most joyous magnitude, when gay Americans are accorded every right and dignity that *all* people are meant to enjoy, life for gay people in this country will continue to be a delicate balancing act between the future and past, hope and memory.

When Arnie Kantrowitz describes his own life, years after the giddiness and promise of the seventies and several lifetimes' worth of experience later, he talks about how the AIDS epidemic has reshaped his world, particularly because of the losses of Vito Russo and Jim Owles, his two best friends from their days together in Gay Activists Alliance in the early seventies. "There's some part of me that has never been able to deal with a certain level of it," he told me. "It's as if I just quietly had to accept that major pieces of my life were ripped out, and I had to keep walking, with no choice." Kantrowitz keeps a huge picture of Russo in his living room, and a photo of Owles on his desk. He wears the gold lambda ring GAA gave to Owles after his first year as president, the one Owles on his deathbed asked him to wear because he had been Owles' vice president.

For Kantrowitz AIDS has changed even the physical landscape of New York City, creating what he calls "hot spots." He explained, "I don't go near the block where Vito lived. I don't go near the block where Jim lived. I once walked past Jim's house, and it's very strong, like this magnetic, intense feeling. I get it each time I walk past the hospital where he died." Greenwich Village, with its promise of liberation, has become a kind of ghost town haunted by the spirits of departed friends. "Now when I walk around the Village," said Kantrowitz, "I'm constantly seeing the spot where I last said goodbye to this one, the window where so-and-so used to live, the street where that one lived and this or that event went on."

It's gotten better, but not much. "I still know some people who are HIV-positive or even AIDS diagnosed," said Kantrowitz, "but no one I know is expected to die in the next year. So I think I've relaxed about it on one level." But on another level, he added, "I'm still in pain talking about it. I still light candles for my dead friends. I do my own rituals. I keep in contact with friends of friends. And I still cry."[148]

Notes

CHAPTER ONE

1. Arnie Kantrowitz, telephone interview with author, 22 November 1996.
2. Arnie Kantrowitz, *Under the Rainbow: Growing Up Gay* (New York: William Morrow, 1977, expanded and reissued by St. Martin's Press, 1996), 115.
3. Ibid., 100.
4. Warren J. Blumenfeld and Diane Raymond, *Looking at Gay and Lesbian Life* (Boston: Beacon Press, 1988), 302.
5. John D'Emilio, *Sexual Politics, Sexual Communities* (Chicago: University of Chicago Press, 1983), 235.
6. Paul Boneberg, interview with author, Washington, D.C., 17 August 1995.
7. Leigh W. Rutledge, *Gay Decades* (New York: Penguin Books, 1992), 139.
8. Rodger Streitmatter, *Unspeakable: The Rise of the Gay and Lesbian Press in America* (Boston: Faber and Faber, 1995), 222.
9. Ibid., 219.
10. Blumenfeld and Raymond, 311.
11. Edmund White, *States of Desire: Travels in Gay America* (New York: E.P. Dutton, 1980), 292.
12. Sidney Brinkley, "Black Gay History in the Making," *Washington Blade* (7 February 1997), 12.
13. Brian McNaught, *On Being Gay* (New York: St. Martin's Press, 1988), 59–60.
14. Eric Rofes, telephone interview with author, 21 June 1996.
15. Ibid., 7 July 1995.
16. Urvashi Vaid, *Virtual Equality: The Mainstreaming of Gay and Lesbian Liberation* (New York: Anchor Books, 1995), 67.
17. Armistead Maupin, telephone interview with author, 23 December 1996.
18. Vaid, *Virtual Equality*, 210–11.
19. Maupin interview.
20. D'Emilio, *Sexual Politics*, 2.
21. Pat Norman, telephone interview with author, 12 September 1995.
22. John D'Emilio, interview with author, Washington, D.C., 24 May 1996.
23. Randy Shilts, *And the Band Played On* (New York: St. Martin's Press, 1987), 15.
24. Carl Wittman, *A Gay Manifesto*, reprinted in Karla Jay and Allen Young, eds., *Out of the Closet: Voices of Gay Liberation* (New York: Douglas Books, 1972), 330–42.

25. White, *States of Desire*, 34–35.

26. Randy Shilts, *The Mayor of Castro Street: The Life and Times of Harvey Milk* (New York: St. Martin's Press, 1982), 226.

27. White, *States of Desire*, 28–64.

28. Ian Young, *The Stonewall Experiment* (London: Cassell, 1995), 63.

29. Harry Hay, "A Separate People Whose Time Has Come." In Mark Thompson, ed., *Gay Spirit: Myth and Meaning* (New York: St. Martin's Press, 1987), 279–91.

30. Stuart Timmons, *The Trouble With Harry Hay, Founder of the Modern Gay Movement* (Boston: Alyson Publications, 1990), 292.

31. John Rechy, *The Sexual Outlaw: A Documentary* (New York: Grove Press, 1977), 31.

32. Young, *The Stonewall Experiment*, 64.

33. Kantrowitz interview.

34. Chuck Frutchey, telephone interview with author, 14 August 1995.

35. Michael Callen, *Surviving AIDS* (New York: HarperCollins, 1990), 3–4.

36. Kantrowitz, *Under the Rainbow*, 133.

37. Maupin interview.

38. Maupin, quoted in Lon G. Nungesser, *Epidemic of Courage: Facing AIDS in America* (New York: St. Martin's Press, 1986), 215.

39. Douglas Sadownick, *Sex Between Men: An Intimate History of the Sex Lives of Gay Men Postwar to Present* (San Francisco: HarperSanFrancisco, 1996), 123.

40. Young, *The Stonewall Experiment*, 170.

41. Ibid., 104.

42. Larry Kramer, "A Good News/Bad News AIDS Joke," *New York Times Magazine* (14 July 1996), 28.

43. Kantrowitz interview.

44. Kantrowitz, *Under the Rainbow*, 119.

45. Andrew Holleran, *Dancer from the Dance* (New York: William Morrow, 1978), 40.

46. Ibid., 207.

47. Ibid., 219.

48. Larry Kramer, *Faggots* (New York: Random House, 1978), 335, 337.

49. Larry Kramer, *Reports from the holocaust: The Making of an AIDS Activist* (New York: St. Martin's Press, 1989), 5.

50. Arnie Kantrowitz, "An Enemy of the People," in Lawrence D. Mass, ed., *We Must Love One Another or Die: The Life and Legacies of Larry Kramer* (New York: St. Martin's Press, 1997), 102.

51. Larry Kramer, interview with author, New York City, 4 March 1995.

52. Kantrowitz, *Under the Rainbow*, 189.

53. John-Manuel Andriote, "Shrinking Opposition," *10 Percent* (Fall 1993), 61. Note that this section on the relationship of homosexuals and psychiatry is based largely upon this article.

54. Richard A. Isay, M.D., *Being Homosexual: Gay Men and Their Development* (New York: Farrar Strauss & Giroux, 1989).

55. Alfred Kinsey, *Sexual Behavior in the Human Male* (Philadelphia: W.B. Saunders, 1948).

56. Evelyn Hooker, "The Adjustment of the Male Overt Homosexual," *Journal of Projective Techniques* 21 (1957): 18–31.

57. *New York Times,* 17 December 1963.

58. Franklin E. Kameny, "Emphasis on Research Has Had Its Day," *The Ladder: A Lesbian Review* (October 1965), 11.

59. Franklin E. Kameny, telephone interview with author, 27 March 1993.

60. Barbara Gittings, telephone interview with author, 8 April 1993.

61. "Psychiatrists Blast Colleagues' Prejudice Against Homosexuals," *Psychiatric News* (7 June 1972), 6.

62. Robert L. Spitzer, M.D., "The Homosexuality Decision—A Background Paper," *Psychiatric News* (16 January 1974), 11.

63. Charles Hite, "APA Rules Homosexuality Not Necessarily a Disorder," *Psychiatric News* (2 January 1974), 1.

64. Irving Bieber, "Against Trustees' Action: A Statement by Irving Bieber," *Psychiatric News* (6 February 1974), 1.

65. Lawrence D. Mass, M.D., interview with author, New York City, 28 April 1995.

66. Howard Brown, M.D., *Familiar Faces, Hidden Lives: The Story of Homosexual Men in America Today* (New York: Harcourt Brace Jovanovich, 1976), 204, 201.

67. Laurie Garrett, *The Coming Plague: Newly Emerging Diseases in a World Out of Balance* (New York: Penguin Books, 1994), 30.

68. Krause quoted in ibid., 5.

69. Mirko D. Grmek, M.D., Ph.D. *History of AIDS: Emergence and Origin of a Modern Pandemic.* Translated by Russell C. Maulitz and Jacalyn Duffin (Princeton, N.J.: Princeton University Press, 1990), 41.

70. Warren E. Leary, "U.S.'s Rate of Sexual Disease Is Highest in Developed World," *New York Times* (20 November 1996), D20; Ethan Bronner, "No Sexology, Please. We're Americans," *New York Times,* "Week in Review" (1 February 1998), 6.

71. Frank Browning, *The Culture of Desire: Paradox and Perversity in Gay Lives Today* (New York: Crown Publishers, 1993), 113.

72. Shilts, *And the Band Played On,* 48.

73. Ibid., 39.

74. Lawrence D. Mass, M.D., *Homosexuality and Sexuality: Dialogues of the Sexual Revolution,* vol. 1 (New York: Harrington Park Press, 1990), 133–34.

75. Dennis Altman, *AIDS in the Mind of America* (New York: Anchor Press/Doubleday, 1986), 143.

76. Callen, *Surviving AIDS,* 4.

77. Mass interview.

78. Norman interview.

79. Gary Remafedi, M.D., telephone interview with author, 14 July 1995.

80. Robert L. Rowan, M.D. and Paul J. Gillette, Ph.D. *The Gay Health Guide: A Complete Medical Reference for Homosexually Active Men and Women* (Boston: Little, Brown, 1978), 3, 7.

81. Callen, *Surviving AIDS,* 4.

82. Shilts, *And the Band Played On,* 38.

83. Young, *The Stonewall Experiment,* 166.

84. Altman, *AIDS*, 143.

85. Callen, *Surviving AIDS*, 12.

86. David G. Ostrow, M.D., interview with author, Chicago, 3 June 1995.

87. Kenneth Mayer, M.D., interview with author, Boston, 25 July 1995.

88. Mayer interview.

89. Walter Lear, M.D., "The National Gay Health Coalition," *Lesbian & Gay Health* (Newsletter of the National Gay Health Education Foundation), January 1984.

90. Lawrence "Bopper" Deyton, M.D., interview with author, Rockville, Md., 24 September 1996.

91. Ostrow interview.

92. Donald P. Francis, M.D., Ph.D., interview with author, Washington, D.C., 9 February 1995.

93. Mayer interview.

94. Ostrow interview.

CHAPTER TWO

1. Donald I. Abrams, M.D., telephone interview with author, 17 July 1995.

2. Edward Alwood, *Straight News: Gays, Lesbians, and the News Media* (New York: Columbia University Press, 1996), 212.

3. Ibid. The first mainstream news account to view the Stonewall rebellion as a major step forward in the gay liberation movement was a cover story by Lucian Truscott IV, in the *Village Voice* on 3 July 1969.

4. Lawrence D. Mass, M.D., "Cancer in the Gay Community," *New York Native* (27 July 1981), 1.

5. Ibid.

6. Dennis Altman, *AIDS in the Mind of America* (Garden City, N.Y.: Anchor Press/Doubleday, 1986), 43.

7. Lawrence D. Mass, M.D., "The Epidemic Continues: Facing a New Case Every Day, Researchers Are Still Bewildered," *New York Native* (29 March 1982), 1.

8. Mass, "Cancer in the Gay Community."

9. David T. Durack, "Opportunistic Infections and Kaposi's Sarcoma in Homosexual Men," *New England Journal of Medicine* 305 (1981): 1465–67.

10. Laurie Garrett, *The Coming Plague: Newly Emerging Diseases in a World Out of Balance* (New York: Penguin Books, 1994), 389.

11. Michael Ver Meulen, "The Gay Plague," *New York* (31 May 1982), 54.

12. In Lon G. Nungesser, *Epidemic of Courage: Facing AIDS in America* (New York: St. Martin's Press, 1986), 136.

13. Larry Kramer, "A Personal Appeal from Larry Kramer," *New York Native* (24 August 1981).

14. See Ver Meulen, "The Gay Plague," 62.

15. Garrett, *The Coming Plague*, 306.

16. Randy Shilts, *And the Band Played On* (New York: St. Martin's Press, 1987), 147, 149, 171.

17. Hank Wilson, interview with author, San Francisco, 30 January 1995.

18. All direct quotations about the BAPHR symposium are borrowed from

Lawrence D. Mass, M.D., "Creative Sex, Creative Medicine: Gay Physicians Meet for a Health Conference," *New York Native* (19 July 1982), 11, 13.

19. Lucia Valeska, "AID: The Appropriate Response." *Task Force Report* (Newsletter of the National Gay Task Force) 9 (August/September 1982).

20. Lawrence D. Mass, M.D., "A Major Meeting on the Epidemic," *New York Native* (2 August 1982).

21. Lawrence D. Mass, M.D., "Time for Prevention: Devising Ways of Evading AID, *New York Native* (16 August 1982), 31.

22. Mass, "The Epidemic Continues."

23. Charles Perrow, Mauro F. Guillén, *The AIDS Disaster: The Failure of Organizations in New York and the Nation* (New Haven: Yale University Press, 1990), 38.

24. Shilts, *And the Band Played On,* 222.

25. Donald P. Francis, M.D., Ph.D., interview with author, Washington, D.C., 9 February 1995.

26. Francis, telephone conversation with author, 24 January 1995.

27. Virginia Apuzzo, telephone interview with author, 8 August 1995.

28. Pat Norman, telephone interview with author, 12 September 1995.

29. Peter Page, M.D., interview with author, Washington, D.C., 2 October 1995.

30. Lawrence D. Mass, M.D., *Dialogues of the Sexual Revolution,* vol. 1, *Homosexuality and Sexuality* (New York: Harrington Park Press, 1990), 144, 152–53.

31. Shilts, *And the Band Played On,* 238.

32. Donald P. Francis and James Chin, "The Prevention of Acquired Immunodeficiency Syndrome in the United States," *Journal of the American Medical Association,* 257 (13 March 1987): 1357–66.

33. John C. Petricciani and Jay S. Epstein, "The Effects of the AIDS Epidemic on the Safety of the Nation's Blood Supply," *Public Health Reports* (May–June 1988): 236–41.

34. Sally Squires, "Blood Banks Adopt Stricter AIDS Test," *Washington Post* (2 April 1996), Health section.

35. Associated Press, "AIDS Risk in Transfusion Said to be 2 in 1 Million," *Washington Post* (27 June 1996), A16.

36. Associated Press, "Settlement Is Approved in Hemophiliac Suit," *New York Times* (15 August 1996), D5.

37. Howard Schneider, "Canada Reduces Red Cross's Authority," *Washington Post* (12 September 1996), A23.

38. Michael Daly, "AIDS Anxiety," *New York* (20 June 1983), 25–29.

39. Altman, *AIDS,* 74.

40. James Kinsella, *Covering the Plague: AIDS and the American Media* (New Brunswick, N.J.: Rutgers University Press, 1989), 71.

41. Altman, *AIDS,* 74.

42. Gil Gerald, telephone interview with author, 25 August 1995.

43. Rodger Streitmatter, *Unspeakable: The Rise of the Gay and Lesbian Press in America* (Boston: Faber and Faber, 1995), 261.

44. Cindy Patton, *Sex & Germs: The Politics of AIDS* (Boston: South End Press, 1985), 97.

45. Shilts, *And the Band Played On,* 347–48.

46. American Family Association letter (undated, circa winter 1983), quoted in Patton, *Sex & Germs*, 85.

47. John Fortunato, *AIDS, the Spiritual Dilemma* (New York: Harper & Row, 1987), 86.

48. James Holm, letter to author, 15 September 1994.

49. Charles Krauthammer, "The Politics of a Plague: Illness as Metaphor Revisited." *The New Republic* (1 August 1983), 18.

50. Streitmatter, *Unspeakable*, 262.

51. Tom Morganthau et al., "Gay America in Transition," *Newsweek* (8 August 1983), 30.

52. Altman, *AIDS*, 69.

53. Lawrence D. Mass, M.D., interview with author, New York City, 28 April 1995.

54. Alice Foley, interview with author, Provincetown, Mass., 30 July 1995.

55. Francis interview.

56. Noted in Mass, *Homosexuality and Sexuality: Dialogues of the Sexual Revolution*, vol. 1, 116.

57. Mass interview.

58. Quoted in Michael Callen, *Surviving AIDS* (New York: HarperCollins, 1990), 4.

59. Michael Callen and Richard Berkowitz, "We Know Who We Are: Two Gay Men Declare War on Promiscuity," *New York Native* (8–21 November 1982). Quoted in Callen, *Surviving AIDS*, 6–7.

60. Cindy Patton, *Fatal Advice: How Safe-Sex Education Went Wrong* (Durham, N.C.: Duke University Press, 1996), 11.

61. Quotation is from Peter A. Seitzman, M.D., "Guilt and AIDS," *New York Native* (3–16 January 1983). In Callen, *Surviving AIDS*, 7.

62. Larry Kramer, "1,112 and Counting," *New York Native* (14–27 March 1983).

63. Quoted in Shilts, *And the Band Played On*, 259–60.

64. Cleve Jones, speaking on an "oral history" panel of longtime AIDS activists, at the National Skills Building Conference, sponsored by the National Minority AIDS Council, National Association of People with AIDS, and AIDS National Interfaith Network, in Atlanta, 31 October 1994.

65. Norman interview.

66. Streitmatter, *Unspeakable*, 252–59.

67. Lawrence D. Mass, M.D., "Early Warnings: 1981." In Mark Thompson, ed., *Long Road to Freedom: The Advocate History of the Gay and Lesbian Movement* (New York: St. Martin's Press, 1994), 211.

68. Randy Shilts, "Gay Freedom Day Raises AIDS Worries," *San Francisco Chronicle* (27 May 1983).

69. Quoted in Kinsella, *Covering the Plague*, 173.

70. Altman, *AIDS*, 149.

71. "Garage Sale Marks Closing of Baths," *Gay Community News* (10 September 1983), 2.

72. Shilts, *And the Band Played On*, 416.

73. John Leo, "The Revolution Is Over: In the '80s, Caution and Commitment are the Watchwords," *Time* (9 April 1984).

74. Mervyn Silverman, M.D., telephone interview with author, 15 February 1995.

75. Brian Jones, "Community Plan to Regulate Baths," *Bay Area Reporter* (27 September 1984).

76. Shilts, *And the Band Played On,* 489.

77. Ibid., 306.

78. David G. Ostrow, M.D., interview with author, Chicago, 3 June 1995.

79. Shilts, *And the Band Played On,* 415.

CHAPTER THREE

1. Margaret Kisliuk, interview with author, San Francisco, 3 February 1995.

2. Peter Nardoza, interview with author, San Francisco, 29 January 1995.

3. Stephen C. Joseph, M.D., *Dragon Within the Gates: The Once and Future AIDS Epidemic* (New York: Carroll and Graf, 1992), 69.

4. Randy Shilts, *And the Band Played On* (New York: St. Martin's Press, 1987), 310, 533.

5. Larry Kramer, "The AIDS Network Letter to Mayor Koch," in *Reports from the holocaust: The Making of an AIDS Activist* (New York: St. Martin's Press, 1989), 53.

6. Dennis Altman, *AIDS in the Mind of America* (Garden City, N.Y.: Anchor Press/Doubleday, 1986), 129.

7. Shilts, *And the Band Played On,* 311.

8. Kramer, *Reports from the holocaust,* 9.

9. Larry Kramer, interview with author, New York City, 4 March 1995.

10. Kramer, *Reports from the holocaust,* 30.

11. Lawrence D. Mass, M.D., interview with author, New York City, 28 April 1995.

12. Kramer interview.

13. Larry Kramer, *The Normal Heart* (New York: Penguin Books, 1985).

14. Marcus Conant, M.D., interview with author, Washington, D.C., 13 July 1995.

15. Cleve Jones, interview with author, San Francisco, 2 February 1995.

16. Charles Garfield, telephone conversation with author, 17 November 1995.

17. Helen Schietinger, interview with author, Washington, D.C., 26 September 1995.

18. John Hannay, telephone interview with author, 16 July 1995.

19. Jim Graham, interview with author, Washington, D.C., 29 March 1995.

20. Jane Silver, interview with author, Washington, D.C., 13 March 1995.

21. Caitlin Conor Ryan, interview with author, Washington, D.C., 23 April 1995.

22. David G. Ostrow, M.D., interview with author, Chicago, 3 June 1995.

23. Larry Kessler, interview with author, Boston, 24 July 1995.

24. Eric Rofes, telephone interview with author, 7 July 1995.

25. Bill Meisenheimer, telephone interview with author, 6 June 1995.

26. Paula Van Ness, interview with author, Washington, D.C., 25 April 1995.

27. Graham interview.

28. James Holm, letter to the author, 29 August 1994.

29. Robert W. Wood, M.D., interview with author, Washington, D.C., 28 September 1995.

30. Bea Kalleigh, telephone interview with author, 5 October 1995.

31. Kristine Gebbie, interview with author, Washington, D.C., 15 March 1995.

32. Larry Prater, M.D., interview with author, Miami Beach, 20 May 1995.

33. Ronald Thompson, telephone interview with author, 15 July 1995.

34. George Bellinger, Jr., interview with author, New York City, 2 March 1995.

35. William Raspberry, "AIDS Is Becoming a Black Disease," *Washington Post* (11 October 1996), A25.

36. Gil Gerald, telephone interview with author, 25 August 1995.

37. Rev. Carl Bean, interview with author, Washington, D.C., 16 November 1995.

38. Ernesto Hinojos, interview with author, New York City, 2 March 1995.

39. Bruce Patterson, interview with author, New York City, 2 March 1995.

40. Virginia Apuzzo, telephone interview with author, 8 August 1995.

41. Lewis Katoff, "Community-Based Services for People with AIDS," *Primary Care* 19 (March 1992): 231–43.

42. Schietinger interview.

43. Ann Thérèse Carlozza, "Ruth Brinker's Spirit Sustains 'Open Hand,'" *The NAN Monitor* (Washington, D.C.: National AIDS Network, Fall 1988).

44. Centers for Disease Control, *HIV/AIDS Surveillance Report* 8 (June 1996).

45. Stephen F. Morin, Kenneth A. Charles, Alan K. Malyon, "The Psychological Impact of AIDS on Gay Men," *American Psychologist* 39 (November 1984): 1288-93.

46. Brian McNaught, telephone interview with author, 25 August 1995.

47. W. H. Auden, "September 1, 1939." Larry Kramer derived the title of his play, *The Normal Heart,* from this poem, and its last line, "We must love one another or die," is the title of an anthology about Kramer, edited by Lawrence D. Mass.

48. Peter X. Lee, telephone interview with author, 2 September 1995.

49. John Paul Barnich, telephone interview with author, 1 October 1995.

50. Alice Foley, interview with author, Provincetown, Mass., 30 July 1995.

51. Lawrence Millhofer, M.D., interview with author, Provincetown, Mass., 30 July 1995.

52. Millhofer interview.

53. Kenneth Mayer, M.D., interview with author, Boston, 25 July 1995.

54. Donald I. Abrams, M.D., telephone interview with author, 17 July 1995.

55. "Visiting Rights Urged for Gay Partners," *San Francisco Chronicle* (20 June 1990), A:20.

56. Cliff Morrison, telephone interview with author, 15 August 1995.

57. Morrison interview.

58. Sandi Feinblum, interview with author, New York City, 26 April 1995.

59. Catherine G. Lynch, interview with author, Miami, 19 May 1995.

60. Charles Garfield, *Sometimes My Heart Goes Numb: Love and Caregiving in a Time of AIDS* (San Francisco: Jossey-Bass, 1995), 8.

61. Robert Washington, interview with author, Washington, D.C., 25 March 1995.

62. Philip M. Kayal, *Bearing Witness: Gay Men's Health Crisis and the Politics of AIDS* (Boulder, Colo.: Westview Press, 1993), xv.

63. Suzanne Ouelette, interview with author, New York City, 27 April 1995.

CHAPTER FOUR

1. Edmund White, "Paradise Found," *Mother Jones,* June 1983, 10–16.

2. Gabriel Rotello, *Sexual Ecology: AIDS and the Destiny of Gay Men* (New York: Dutton, 1997), 224–25.

3. Marshall Forstein, M.D., interview with author, Washington, D.C., 13 September 1995.

4. Bruce Ward, "Decade" (unpublished play), 1992.

5. Conference program, The Fifth National Lesbian/Gay Health Conference, Denver, Colorado, 9–12 June 1983. Sponsored by the National Gay Health Education Foundation, American Association of Physicians for Human Rights, and the Gay and Lesbian Health Alliance of Denver.

6. Stephen Morin, interview with author, Washington, D.C., 20 March 1995.

7. Jackson Peyton, "AIDS Prevention for Gay Men: A Selected History and Analysis of the San Francisco Experience, 1982–1987" (San Francisco: San Francisco AIDS Foundation, 1989).

8. Rodger McFarlane, interview with author, New York City, 4 March 1995.

9. Larry Kramer, "An Open Letter to Richard Dunne/1987." In *Reports from the holocaust* (New York: St. Martin's Press, 1989), 103.

10. Dennis Altman, *AIDS in the Mind of America* (New York: Anchor Press/ Doubleday, 1986), 164.

11. Peyton, "AIDS Prevention for Gay Men."

12. Leon McKusick, William Horstman, Thomas J. Coates, "AIDS and Sexual Behavior Reported by Gay Men in San Francisco," *American Journal of Public Health* 75 (May 1985), 493–96.

13. San Francisco AIDS Foundation, *A Comprehensive AIDS Education/Prevention Plan for Fiscal Year 1984–85,* 18 June 1984.

14. Jackson Peyton, interview with author, Washington, D.C., 20 February 1995.

15. Bruce Ward, interview with author, Boston, 24 July 1995.

16. John L. Martin, "The Impact of AIDS on Gay Male Sexual Behavior Patterns in New York City," *American Journal of Public Health* 77 (May 1987), 578–81.

17. Curtis Decker, interview with author, Washington, D.C., 13 February 1995.

18. R. A. Kaslow, D. G. Ostrow, R. Detels, J. P. Phair, B. F. Polk, C. R. Rinaldo Jr., "The Multicenter AIDS Cohort Study: rationale, organization, and selected characteristics of the participants, *American Journal of Epidemiology* (1987), 310–18.

19. Cindy Patton, *Sex and Germs* (Boston: South End Press, 1985), 44.

20. Bruce Voeller, "Take the Test!" *The Advocate* (30 April 1985).

21. Paul Berg, "To Know You've Been Exposed," *Washington Post* (4 September 1985), Health section, 11.

22. Warren Winkelstein, Jr., et al., "The San Francisco Men's Health Study: III. Reduction in HIV transmission among homosexual/bisexual men," *American Journal of Public Health* 76 (June 1987), 685-89.

23. Randy Shilts, *Conduct Unbecoming: Gays & Lesbians in the U.S. Military* (New York: St. Martin's Press, 1993), 504.

24. National Research Council, *The Social Impact of AIDS in the United States* (Washington, D.C.: National Academy Press, 1993), 263.

25. Winkelstein et al., *San Francisco Men's Health Study.*

26. "Declining Rates of Rectal and Pharyngeal Gonorrhea Among Males— New York City," *Morbidity and Mortality Weekly Report* 33 (1 June 1984): 295-97.

27. Kathleen McAuliffe et al., "AIDS: At the Dawn of Fear," *U.S. News & World Report* (12 January 1987), 60–70.

28. Barbara Kantrowitz, "Fear of Sex," *Newsweek* (24 November 1986), 40, 42.

29. Clifton C. Jones et al., "Persistence of High-Risk Sexual Activity Among Homosexual Men in an Area of Low Incidence of the Acquired Immunodeficiency Syndrome." *Sexually Transmitted Diseases* (April–June 1987): 79–82.

30. Daniel Wohlfeiler, telephone interview with author, 15 February 1995.

31. Marvin E. Bailey, "Community-based Organizations and CDC as Partners in HIV Education and Prevention," *Public Health Reports* 106 (1991): 702–8.

32. U.S. Congress, Office of Technology Assessment, *Review of the Public Health Service Response to AIDS* (Washington, D.C.: OTA, 1985).

33. David Talbot and Larry Bush, "At Risk," *Mother Jones* (April 1985), 29–37.

34. Alan E. Gambrell, interview with author, Washington, D.C., 25 February 1995.

35. "Coolfont Report: A PHS Plan for Prevention and Control of AIDS and the AIDS Virus," *Public Health Reports* 101 (July–August 1986): 341–48.

36. Lisa Keen, "Hardwick Revisited." *Washington Blade* (5 July 1996), 1.

37. Leigh W. Rutledge, *Gay Decades* (New York: Penguin Books, 1992), 254.

38. Arnie Kantrowitz, *Under the Rainbow: Growing Up Gay* (New York: St. Martin's, 1996), 206.

39. C. Everett Koop, M.D., Surgeon General, "Introductory Statement, Report on AIDS" (Rockville, Md.: U.S. Government Printing Office, 22 October 1986).

40. Institute of Medicine/National Academy of Sciences, *Confronting AIDS: Directions for Public Health, Health Care, and Research* (Washington, D.C.: National Academy Press, 1986), see especially 95–105.

41. "SF Anger Over 'Jokes' at White House," *San Francisco Chronicle* (3 October 1986). Noted in James Kinsella, *Covering the Plague: AIDS and the American Media* (New Brunswick, N.J.: Rutgers University Press, 1987), 3.

42. Quoted in Nicholas Freudenberg, *Preventing AIDS: A Guide to Effective Education for the Prevention of HIV Infection* (Washington, D.C.: American Public Health Association, 1989), 115.

43. Julie Kosterlitz, "Educating About AIDS," *National Journal* (30 August 1986), 2044.

44. Institute of Medicine, *Confronting AIDS* (Washington, D.C.: National Academy Press, 1986), 99.

45. Tom Morganthau et al., "Future Shock," *Newsweek* (24 November 1986), 30–39.

46. McAuliffe et al., "AIDS: At the Dawn of Fear."

47. Donald P. Francis, M.D., Ph.D., interview with author, Washington, D.C., 9 February 1995.

48. "The Federal Response to the AIDS Epidemic: Information and Public Education," hearing before a subcommittee of the Committee on Government Operations, House of Representatives, 16 March 1987. Noted in *"The Politics of AIDS Prevention: Science Takes a Time Out,"* report of the Committee on Government Operations, U.S. House of Representatives. (Washington, D.C.: U.S. Government Printing Office, 1992).

49. Unsigned editorial, "Mr. Reagan's AIDS Test," *New York Times* (2 June 1987).

50. Priscilla B. Holman et al., "Increasing the Involvement of National and Regional Racial and Ethnic Minority Organizations in HIV Information and Education," *Public Health Reports* 106 (November–December 1991): 687–94.

51. Jacqueline Bowles and William A. Robinson, "PHS Grants for Minority Group HIV Infection Education and Prevention Efforts," *Public Health Reports* 104 (November–December 1989): 552–59.

52. Department of Health and Human Services, Office of Minority Health, *Prevention and Beyond: A Framework for Collective Action (A National Conference on HIV Infection and AIDS Among Racial and Ethnic Populations),* 1989.

53. Reginald Williams, telephone interview with author, 25 August 1995.

54. Randy Miller, interview with author, San Francisco, 31 January 1995.

55. Williams interview.

56. Richard Stengel, "The Changing Face of AIDS," *Time* (17 August 1987), 12–14.

57. Lawrence K. Altman, "Obstacle-Strewn Road to Rethinking the Numbers on AIDS," *New York Times* (1 March 1994), C3.

58. Richard Tagle and Gil Gerald, *Assessing the HIV Prevention Needs of Gay and Bisexual Men of Color* (Washington, D.C.: U.S. Conference of Mayors, 1993).

59. Ibid.

60. National Commission on AIDS, *The Challenge of HIV/AIDS in Communities of Color* (Washington, D.C.: National Commission on AIDS, 1992).

61. Centers for Disease Control and Prevention. *HIV/AIDS Surveillance Report* 7(2) (1995): 10.

62. Thomas J. Coates and Pamela DeCarlo, "Fifteen Years Later, Prevention Still Falls Short," *Washington Blade* (28 June 1996), 39.

63. "HIV Prevention Efforts Fall Short," *San Francisco Sentinel* (29 March 1995), 18.

64. *Surgeon General's Report to the American Public on HIV Infection and AIDS* (Rockville, Md.: U.S. Government Printing Office, June 1993), 1.

65. *CDC National AIDS Clearinghouse. Catalog of HIV and AIDS Education and Prevention Materials* (Washington, D.C.: U.S. Department of Health and Human Services, January 1993).

66. An Internet search on 4 May 1998 found that AEGIS, at <www.aegis. com> lists every "group" of people at risk for or affected by HIV/AIDS, except "men who have sex with men," as the CDC designates gay and bisexual men. AEGIS operates as a religiously affiliated, nonprofit California organization. When I inquired about this startling omission, given the epidemiology of the epidemic in the U.S., I was barraged with e-mail messages from Rick M. Wagner and someone else at AEGIS called "Wynn." In a message dated 4 May 1998, Wagner wrote: "Unfortunately to those people who need to see the words GAY, HOMOSEXUAL, QUEER (whatever) plastered all over the web site, I can only suspect that the topic of HIV/AIDS is secondary to their own sexual identity." Both men identified themselves as gay, yet they dismissed my questions and defended themselves vociferously in personal, patronizing attacks. They threatened me with a libel suit for "defaming" what Wagner called their "great service."

67. Sari Staver, "CDC Advised to Refocus Its HIV Prevention Efforts," *American Medical News* (13 December 1993), 10.

68. Ibid.

69. Gina Kolata, "Targeting Urged In Attack on AIDS," *New York Times* (8 March 1993), 1.

70. U.S. House of Representatives, *"The Politics of AIDS Prevention: Science Takes a Time Out"* (1992).

71. Laurie Jones, "New Ads Say AIDS Can Hit Anywhere," *American Medical News* (13 April 1992), 3.

72. Ibid.

73. Unsigned editorial, "A Deathly Silence," *New York Times* (2 August 1994).

74. Jeffrey A. Kelly, Janet S. St. Lawrence, Ted L. Brasfield, "Predictors of Vulnerability to AIDS Risk Behavior Relapse," *Journal of Consulting and Clinical Psychology* 59 (1991): 163–66.

75. Jane Gross, "Second Wave of AIDS Feared By Officials in San Francisco," *New York Times* (11 December 1993).

76. Ibid.

77. Michael Munzell, "Dancing with Death," *Image* (23 August 1992), 23–27.

78. John-Manuel Andriote, "Gay Men and Unsafe Sex," *Washington Post*, "Health" supplement (10 August 1993).

79. Abraham Verghese, *My Own Country: A Doctor's Story* (New York: Vintage Books, 1994), 133.

80. Eric Rofes, *Reviving the Tribe: Regenerating Gay Men's Sexuality and Culture in the Ongoing Epidemic* (New York: The Harrington Park Press, 1995), 145.

81. Ibid., 119, 126.

82. Charles Holmes, telephone interview with author, 7 April 1995.

83. Cindy Patton, *Fatal Advice: How Safe Sex Education Went Wrong* (Durham, N.C.: Duke University Press, 1996), 124–27.

84. David G. Ostrow, M.D., interview with author, Chicago, 3 June 1995.

85. Amy Goldstein, "Gay Social Club in DC Raises Health Concerns," *Washington Post* (17 April 1995), 1; Unsigned editorial, "Why Another Bathhouse in DC?" *Washington Post,* (20 April 1995).

86. Sara Miles, "And the Bathhouse Plays On," *Out* (July/August 1995).

87. Ibid.

88. David France, "Second Wave, Second Thoughts," *POZ* (June/July 1995).

89. Miles, "And the Bathhouse Plays On."

90. Ibid.

91. Michelangelo Signorile, "All Unsafe Sex Isn't Created Equal," *Out* (October 1995), 30–33, 138.

92. Bob Warfel, "The Bottom Line" (Readers Forum), *Washington Blade* (26 May 1995), 43.

93. Gay and Lesbian Medical Association, *The Silent Crisis: Ongoing HIV Infections Among Gay Men, Bisexuals and Lesbians at Risk.* Report of the GLMA/AAPHR Summit on HIV Prevention for Gay Men, Bisexuals and Lesbians at Risk, Dallas, Texas, 15–17 July 1994.

94. Walter Odets, interview with author, Chicago, 2 June 1995.

95. Thomas J. Coates, interview with author, Washington, D.C., 16 May 1995.

96. Robert Paul Cabaj, M.D., interview with author, San Francisco, 4 February 1995.

97. Sidney Brinkley, "Letter from San Francisco: Getting the Message Out," *Washington Blade* (7 April 1995), 14.

98. Cabaj interview.

99. Office of National AIDS Policy, *Youth & HIV/AIDS: An American Agenda* (Washington, D.C.: Office of National AIDS Policy, March 1996).

100. Patricia Fleming, telephone conversation with author, 22 March 1995.

101. Chris Bull and John Gallagher, "The Lost Generation," *The Advocate* (31 May 1994), 36–40.

102. Gary Remafedi, M.D., telephone interview with author, 14 July 1995.

103. Martina Morris, Jane Zavisca, Laura Dean, "Social and Sexual Networks: Their Role in the Spread of HIV/AIDS Among Young Gay Men," *AIDS Prevention and Education* 7 (1995): 24–35.

104. Ilan H. Meyer and Laura Dean. "Patterns of Sexual Behavior and Risk Taking Among Young New York City Gay Men," *AIDS Prevention and Education* 7 (1995): 13–23.

105. Walter Odets, *In the Shadow of the Epidemic: Being HIV-Negative in the Age of AIDS* (Durham: Duke University Press, 1995), 102.

106. Cynthia Laird, "UCSF AIDS Fighters Talk About Their Work," *Bay Area Reporter* (19 September 1996), 26.

CHAPTER FIVE

1. Michael Callen and Dan Turner, "A History of the People with AIDS Self-Empowerment Movement." In Michael Shernoff, William A. Scott, eds., *The*

Sourcebook on Lesbian/Gay Health Care (Washington, D.C.: National Lesbian/Gay Health Foundation, 1988), 187–92.

2. Lon G. Nungesser, *Epidemic of Courage: Facing AIDS in America* (New York: St. Martin's Press, 1986), 119.

3. Lawrence D. Mass, *Dialogues of the Sexual Revolution*, vol. 1 (New York: The Haworth Press, 1990), 139.

4. Martin Delaney, telephone interview with author, 7 February 1995.

5. Sidney Brinkley, "Helping People Save Their Lives," *Washington Blade* (3 June 1994), 18.

6. Mervyn Silverman, M.D., telephone interview with author, 15 February 1995.

7. Stosh Ostrow, M.D., telephone interview with author, 23 September 1995.

8. Dennis Altman, *AIDS in the Mind of America* (New York: Anchor Press/Doubleday, 1986), 96.

9. Albert R. Jonsen and Jeff Stryker, eds., *The Social Impact of AIDS in the United States* (Washington, D.C.: National Academy Press, 1993), 91.

10. Michael Callen, Remarks, 24 April 1987.

11. Ibid.

12. Sally Cooper, interview with author, New York City, 29 April 1995.

13. Derek Hodel, interview with author, New York City, 27 April 1995.

14. Matthew Sharp, interview with author, San Francisco, 1 February 1995.

15. Tom Blount, telephone interview with author, 27 September 1995.

16. National Association of People with AIDS, *Community Report FY 95* (Washington, D.C.: NAPWA, 1995).

17. Brian O'Connell, "NAPWA Budget Woes Force Layoffs," *Washington Blade* (4 October 1996), 1.

18. National Association of People with AIDS, *HIV in America: A Profile of the Challenges Facing Americans Living with HIV* (Washington, D.C.: NAPWA, 1992).

19. A. Cornelius Baker, interview with author, Washington, D.C., 21 March 1995.

20. Michael Callen, *Surviving AIDS* (New York: HarperCollins, 1990), 121.

21. Peter S. Arno and Karyn L. Feiden, *Against the Odds: The Story of Drug Development, Politics, and Profits* (New York: HarperCollins, 1992), 42.

22. Margaret A. Fischl, M.D., et al., "The Efficacy of Azidothymidine (AZT) in the Treatment of Patients with AIDS and AIDS-Related Complex: A Double-Blind, Placebo-Controlled Trial," *New England Journal of Medicine* 317 (1987): 185–91.

23. Ellen Cooper, M.D., interview with author, Bethesda, Md., 4 December 1996.

24. Sari Staver, "AZT Turnaround," *American Medical News* (20 February 1987), 14.

25. Larry Kramer, *Reports from the holocaust* (New York: St. Martin's Press, 1989), 127–39.

26. Ibid., 140–44.

27. Douglas Crimp with Adam Rolston, *AIDS DemoGraphics* (Seattle: Bay Press, 1990), 28, 37.

28. Ibid.

29. A 1988 report by the U.S. House of Representatives Committee on Government Operations (*AIDS Drugs: Where Are They?*) notes, "NCI [National Cancer Institute], along with NIAID [National Institute of Allergy and Infectious Diseases], not only participated heavily in the development of the drug [AZT], but also supplied Burroughs Wellcome with large amounts of thymidine, a scarce and expensive ingredient. However, because the federal government has granted the company an exclusive patent on AZT, the government will not share in profits from its sale, nor is it in a position, under current law, to affect the cost of the drug to the public."

30. Arno and Feiden, *Against the Odds,* 60.

31. Crimp and Rolston, *AIDS DemoGraphics,* 76–83.

32. Robert Bray, interview with author, San Francisco, 2 February 1995.

33. Steven Epstein, *Impure Science: AIDS, Activism, and the Politics of Knowledge* (Berkeley: University of California Press, 1996), 226.

34. Donald Abrams, M.D., telephone interview with author, 17 July 1995.

35. Kramer, *Reports from the holocaust,* 209.

36. Callen, *Surviving AIDS,* 10.

37. Callen, quoted in Arno and Feiden, *Against the Odds,* 118.

38. Ellen Cooper interview.

39. Arno and Feiden, *Against the Odds,* 124.

40. U.S. House of Representatives, Committee on Government Operations, *AIDS Drugs: Where Are They?* (Washington, D.C.: Government Printing Office, 1988).

41. AIDS Clinical Trials Advisory Group, *Final Report* (January 22, 1988), 4.

42. U.S. House of Representatives, Committee on Government Operations, *AIDS Drugs: Where Are They?*

43. Delaney interview.

44. Calvin Cohen, Abby Shevitz, Kenneth Mayer, "Expanding Access to Investigational New Therapies," *Primary Care* 19 (March 1992): 87–96.

45. Arno and Feiden, *Against the Odds,* 209.

46. Ibid., 213.

47. Ellen Cooper interview.

48. Delaney interview.

49. Philip J. Hilts, "Drug Said to Help AIDS Cases with Virus but No Symptoms," *New York Times* (18 August 1989), A1.

50. Ibid.

51. My information about the 14 September 1989 ACT-UP demonstration on Wall Street is derived from Arno and Feiden, *Against the Odds,* 135–38, and Crimp and Rolston, *AIDS DemoGraphics,* 114–19.

52. Kramer, *Reports from the holocaust.* 287–88.

53. Larry Kramer, *Reports from the holocaust: The Story of an AIDS Activist* (updated and expanded, New York: St. Martin's Press, 1994), 347.

54. Lawrence "Bopper" Deyton, M.D., interview with author, Rockville, Md., 24 September 1996.

55. Jack Killen, M.D., interview with author, Rockville, Md., 28 March 1995.

56. James Hill, interview with author, Washington, D.C., 24 June 1995.

57. Anthony Fauci, M.D., interview with author, Bethesda, Md., 14 April 1995.

58. Ibid.

59. Jonsen and Stryker, *The Social Impact of AIDS,* 96.

60. Fauci interview.

61. Larry Kramer, *The Destiny of Me* (New York: Penguin, 1993), 17.

62. Epstein, *Impure Science,* 292.

63. Ibid.

64. John James, interview with author, San Francisco, 4 February 1995.

65. Spencer Cox, telephone interview with author, 21 November 1996.

66. David Brown, "Popular U.S. Treatment for HIV is Challenged By European Study," *Washington Post* (9 June 1993), A4.

67. Moisés Agosto, interview with author, Washington, D.C., 5 September 1995.

68. Ellen Cooper interview.

69. Kramer, *Reports from the holocaust* (1994 edition), 303.

70. Bill Bahlman, interview with author, New York City, 3 March 1995.

71. James interview.

72. Peter Staley, "Start Making Sense," *POZ* (August–September 1995), 40.

73. Tim Horn, "Protease Inhibited," *POZ* (April 1996), 64.

74. Agosto interview.

75. Felicia R. Lee, "U.S. Cuts AIDS Research Grants in New York City," *New York Times* (8 November 1994), A1.

76. Ibid.

77. Ellen Cooper interview.

78. Robert M. Wachter, M.D., "AIDS, Activism, and the Politics of Health," *New England Journal of Medicine* 326 (9 January 1992): 128–32.

CHAPTER SIX

1. Larry Kramer, "1,112 and Counting," *New York Native* (14–27 March 1983). In *Reports from the holocaust: The Making of an AIDS Activist* (New York: St. Martin's Press, 1989), 33–51.

2. Larry Kramer, "The AIDS Network Letter to Mayor Koch." In *Reports from the holocaust,* 52–59.

3. Randy Shilts, *And the Band Played On* (New York: St. Martin's Press, 1987), 245.

4. Larry Kramer, "Where Are We Now?" *GMHC Newsletter,* No. 2, February 1983. In *Reports from the holocaust,* 27.

5. Larry Kramer, interview with author, New York City, 4 March 1995.

6. Shilts, *And the Band Played On,* 131.

7. James Kinsella, *Covering the Plague: AIDS and the American Media* (New Brunswick, N.J.: Rutgers University Press, 1989), 262, 263.

8. Shilts, *And the Band Played On,* 467.

9. Michael J. Ybarra, "Nature and Apathy Destroy AIDS Vigil," *New York Times* (22 December 1995), A22.

10. Paul Boneberg, interview with author, Washington, D.C., 17 August 1995.

11. Bill Bahlman, interview with author, New York City, 3 March 1995.

12. John-Manuel Andriote, "AIDSweek: May 31–June 5," *Washington City Paper* (June 12, 1987), 6–11.

13. Bahlman interview.

14. Paul Akio Kawata, ed., *Americans Who Care: Volunteers Working in the Battle Against AIDS* (Washington, D.C.: National AIDS Network, 1987), 77.

15. Kramer interview.

16. Larry Kramer, "The Beginning of ACTing Up/1987." In *Reports from the holocaust*, 128, 135.

17. David B. Feinberg, *Queer and Loathing: Rants and Raves of a Raging AIDS Clone* (New York: Penguin Books, 1994), 10.

18. Bahlman interview.

19. Ibid.

20. B. Michael Hunter, "Allan Robinson, AIDS Activist." In B. Michael Hunter, ed., *Sojourner: Black Gay Voices in the Age of AIDS* (New York: Other Countries Press, 1993), 54–61.

21. Douglas Crimp and Adam Rolston, *AIDS DemoGraphics* (Seattle: Bay Press, 1990), 26–30. Note: Crimp and Rolston say this first ACT UP demonstration took place on Thursday, 24 March 1987; however, 24 March 1987 was a Tuesday—exactly two weeks after Larry Kramer's 10 March speech at the Gay and Lesbian Community Center, in New York, which is credited as having launched ACT UP.

22. Hank Wilson, interview with author, San Francisco, 30 January 1995.

23. Jeff Graham, telephone interview with author, 13 September 1995.

24. Michael Petrelis, "ACT UP Isn't 'Gay,' " *Wall Street Journal* (21 February 1992), A-15.

25. Crimp and Rolston, *AIDS DemoGraphics* (p. 76) call the FDA action "the most significant demonstration of the AIDS activist movement's first two years" without regard to the fact that AIDS activism, as I have demonstrated in this chapter, had been underway, particularly in New York and San Francisco, for at least the previous five years. As I note further in the chapter, this solipsism would prove to be one of ACT UP's fatal flaws.

26. Michelangelo Signorile, *Queer in America: Sex, the Media, and the Closets of Power* (New York: Anchor Books, 1993), 4, 5.

27. Ibid., 10.

28. Ibid., 12.

29. Ibid., 16.

30. Timothy Westmoreland, interview with author, Washington, D.C., 18 July 1995.

31. Shilts, *And the Band Played On*, 143.

32. Urvashi Vaid, *Virtual Equality: The Mainstreaming of Gay and Lesbian Liberation* (New York: Anchor Books/Doubleday, 1995), 7.

33. Virginia Apuzzo, telephone interview with author, 8 August 1995.

34. Westmoreland interview.

35. Jeffrey Levi, interview with author, Washington, D.C., 24 February 1995.

36. Shilts, *And the Band Played On*, 359.

37. Apuzzo read this list of failures from a press release issued by the National Gay Task Force on 1 August 1983, the day of the hearings sponsored by New

York Representative Ted Weiss's Government Operations Subcommittee on Intergovernmental Relations and Human Resources.

38. Shilts, *And the Band Played On,* 466–67.

39. Ibid., 466.

40. Gary MacDonald, interview with author, Washington, D.C., 7 February 1995.

41. MacDonald interview.

42. Pat Christen, telephone interview with author, 20 September 1995.

43. Timothy Sweeney, interview with author, New York City, 2 March 1995.

44. Daniel Bross, interview with author, Washington, D.C., 17 February 1995.

45. Jean McGuire, interview with author, Cambridge, Mass., 25 July 1995.

46. Vic Basile, interview with author, Washington, D.C., 8 July 1996.

47. Thomas Sheridan, interview with author, Washington, D.C., 24 February 1995.

48. Basile interview.

49. Sheridan interview.

50. Aras van Hertum, "Bill Bailey, Influential Lobbyist on AIDS, Dies at 34," *Washington Blade* (29 April 1994), 31.

51. Chai Feldblum, interview with author, Washington, D.C., 12 April 1996.

52. Sue Fox, "While Signing CARE Act, Clinton Calls for Educating Gay Youth," *Washington Blade* (24 May 1996), 14.

53. See Chai R. Feldblum, "Antidiscrimination Requirements of the ADA." In Lawrence O. Gostin, Henry A. Bayer, eds., *Implementing the Americans with Disabilities Act: Rights and Responsibilities of All Americans* (Baltimore, Md.: Paul H. Brookes Publishing Co., 1993), 35–54.

54. Diane M. Gianelli, "High Court Ruling Gives Basis for AIDS Bias Suits," *American Medical News* (13 March 1987), 1.

55. Joan Biskupic and Amy Goldstein, "Disability Law Covers HIV, Justices Rule," *Washington Post* (26 June 1998), 1. The case before the court, Bragdon v. Abbott, was brought by Sidney Abbott after a Bangor, Maine, dentist, Randon Bragdon, refused to fill a cavity for her after Abbott checked off "yes" to the question of whether she was infected with HIV on a routine questionnaire in the dentist's office. Bragdon claimed Abbott was not protected by the ADA because she was merely HIV-positive and had no AIDS-defining conditions. Abbott claimed that indeed she was "substantially limited" in a major life activity—a criterion for a condition's being considered a disability under the ADA—in that her reproductive choices were affected by her fear of transmitting HIV to a child and not living long enough to rear it. The court made clear that HIV-positive Americans are protected from discrimination from the moment they become infected.

56. Curtis Decker, interview with author, Washington, D.C., 13 February 1995.

57. Decker interview.

58. Feldblum interview.

59. Martha M. McKinney, "Consortium Approaches to HIV Services Delivery Under the Ryan White CARE Act" (Washington, D.C.: U.S. Department of Health and Human Services, 1993), iii.

60. McGuire interview.

61. Vaid, *Virtual Equality*, 75.

62. Timothy McFeeley, interview with author, Washington, D.C., 26 June 1995.

63. I have based this reporting on several articles: Al Kamen, "Guards Don Gloves as Gay Officials Visit White House," *Washington Post* (15 June 1995), 1; Lou Chibarro, Jr., "Secret Service Dons Rubber Gloves to Search Officials," *Washington Blade* (16 June 1995), 1; Frank Rich, "The Gloved Ones," *New York Times* (18 June 1995); Lou Chibarro, Jr., "Clinton Apologizes for Glove Incident," *Washington Blade* (23 June 1995), 1; Linda Greenhouse, "Gay Rights Laws Can't Be Banned, High Court Rules," *New York Times* (21 May 1996), 1; Frank Rich, "A Gay-Rights Victory Muffled," *New York Times* (22 May 1996), A17; and David W. Dunlap, "Clinton Names First Liaison to Gay and Lesbian Groups," *New York Times* (14 June 1995).

64. Quoted in David Mixner, *Stranger Among Friends* (New York: Bantam, 1996), 239.

65. Vaid, *Virtual Equality*, 129.

66. Benjamin Schatz, interview with author, San Francisco, 2 February 1995.

67. Darrell Yates Rist, "AIDS as Apocalypse: The Deadly Costs of an Obsession," *The Nation* (13 February 1989), 181.

68. Eric Rofes, "Gay Groups vs. AIDS Groups: Averting Civil War in the 90s," *Out/Look* (Spring 1990).

69. Vaid interview.

70. Jeffrey Schmalz, "Whatever Happened to AIDS?" *New York Times Magazine* (28 November 1993).

71. Boneberg interview.

72. John D'Emilio, interview with author, Washington, D.C., 24 May 1996.

73. Dennis Altman, "Legitimation through Disaster: AIDS and the Gay Movement." In Elizabeth Fee, Daniel M. Fox, eds., *AIDS: The Burdens of History* (Berkeley: University of California Press, 1988), 309.

74. "AIDS Action Executive Director," quarter-page advertisement in *Washington Blade* (31 May 1996), 32.

75. Vaid, *Virtual Equality*, 101.

76. Levi interview.

77. Kramer, "What Are You Doing to Save My Fucking Life?" In *Reports from the holocaust*, 309-13.

78. Feldblum interview.

79. Kristine Gebbie, interview with author, Washington, D.C., 15 March 1995.

80. Patricia Fleming, interview with author, Washington, D.C., 22 March 1995.

81. McFeeley interview.

82. "Bush: The Law Must Protect Rights of PWAs," *Au Courant* (16 April 1990), 10.

83. Basile interview.

84. Vaid interview.

85. Kramer, *Reports from the holocaust* (1994 edition), 314.

86. Marilyn Chase, "Demonstrations and Boycott Over Travel Curbs Threaten to Disrupt International AIDS Meeting," *Wall Street Journal* (8 May 1990), A26.

87. Crimp and Rolston, *AIDS DemoGraphics*, 138.

88. Cited in Robert M. Wachter, *The Fragile Coalition: Scientists, Activists, and AIDS* (New York: St. Martin's Press, 1991), 63.

89. Ibid., 103.

90. Elinor Burkett, *The Gravest Show On Earth: America in the Age of AIDS* (New York: Houghton Mifflin, 1995), 20.

91. Boneberg interview.

92. Wachter, *The Fragile Coalition*, 169.

93. Ibid., 216–17.

94. Ibid., 227.

95. Kramer interview.

96. Donna Minkowitz, "ACT UP at a Crossroads," *Village Voice* (5 July 1990), 19–22.

97. Peter Staley, "Has the Direct-Action Group ACT UP Gone Astray?" *The Advocate* (30 July 1991), 98.

98. Westmoreland interview.

99. Graham interview.

100. Eugene Harrington, telephone interview with author, 20 October 1995.

101. Vaid, *Virtual Equality*, 364, 385.

102. Vaid interview.

103. Kramer interview.

104. Kramer interview.

105. Susan Ryan-Vollmar, "Ignoring the Skeptics, Activist Steve Michael Runs for President," *Bay Windows* (19 October 1995), 3.

106. Wendy Johnson, "ACT UP Fouls Forum with Kitty Litter," *Washington Blade* (8 November 1996), 14.

107. Alex Witchel, "When a Roaring Lion Learns to Purr," *New York Times* (12 January 1995), C1.

108. Kramer interview.

CHAPTER SEVEN

1. Paula Van Ness, interview with author, Washington, D.C., 25 April 1995.

2. Gary MacDonald, interview with author, Washington, D.C., 7 February 1995.

3. Paul Akio Kawata, interview with author, Washington, D.C., 24 March 1995.

4. John Paul Barnich, telephone interview with author, 1 October 1995.

5. Jim Graham, interview with author, Washington, D.C., 29 March 1995.

6. Timothy Wolfred, telephone interview with author, 30 September 1995.

7. Michael E. Carbine and Peter Lee, *AIDS Into the 90s: Strategies for an Integrated Response to the AIDS Epidemic* (Washington, D.C.: National AIDS Network, 1988).

8. Peter X. Lee, telephone interview with author, 2 September 1995.

9. John-Manuel Andriote, "NAN to House National Philanthropic Fund," *NAN Network News* (Washington, D.C.: National AIDS Network, 1 May 1988).

10. Jean McGuire, interview with author, Cambridge, Mass., 25 July 1995.

11. National AIDS Network, *Conference Chronicle: The Publication of the*

1988 NAN Skills Building Conference 2 (Washington, D.C.: National AIDS Network, 1988).

12. "NAN Executive Director to Move On." News release from the National AIDS Network (18 February 1989).

13. William J. Freeman, interview with author, Washington, D.C., 13 February 1995.

14. James Holm, telephone interview with author, 17 September 1995.

15. Ibid.

16. Julie Brienza, "National AIDS Network Hits Hard Times," *Washington Blade* (16 March 1990), 1.

17. David Anger, " 'The End Was Chaos': The Rise and Fall of AIDS Activist Eric Engstrom," *Twin Cities Reader* (13 November 1990), 6–9.

18. Rodger McFarlane, "Who's Driving the Bus? The Leadership Crisis in AIDS Service Organizations," *Village Voice* (4 September 1990), 18.

19. Elizabeth Greene, "A Worrisome Shutdown," *The Chronicle of Philanthropy* (10 July 1990), 17.

20. Pat Norman, telephone interview with author, 12 September 1995.

21. Lewis Katoff, "Community-Based Services for People with AIDS," *Primary Care* 19 (March 1992): 231–43.

22. Paul Jellinek, telephone interview with author, 10 February 1995.

23. Mervyn F. Silverman, M.D., "The Robert Wood Johnson Foundation AIDS Health Services Program." In Vivian E. Fransen, ed., *Proceedings: AIDS Prevention and Services Workshop, February 15–16, 1990* (Princeton, N.J.: Robert Wood Johnson Foundation, June 1990), 37.

24. Ruby P. Hearn, "An Overview of AIDS Programs Receiving Support from the Robert Wood Johnson Foundation," in Fransen, *Proceedings*. Also Victoria D. Weisfield, ed., *AIDS Health Services at the Crossroads: Lessons for Community Care* (Princeton, N.J.: Robert Wood Johnson Foundation, 1991).

25. Mervyn F. Silverman, M.D., telephone interview with author, 15 February 1995.

26. Cliff Morrison, telephone interview with author, 15 August 1995.

27. Peter S. Arno, "The Nonprofit Sector's Response to the AIDS Epidemic: Community-based Services in San Francisco," *American Journal of Public Health* 76 (1986): 1325–30.

28. Silverman interview.

29. Jesse Peel, M.D., telephone interview with author, 13 September 1995.

30. Bea Kalleigh, telephone interview with author, 5 October 1995.

31. Quoted in Weisfield, *AIDS Health Services at the Crossroads: Lessons for Community Care*.

32. Embry M. Howell, "The Role of Community-based Organizations in Responding to the AIDS Epidemic: Examples from the HRSA Service Demonstrations," *Journal of Public Health Policy* (Summer 1991): 165–74.

33. From O'Neill's opening remarks to the Special Projects of National Significance "Objective Review Panels" review of grant proposals, at the Radisson-Barcelo Hotel, Washington, D.C., 26 June 1996.

34. *HIV/AIDS Programs Expenditures and Accomplishments: FY91–FY95 State Profiles* (Rockville, Md.: Health Resources and Services Administration, May 1995).

35. Stephen Bowen, M.D., telephone interview with author, 5 July 1995.

36. Miguel Gomez, interview with author, Washington, D.C., 13 April 1995.

37. Kawata interview.

38. Joseph O'Neill, M.D., interview with author, Washington, D.C., 29 August 1995.

39. Mark Barnes, "Cooperation Needed to Pass Ryan White Bill," *Washington Blade* (14 April 1995), 45.

40. Ernest Hopkins, "Sound Strategy Needed to Pass Ryan White Act," *Washington Blade* (21 April 1995), 43.

41. José Zuniga, "Departure Signals Rift in Ranks at AIDS Group," *Washington Blade* (23 June 1995), 1.

42. Pat Christen, telephone interview with author, 20 September 1995.

43. Thomas Sheridan, interview with author, Washington, D.C., 24 February 1995.

44. José Zuniga, "Departure Signals Rift in Ranks at AIDS Groups."

45. Ralph Payne, interview with author, Washington, D.C., 24 September 1995.

46. Westmoreland made these remarks during a 14 February 1995 breakfast "roundtable" at the offices of the National Gay and Lesbian Task Force (NGLTF), in Washington, D.C.

47. Mark Barnes, "Medicaid Proposal Spells Out Deadly Reform," *Washington Blade* (13 October 1995), 33.

48. Payne interview.

49. McGuire interview.

50. Jane Silver, interview with author, Washington, D.C., 13 March 1995.

51. McGuire interview.

52. Thomas McNaught, interview with author, Boston, 24 July 1995.

53. Larry Kessler, interview with author, Boston, 24 July 1995.

54. Joseph Fera, interview with author, San Francisco, 30 January 1995.

55. Eileen Dirkin, interview with author, Chicago, 1 June 1995.

56. Karl Mathiasen, III, interview with author, Washington, D.C., 4 April 1995.

57. Torie Osborn, interview with author, Washington, D.C., 15 February 1995.

58. Timothy Sweeney, interview with author, New York City, 2 March 1995.

59. Wolfred interview.

60. Alan Flippen, "The $195,000 Question," *The Advocate* (7 July 1998), 41.

61. Christen interview.

62. Flippen, "The $195,000 Question," 41.

63. Jeffrey Graham, telephone interview with author, 13 September 1995.

64. Fera interview.

65. Derek Hodel, interview with author, New York City, 27 April 1995.

66. Suzanne C. Ouelette, interview with author, New York City, 27 April 1995.

CHAPTER EIGHT

1. "A Beach Boogie Benefit," *New York Times* (27 August 1995), "Styles" section, 42.

2. Larry Kramer, *Reports from the holocaust: The Making of an AIDS Activist* (New York: St. Martin's Press, 1989), 14–15.

3. Randy Shilts, *And the Band Played On* (New York: St. Martin's Press, 1987), 134–135.

4. Larry Kramer, interview with author, New York City, 4 March 1995.

5. Shilts, *And the Band Played On*, 282–83.

6. Rodger McFarlane, interview with author, New York City, 4 March 1995.

7. Shilts, *And the Band Played On*, 331.

8. Cleve Jones, interview with author, San Francisco, 2 February 1995.

9. Jesse Peel, M.D., telephone interview with author, 13 September 1995.

10. Sally Dodds, telephone interview with author, 5 July 1995.

11. Bill Meisenheimer, telephone interview with author, 6 June 1995.

12. Shilts, *And the Band Played On*, 579.

13. Ann Maguire, interview with author, Provincetown, Mass., 28 July 1995.

14. Anthony Braswell, telephone interview with author, 19 September 1995.

15. Paul Akio Kawata, interview with author, Washington, D.C., 24 March 1995.

16. Bernard Weinraub, "Stars Flock to Be in HBO Film About the Early Years of AIDS," *New York Times* (11 January 1993), C11.

17. Clifford Rothman, " 'Philadelphia': Oscar Gives Way to Elegy," *New York Times* (1 January 1995), H9.

18. "Q&A: Tom Hanks: There Are 'A Zillion More Stories' Hollywood Should Be Telling," *Washington Blade* (28 July 1995), 43.

19. Ingrid Sischy, "Elton John: 150% Involved," *Interview* (April 1995), 74.

20. Greg Louganis, with Eric Marcus, *Breaking the Surface* (New York: Random House, 1995), 272.

21. Chronicle: "Deborah Harry in a Summer's-End AIDS Event," *New York Times* (22 August 1995), B2.

22. "Cyndi Lauper to Perform at AIDSWALK Concert; Diane Reeves to Round Out Closing Ceremonies," *Washington Blade* (15 September 1995), 2.

23. Chronicle: "For Rosie Perez, a 10-Kilometer Act of Penance in Memory of a Friend," *New York Times* (11 September 1995), B-12.

24. Kathy Spahn, telephone conversation with author, 17 August 1998.

25. John-Manuel Andriote, "Society Gets AIDS," *Washington Dossier* (December 1990), 32-35.

26. Michelangelo Signorile, *Queer in America: Sex, the Media, and the Closets of Power* (New York: Anchor Books/Doubleday, 1993), 302–309.

27. David J. Fox, "Geffen Gives $1 Million to AIDS Group for New Office Space," *Los Angeles Times* (3 March 1992), B1.

28. Timothy Wolfred, telephone interview with author, 30 September 1995.

29. Urvashi Vaid, *Virtual Equality: The Mainstreaming of Gay & Lesbian Liberation* (New York: Anchor Books/Doubleday, 1995), 77.

30. Donald Smith, telephone interview with author, 16 September 1995.

31. Seltzer interview.

32. John Clinton, ed., *AIDS Funding: A Guide to Giving by Foundations and Charitable Organizations* (Washington, D.C.: The Foundation Center, 1988).

33. Paul Jellinek, telephone interview with author, 10 February 1995.

34. Vivian E. Fransen, ed., *Proceedings: AIDS Prevention and Services Work-*

shop, February 15–16, 1990 (Princeton: Robert Wood Johnson Foundation, 1990).

35. Jellinek interview.

36. Daniel M. Fox, "AIDS and the American Health Polity: The History and Prospects of a Crisis of Authority." In Elizabeth Fee and Daniel M. Fox, eds., *AIDS: The Burdens of History* (Berkeley: University of California Press, 1988), 333.

37. Paula Van Ness, interview with author, Washington, D.C., 25 April 1995.

38. National AIDS Fund, "Why You Should Support the National AIDS Fund's 10th Anniversary Campaign" fact sheet, 1998.

39. Van Ness interview.

40. Drawn from a DIFFA advertising supplement to the *New York Times Magazine* (26 June 1994).

41. Ibid.

42. Nick Steele, "Design for Dignity: DIFFA's Innovative Decade in the War Against AIDS," *Art & Understanding* (January/February 1995), 25.

43. Ibid.

44. U.S. Congress, Office of Technology Assessment, *Review of the Public Health Service Response to AIDS* (Washington, D.C.: OTA, 1985).

45. Fee and Fox, *AIDS,* 330.

46. Meisenheimer interview.

47. Mervyn P. Silverman, M.D., telephone interview with author, 15 February 1995.

48. John-Manuel Andriote, "AIDSweek: May 31–June 5," *Washington City Paper* (12 June 1987).

49. *Report of the Presidential Commission on the Human Immunodeficiency Virus Epidemic* (Washington, D.C.: Government Printing Office, 24 June 1988), 117.

50. Steve Friess, "Are Gays Really Rich?" *The Advocate* (28 April 1998), 37.

51. Larry Kessler, interview with author, Boston, 24 July 1995.

52. Eileen Dirkin, interview with author, Chicago, 1 June 1995.

53. Joseph O'Neill, M.D., interview with author, Washington, D.C., 29 August 1995.

54. Frank Pieri, M.D., interview with author, Chicago, 3 June 1995.

55. Timothy Sweeney, interview with author, New York City, 2 March 1995.

56. Lorri L. Jean, telephone interview with author, 26 October 1995.

57. Rev. Carl Bean, interview with author, Washington, D.C., 16 November 1995.

58. Linda Campbell, interview with author, New York City, 28 April 1995.

59. George Bellinger, Jr., interview with author, New York City, 2 March 1995.

60. Lou Chibbaro, Jr., "IMPACT Misses Deadline: Three-Minute Delay Costs Group About $130,000 in Federal Funds," *Washington Blade* (6 May 1994), 1.

61. John-Manuel Andriote, "The New AIDS War," *10 Percent* (January/February 1994), 51.

62. Ibid.

63. Pieri interview.

64. Richard Cohen, "Federal Money for Racists," *Washington Post* (29 July 1993), A25.

65. Jim Graham, interview with author, Washington, D.C., 30 August 1993.

66. Andriote, "The New AIDS War."

67. Corrections, *Washington Post* (15 July 1993), A3.

68. Joann Byrd, "The Flawed Column," *Washington Post* (25 July 1993), C6; Joann Byrd, "The Flawed Column (Part II)," *Washington Post* (1 August 1993), C6.

69. Courtland Milloy, "War on AIDS is Victim of Friendly Fire," *Washington Post* (7 July 1993), D1.

70. Caitlin Conor Ryan, interview with author, Washington, D.C., 21 August 1993.

71. Lou Chibbaro, Jr., "Black Gays Debate Abundant Life Role in AIDS Coalition," *Washington Blade* (3 September 1993), 1.

72. Julian K. Tolver, "Fighting for African Americans' Survival," *Washington Blade* (17 September 1993), 41.

73. Amy Goldstein, "City Giving AIDS Clinic $1.2 Million," *Washington Post* (16 June 1994), D1.

74. Andriote, "The New AIDS War."

75. Felicia R. Lee, "Blacks' Dollars Seem Scarce in AIDS Fight," *New York Times* (20 August 1995), 35.

76. Dennis Altman, *Power and Community: Organizational and Cultural Responses to AIDS* (London: Taylor & Francis, 1994), 116.

77. National Task Force on AIDS Prevention, *Report on Standards As Set Forth at the Gay Men of Color AIDS Summit, August 31–September 3, 1995* (San Francisco: National Task Force on AIDS Prevention, 1995).

78. Lee, "Blacks' Dollars Seem Scarce in AIDS Fight."

79. Peter Frieberg, "DIFFA Loses $30,000 on Stonewall 25 Fundraiser," *Washington Blade* (12 August 1994), 21.

80. José Zuniga, "Face of AIDS Groups Changes," *Washington Blade* (21 July 1995), 1.

81. José Zuniga, "AmFAR Closes Rockville Office: Budget Woes Force Layoffs for Nation's Largest AIDS Group," *Washington Blade* (16 June 1995), 6.

82. Aras van Hertum, "AIDS Action Foundation's Donations Drop $342,000," *Washington Blade* (8 July 1994), 27.

83. Jane Lowers, "The Funding Crunch: AIDS, Gay and Lesbian Organizations Compete for Limited Resources," *Outlines* (June 1995), 16.

84. Seltzer interview.

85. Fred Bayles, "AIDS Organizations Feeling the Brunt of General Public's 'Compassion Fatigue,'" *Bay Windows* (10 August 1995).

86. Kiki Mason, "Black Tie Lies," *POZ* (February/March 1995), 48.

87. Sue Fox, "Consultant Producing AIDSWALK 1996," *Washington Blade* (15 December 1995).

88. James F. Smith, "Bottom Line Questions," *Washington Blade* (5 July 1996), 29.

89. Lou Chibbaro, Jr., "Philly Groups Pull Out of AIDS Ride," *Washington Blade* (13 September 1996), 5.

90. Scott A. Giordano, "Pa. Attorney General Began Ride Investigation in April," *Philadelphia Gay News* (30 August–5 September 1996), 14.

91. Editorial, "A Few Words About the AIDS Ride," *Philadelphia Gay News* (30 August–5 September 1996), 13.

92. Advertisement in *Washington Post*, "Weekend" (27 September 1996).

93. Lou Chibbaro, Jr., "Philly is Bumped From AIDS Ride," *Washington Blade* (27 September 1996), 5.

94. Lou Chibbaro, Jr., "AIDS Ride Organizer to Pay Fine," *Washington Blade* (25 April 1997), 1.

95. Sue Rich, "Taken for a Ride," *Minneapolis City Paper* (2 July 1997), 8.

96. Lou Chibbaro, Jr., "Florida AIDS Groups Drop Promoter," *Washington Blade* (13 June 1997), 16.

97. Timothy Cwiek, "PCHA Plans 'Low-Key' Bike Ride as Fund-Raiser," *Philadelphia Gay News*, 20–26 June 1997), 8.

98. Rick Weiss, "Questions on Overhead Dog AIDS Bike-Trip Organizer," *Washington Post* (9 June 1997), A6.

99. Christopher Jones, "AIDS Ride Distributes $2 Million to Charities," *Washington Blade* (12 September 1997), 1.

100. Peter Frieberg, "Mixing Politics and Profits: Entrepreneur Sean O'Brien Strub Says He's an Activist at Heart," *Washington Blade* (19 July 1996), 14.

101. Seltzer interview.

CHAPTER NINE

1. Larry Kramer, *Reports from the holocaust* (New York: St. Martin's Press, expanded and reissued 1994), 137. Kramer notes that two days after his speech on Tuesday, 10 March 1987, "The gay grapevine functioned remarkably well, for some three hundred or more showed up that Thursday night, and the result was the establishment of ACT UP—the AIDS Coalition to Unleash Power—an ad hoc community protest group that, originally, was pledged to concentrate on fighting for the release of experimental drugs."

2. Ellen Graham and Roger Ricklefs, "AIDS Has Been Cruel to Greenwich Village and Its Homosexuals," *Wall Street Journal* (13 March 1987), 1.

3. Randy Shilts, *And the Band Played On* (New York: St. Martin's Press, 1987), 589.

4. Diane M. Gianelli, "High Court Ruling Gives Basis for AIDS Bias Suits," *American Medical News* (13 March 1987), 1.

5. Cleve Jones, in Joe Brown, ed., *A Promise to Remember: The NAMES Project Book of Letters* (New York: Avon Books, 1992), vi.

6. Fenton Johnson, "Death Into Life," *New York Times* (24 December 1994).

7. *Projections of the AIDS Epidemic in San Francisco: 1994–1997* (San Francisco: Department of Public Health, 15 February 1994). Noted in Eric Rofes, *Reviving the Tribe: Regenerating Gay Men's Sexuality and Culture in the Ongoing Epidemic* (New York: The Harrington Park Press, 1995), 169. Rofes explains that he arrived at the figure of 75,000 gay men in San Francisco in 1980 by estimating the city's lesbian and gay population at 20 percent of the city's total 1980 population of about 750,000, divided equally between lesbians and gay men.

8. Lisa M. Krieger, "AIDS Loses Urgency in Nation's List of Worries," *San Francisco Examiner* (29 January 1995), 1.

9. Dennis Conkin, "AIDSphobia Hits the SF Airwaves," *Bay Area Reporter* (26 January 1995), 1.

10. Fenton Johnson, interview with author, San Francisco, 31 January 1995.

11. John Preston, ed., *Personal Dispatches: Writers Confront AIDS* (New York: St. Martin's Press, 1988), xv.

12. Rofes, *Reviving the Tribe*, 23, 29.

13. Simon Watney, "Acts of Memory," *Out* (September 1994), 92.

14. Sandra Jacoby Klein, "AIDS-Related Multiple Loss Syndrome," *Illness, Crisis and Loss* 4 (1994): 15.

15. David Firestone, "Life Span Dips for Men Born in New York: AIDS is the Main Reason for Decline, Report Says," *New York Times* (27 April 1996), 25.

16. John Newmeyer, interview with author, San Francisco, 31 January 1995.

17. Andrew Sullivan, "Gay Life, Gay Death," *New Republic* (17 December 1990), 19–25.

18. Stephen F. Morin, Kenneth A. Charles, Alan K. Malyon, "The Psychological Impact of AIDS on Gay Men," *American Psychologist* 39 (November 1984): 1288–93.

19. Chris Glaser, "AIDS and A-Bomb Disease: Facing a Special Death," *Christianity & Crisis* (28 September 1987).

20. Fred Boykin, "The AIDS Crisis and Gay Male Survivor Guilt," *Smith College Studies in Social Work* (June 1991): 256.

21. Walt Odets, *In the Shadow of the Epidemic: Being HIV-Negative in the Age of AIDS* (Durham, N.C.: Duke University Press, 1995), 42.

22. John L. Martin and Laura Dean, "Effects of AIDS-Related Bereavement and HIV-Related Illness on Psychological Distress Among Gay Men: A 7-year Longitudinal Study, 1985–1991," *Journal of Consulting and Clinical Psychology* 61 (1993): 94–103.

23. Stosh Ostrow, M.D., telephone interview with author, 23 September 1995.

24. Eric Rofes, telephone interview with author, 7 July 1995.

25. Rofes interview.

26. Arnie Kantrowitz, "Friends Gone With the Wind." In John Preston, ed., *Personal Dispatches: Writers Confront AIDS* (New York: St. Martin's Press, 1989), 21.

27. Michael Lassell, *Decade Dance* (Boston: Alyson Publications, 1990), 69.

28. Tony Kushner, "The *Angels in America* Author on Beauty and Remembrance," *Architectural Digest* (November 1995), 28.

29. Rofes, *Reviving the Tribe*, 79.

30. Ibid., 238.

31. John Snow, *Mortal Fear: Meditations on Death and AIDS* (Cambridge, Mass.: Cowley Publications, 1987), 14.

32. James B. Nelson, *Embodiment: An Approach to Sexuality and Christian Theology* (Minneapolis: Augsburg Publishing House, 1978), 204.

33. Jeff Nunokawa, " 'All the Sad Young Men': AIDS and the Work of Mourning," *Yale Journal of Criticism* (Spring 1991): 1–12.

34. Odets, *In the Shadow of the Epidemic*, 74.

35. "The Face of AIDS: One Year in the Epidemic," *Newsweek* (10 August 1987), 22–37.

36. Cindy Patton, *Fatal Advice: How Safe-Sex Education Went Wrong* (Durham, N.C.: Duke University Press, 1996), 64.

37. "And now was acknowledged the presence of the Red Death. He had come like a thief in the night. And one by one dropped the revelers in the blood-bedewed halls of their revel, and died each in the despairing posture of his fall." Edgar Allen Poe's "Masque of the Red Death" is eerily relevant to the denial with which America has handled the AIDS epidemic. See *Tales of Mystery and Imagination By Edgar Allen Poe* (New York: Weathervane Books, 1935).

38. John-Manuel Andriote, "The Survivors: How Do You Grieve the Loss of a Forbidden Love?" *Washington City Paper* (19–25 September 1986), 1.

39. Laura Dean, interview with author, New York City, 29 April 1995.

40. Charles Silverstein, M.D., *Man to Man: Gay Couples in America* (New York: William Morrow, 1981), 265.

41. Philip J. Hilts, "AIDS Deaths Continue to Rise in 25–44 Age Group, U.S. Says," *New York Times* (16 February 1996), A22.

42. Virginia Apuzzo, telephone interview with author, 8 August 1995.

43. John-Manuel Andriote, "Coping with Grief in the Time of AIDS," *Windy City Times* (27 March 1986), 6.

44. Tony Kushner, *Angels in America: A Gay Fantasia on National Themes, Part One: Millennium Approaches* (New York: Theatre Communications Group, 1992), 25, 99.

45. Elisabeth Kübler-Ross, *AIDS: The Ultimate Challenge* (New York: Macmillan, 1987), 11.

46. Andriote, "The Survivors," 1986.

47. Judith Pollatsek, "Grief, Multiple Loss, and Burnout: Care for the Caregiver." Speech presented at the National HIV Frontline Forum, 1994, and published in *Multimedia Self-Study Kit for Professionals Who Counsel People Living with HIV* (New York: NCM Publishers, 1994).

48. Howard Brown, M.D., *Familiar Faces, Hidden Lives: The Story of Homosexual Men in America Today* (New York: Harcourt Brace Jovanovich, 1976), 140–41.

49. Abraham Verghese, M.D., *My Own Country: A Doctor's Story* (New York: Simon & Schuster, 1994), 223.

50. James Halloran, telephone interview with author, 10 October 1995.

51. Shilts, *And the Band Played On*, 356.

52. Bryan Robinson, Patsy Skeen, Lynda Walters, "The AIDS Epidemic Hits Home," *Psychology Today* (April 1987), 48–52.

53. John Paul Barnich, telephone interview with author, 1 October 1995.

54. Suzanne Benzer, interview with author, New York City, 26 April 1995.

55. Georgia Dullea, "AIDS Mothers' Undying Hope," *New York Times* (20 April 1994), C1.

56. Susan Folkman, Margaret A. Chesney, Anne Christopher-Richards, "Stress and Coping in Caregiving Partners of Men With AIDS," *Psychiatric Clinics of North America* (March 1994), 35–53.

57. Sandi Feinblum, interview with author, New York City, 26 April 1995.

58. Pollatsek, "Grief, Multiple Loss, and Burnout: Care for the Caregiver."

59. Jeffrey Akman, M.D., interview with author, Washington, D.C., 17 March 1995.

60. Fawzy I. Fawzy, Nancy W. Fawzy, Robert O. Pasnau, "Bereavement in AIDS," *Psychiatric Medicine* 9 (1991): 469–82; Caitlin Conor Ryan, "The Social and Clinical Challenges of AIDS," *Smith College Studies in Social Work* 59 (November 1988): 3–20.

61. Gil Tunnell, "Special Issues in Group Psychotherapy for Gay Men With AIDS." In Steven A. Cadwell, Robert A. Burnham, Jr., and Marshall Forstein, eds., *Therapists on the Front Line: Psychotherapy with Gay Men in the Age of AIDS* (Washington, D.C.: American Psychiatric Press, 1994), 239–40.

62. Karl Goodkin, M.D., Ph.D., interview with author, Miami, 19 May 1995.

63. Sister Patrice Murphy, interview with author, New York City, 1 March 1995.

64. Cardinal Joseph Ratzinger, "Letter to the Bishops of the Catholic Church on the Pastoral Care of Homosexual Persons" (The Vatican, 1986). In Jeffrey S. Siker, ed., *Homosexuality in the Church: Both Sides of the Debate* (Louisville: John Knox Press, 1994), 39.

65. Andriote, "Coping with Grief in the Time of AIDS."

66. Richard A. Rasi, telephone interview with author, 13 December 1996.

67. Murphy interview.

68. Shilts, *And the Band Played On,* 284–86.

69. Ibid., 284–86.

70. Paul Boneberg, interview with author, Washington, D.C., 17 August 1995.

71. José Zuniga, "Candlelight Vigil Draws About 1,500," *Washington Blade* (26 May 1995).

72. Larry Prater, M.D., interview with author, Miami Beach, 20 May 1995.

73. Obituaries, "John Howard Martindale, Jr.," *Bay Area Reporter* (26 June 1997), 20.

74. Michael Bronski, "Death and the Erotic Imagination" and "AIDS, Art and Obits," In *Personal Dispatches: Writers Confront AIDS,* 136, 166.

75. Mireya Navarro, "Ritualizing Grief, Love and Politics: AIDS Memorial Services Evolve Into a Distinctive Gay Rite," *New York Times* (30 November 1994), B1.

76. Judith Pollatsek, interview with author, Washington, D.C., 27 February 1995.

77. Ibid.

78. Randy Miller, interview with author, Washington, D.C., 17 August 1995.

79. Richard Neugebauer, et al., "Bereavement Reactions Among Homosexual Men Experiencing Multiple Losses in the AIDS Epidemic," *American Journal of Psychiatry* 149 (October 1992): 1374–79.

80. Elisabeth Rosenthal, "Struggling to Cope With the Losses As AIDS Rips Relationships Apart," *New York Times* (6 December 1992), 1.

81. Douglas Crimp, "Mourning and Militancy," *October* 51 (1989), 3–18.

82. David B. Feinberg, *Queer and Loathing: Rants and Raves of a Raging AIDS Clone* (New York: Penguin Books, 1994), 196, 254–65.

83. Ibid.

84. Armistead Maupin, telephone interview with author, 23 December 1996.

85. Andrew Holleran, *The Beauty of Men* (New York: Penguin Books, 1996), 54.

86. David Ansen, et al. "AIDS and the Arts: A Lost Generation," *Newsweek* (18 January 1993), 16–23.

87. Joseph Papp, in the foreword to Larry Kramer, *The Normal Heart* (New York: Penguin Books, 1985), 29.

88. Cynthia Laird, "AIDS Memorial Grove Designated National Memorial by Congress," *Bay Area Reporter* (10 October 1996), 1.

89. *AIDS Memorial Quilt*, booklet (San Francisco: NAMES Project Foundation, 1996).

90. Cleve Jones. In Joe Brown, ed., *A Promise to Remember: The NAMES Project Book of Letters*, vi.

91. Cleve Jones, interview with author, San Francisco, 2 February 1995.

92. Jones interview.

93. Urvashi Vaid, interview with author, Provincetown, Mass., 29 July 1995.

94. Anthony Turney, interview with author, San Francisco, 1 February 1995.

95. Sheila Walsh, "D.C. Gearing Up for Quilt's Return," *Washington Blade* (16 June 1995), 5.

96. Sue Fox, "Clintons Agree to Chair Upcoming AIDS Quilt Display," *Washington Blade* (12 July 1996), 19.

97. Wendy Johnson, "You Can't See the Quilt Without Being Changed," *Washington Blade* (18 October 1996), 1.

98. Richard D. Mohr, "The Quilt's Celebration of 70,000 Individuals," *Washington Blade* (11 October 1996), 41.

99. Richard D. Mohr, *Gay Ideas: Outing and Other Controversies* (Boston: Beacon Press, 1992), 126.

CHAPTER TEN

1. Lawrence K. Altman, M.D., "Government Panel on HIV Finds the Prospect for Treatment Bleak," *New York Times* (29 June 1993), C3.

2. Lawrence K. Altman, M.D., "Conference Ends with Little Hope for AIDS Cure," *New York Times* (15 June 1993), C1.

3. Cindy Patton, *Sex and Germs: The Politics of AIDS* (Boston: South End Press: 1985), 47.

4. Gina Kolata, "New AIDS Findings on Why Drugs Fail," *New York Times* (12 January 1995), A1.

5. John Schwartz, "FDA Approves First in New Family of AIDS Drugs," *Washington Post* (8 December 1995).

6. Philip J. Hilts, "Drug Agency Acts Quickly on a New AIDS Treatment," *New York Times* (2 March 1996).

7. Lawrence K. Altman, M.D., "AIDS Meeting: Signs of Hope, and Obstacles," *New York Times* (7 July 1996), A1.

8. Unsigned editorial, "Elation, and Deflation, Over AIDS," *New York Times* (13 July 1996), National edition, 14.

9. Jerome Groopman, M.D., "Chasing the Cure," *The New Republic* (12 August 1996), 14, 16.

10. David Sanford, "One Man's AIDS Tale Shows How Quickly the Epidemic Has Turned," *Wall Street Journal* (8 November 1996), 1.

11. Andrew Sullivan, "When AIDS Ends," *New York Times Magazine* (10 November 1996).

12. The United Nations reported 3 million new HIV cases in 1996, for a worldwide total of 23 million HIV-infected people. In the fifteen years since the discovery of AIDS to that point, 6.4 million had died; of those deaths, 1.5 million occurred in 1996. See Lawrence K. Altman, M.D., "U.N. Reports 3 Million New HIV Cases Worldwide for '96," *New York Times* (28 November 1996), A10.

13. Mark Schoofs, "Why It's Too Soon to Declare the End of AIDS," *Washington Post* (15 December 1996), C1.

14. Lawrence K. Altman, M.D., "Deaths from AIDS Decline Sharply in New York City," *New York Times* (25 January 1997), 1.

15. Richard Lacayo, "Hope With an Asterisk," *Time* (30 December 1996–6 January 1997).

16. Bill Bahlman, interview with author, New York City, 16 November 1996.

17. Moisés Agosto, interview with author, Washington, D.C., 5 December 1996.

18. Anne-christine d'Adesky, "Rich Man's Drug," *Out* (August 1996), 62.

19. Larry Kramer, "A Good News/Bad News AIDS Joke," *New York Times Magazine* (14 July 1996), 26.

20. Sean Strub, telephone interview with author, 27 June 1995.

21. Agosto interview.

22. Lawrence K. Altman, M.D., "With AIDS Advance, More Disappointment," *New York Times* (19 January 1997), A1.

23. Lynda Richardson, "An Old Experiment's Legacy: Distrust of New AIDS Drugs," *New York Times* (21 April 1997), A20.

24. Bettina Boxall, "Minorities Missing Out on Revolution in AIDS Drugs," *Los Angeles Times* (Washington edition; 14 April 1998), 1.

25. Sheryl Gay Stolberg, "Eyes Shut, Black America Is Being Ravaged by AIDS, "*New York Times* (29 June 1998).

26. Rhonda Smith, "Black Ministers' Response to HIV Called Too Slow," *Washington Blade* (10 April 1998), 1.

27. Sean Scully, "Black Caucus Calls for AIDS to Get 'Emergency' Attention," *Washington Times* (12 May 1998), A4. In fact, reported the *Washington Post* not long before this book's publication, "Federal health officials are beginning a major initiative to lessen the ravaging effects of AIDS in black and Latino communities, marking a victory for minority lawmakers who have crusaded for stronger defenses against the epidemic in the nation's most vulnerable neighborhoods" (Amy Goldstein, "U.S. to Begin Minority AIDS Initiative," *Washington Post* [29 October 1998], A3). The White House released $156 million for the initiative, which was intended to create HIV-prevention campaigns, place more drug addicts and HIV patients into medical care, and help local health workers and AIDS activists in assessing the needs of sick people.

28. Rhonda Smith, "Latino Leaders Start Work on National Plan to Fight AIDS," *Washington Blade* (8 May 1998), 1.

29. Lawrence K. Altman, "AIDS Deaths Drop 48 Percent in New York,"

New York Times (3 February 1998), 1; Lidia Wasowicz, "California AIDS Deaths Plummet 60 Percent," United Press International news wire (9 January 1998).

30. Associated Press, "Setbacks for Many on Drugs for AIDS," *New York Times* (30 September 1997), C4.

31. Mark Sullivan, "Study Finds Many Miss Doses of HIV Medicine," *Washington Blade* (19 December 1997), 23.

32. Reuters news wire, "U.S. HIV Patients Admit They Don't Take Drugs—Survey Results" (5 May 1998).

33. Sheryl Gay Stolberg, "U.S. Awakes to Epidemic of Sexual Diseases," *New York Times* (9 March 1998), 1.

34. Robert Pear, "New U.N. Estimate Doubles Rate of Spread of AIDS Virus," *New York Times* (26 November 1997).

35. Peter Freiberg, "Viatical Industry in 'Utter Chaos,' " *Washington Blade* (14 February 1997), 1.

36. Lynda Richardson, "A Gap in the Résumé: When HIV Loosens Grip, It's Back to the Job Market," *New York Times* (21 May 1997), A23.

37. Fred Kuhr, "Menino Proposes $250K Increase in Boston AIDS Budget," *Bay Windows* (26 March 1998), 1.

38. Sue Ellen Christian, "Living with AIDS Means Working with It," *Chicago Tribune Online* (27 April 1998).

39. Reporting drawn from Peter Freiberg, "Early Signs of Funding Fatigue?" *Washington Blade* (8 August 1997), 12; John Gallagher, "Cutting Back," *The Advocate* (3 February 1998), 37; Mark Sullivan, "GMHC Executive Director to Step Down," *New York Blade News* (27 March 1998), 1; and Katie Szymanski, "AIDS Walk Donations Drop for Second Year," *New York Blade News* (22 May 1998), 1.

40. Gallagher, "Cutting Back."

41. Freiberg, "Early Signs."

42. Rhonda Smith, "Black Leaders Chided on AIDS," *Washington Blade* (20 March 1998), 1.

43. Albert R. Jonsen and Jeff Stryker, eds., *The Social Impact of AIDS in the United States* (Washington, D.C.: National Academy Press, 1993), 27.

44. Jean McGuire, interview with author, Cambridge, Mass., 25 July 1995.

45. Thomas Sheridan, interview with author, Washington, D.C., 24 February 1995.

46. Mervyn Silverman, M.D., speaking on a panel ("Specialty vs. Integrated Care: Can HIV Clinics and Clinicians Continue to Handle the Load?") at the Seventh National AIDS Update Conference, San Francisco, 3 February 1995.

47. Mervyn Silverman, M.D., telephone interview with author, 15 February 1995.

48. Eileen Dirkin, interview with author, Chicago, 1 June 1995.

49. Frank Pieri, M.D., interview with author, Chicago, 3 June 1995.

50. Kenneth Mayer, M.D., interview with author, Boston, 25 July 1995.

51. Sue Fox, "Whitman-Walker Revisits Its Mission," *Washington Blade* (24 May 1996), 5.

52. Christopher J. Portelli, interview with author, Washington, D.C., 3 April 1995.

53. Lisa Keen, "AMA Urges Doctors to 'Recognize' Gay Patients," *Washington Blade* (3 May 1996), 19.

54. Joseph O'Neill, M.D., interview with author, Washington, D.C., 29 August 1995.

55. Christopher J. Portelli, telephone interview with author, 6 January 1997.

56. Peter T. Kilborn, "Voters' Anger at HMOs Plays as Hot Political Issue," *New York Times* (17 May 1998), 1; Robert Pear, "Government Lags in Steps to Widen Health Coverage," *New York Times* (9 August 1998), 1.

57. Virginia Apuzzo, telephone interview with author, 8 August 1995.

58. Timothy Westmoreland, interview with author, Washington, D.C., 18 July 1995.

59. Daniel Bross, interview with author, Washington, D.C., 17 February 1995.

60. McGuire interview.

61. Paul Jellinek, telephone interview with author, 10 February 1995.

62. Cliff Morrison, telephone interview with author, 15 August 1995.

63. Michael Seltzer, interview with author, New York City, 4 March 1995.

64. Anthony Fauci, M.D., interview with author, Bethesda, Md., 14 April 1995.

65. Timothy Sweeney, interview with author, New York City, 2 March 1995.

66. Paul Boneberg, interview with author, Washington, D.C., 17 August 1995.

67. Centers for Disease Control and Prevention, *Morbidity and Mortality Weekly Report* 47 (24 April 1998). "Men who have sex with men" accounted for 32 percent of new HIV diagnoses between January 1994 and June 1997. An additional 28 percent, overwhelmingly male, are noted as having "unreported" risk. Upon investigation, the CDC has consistently found virtually all of such males to have been infected with HIV via homosexual sex or injection drug use, stigmatized behaviors that are always underreported. Taken together, then, "men who have sex with men" continue to account for well over half the new HIV infections in the U.S.

68. Thomas J. Coates and Michael Shriver, "In the Race for a Cure, Prevention Must Persist," *Washington Blade* (29 November 1996), 31.

69. Donald Abrams, M.D., "A Load Off His Mind," *POZ* (March 1997), 105. Dr. Abrams, assistant director of the University of California–San Francisco AIDS Program at San Francisco General Hospital, noted, "As the drugs have been widely available by prescription for just about a year, the duration of their potency and the real clinical meaning of having HIV RNA loads driven below the level of detection of the assay remains to be seen. One thing's for sure—having an 'undetectable' viral load does not mean an individual is no longer able to transmit HIV to others! For now, an ounce of prevention is still worth a pound of cure."

70. David W. Dunlap, "In Age of AIDS, Love and Hope Can Lead to Risk," *New York Times* (27 July 1996), 7.

71. Walt Odets, interview with author, Chicago, 2 June 1995.

72. Odets interview.

73. Thomas J. Coates, interview with author, Washington, D.C., 16 May 1995.

74. Coates interview.

75. Ronald S. Gold, M. J. Skinner, M. W. Ross, "Unprotected Anal Inter-

course in HIV-Infected and Non-HIV-Infected Gay Men," *Journal of Sex Research* 31 (1994): 59–77.

76. Michelangelo Signorile, "HIV-Positive and Careless," *New York Times* (26 February 1995), E-15.

77. Eric Rofes, *Reviving the Tribe: Regenerating Gay Men's Sexuality and Culture in the Ongoing Epidemic* (New York: The Harrington Park Press, 1995), 197, 199.

78. S. Kippax, J. Crawford, M. Davis, et al. Sustaining Safe Sex: A Longitudinal Study of a Sample of Homosexual Men, *AIDS* 7 (1993): 279–82.

79. The issue of oral sex has engendered considerable argument among AIDS educators, and confusion among ordinary gay men. While Boston's AIDS Action Committee advocated oral sex as a safer alternative to unprotected anal intercourse, Washington, D.C.'s Whitman-Walker Clinic, for example, continued to recommend that men use condoms if they engaged in oral sex. When the Gay and Lesbian Medical Association in March 1996 recommended that oral sex be classified as "low-risk," Benjamin Schatz, the group's executive director, said, "We're not saying [oral sex] is zero risk. We're saying the overwhelming cause of the spread of HIV among gay and bisexual men is unprotected anal intercourse." On the other hand, Dr. Peter Hawley, medical director of Whitman-Walker Clinic, said, "Our stance is that oral sex is a risk." Although he conceded that it "may be qualitatively less risk than anal intercourse," Hawley said the clinic still recommended that gay men use a condom with either oral or anal intercourse. ("Gay Doctors Say Oral Sex Risk is 'Low,'" *Washington Blade*, 30 March 1996, 23). The different emphases of the Boston and Washington, D.C., groups represent the two poles of the debate. AIDS Action Committee recognized the right of gay men to choose their sexual behavior while guiding them toward a safer choice, while Whitman-Walker Clinic continued the widely used approach to prevention education that advocates only absolutes. It is this author's experience, as a long-term resident of Washington, D.C., and observer of both Whitman-Walker Clinic's prevention programs and of gay men's sexual behavior, that the overwhelming majority of gay men in the city have never heeded the clinic's counsel on oral sex, even as they (mostly) use condoms during anal intercourse.

80. Larry Kessler, interview with author, Boston, 24 July 1995.

81. AIDS Action Committee of Massachusetts, "AIDS Action Launches New Statewide Initiative to Stem Tide of New Infections Among Gay Men" (News release, 19 June 1995).

82. Dana Van Gorder, interview with author, San Francisco, 31 January 1995.

83. Dana Van Gorder, "Prevention More than Medical Issue," *San Francisco Sentinel* (11 January 1995), 20.

84. Van Gorder interview.

85. Lawrence D. Mass, M.D., *Homosexuality and Sexuality: Dialogues of the Sexual Revolution*, vol. 1 (New York: Harrington Park Press, 1990), 140.

86. Steve Martz, "A Concluding Word," *Washington Blade* (25 February 1983), 21. Quoted in Rodger Streitmatter, *Unspeakable: The Rise of the Gay and Lesbian Press in America* (Boston: Faber and Faber, 1996), 267.

87. John D'Emilio, interview with author, Washington, D.C., 24 May 1996.

88. Thomas Avena, "Interview: Edmund White." In Thomas Avena, ed., *Life Sentences: Writers, Artists, and AIDS* (San Francisco: Mercury House, 1994), 226.

89. Apuzzo interview.

90. Lorri L. Jean, telephone interview with author, 26 October 1995.

91. Van Gorder interview.

92. Randy Miller, interview with author, Washington, D.C., 17 August 1995.

93. Rev. Carl Bean, interview with author, Washington, D.C., 16 November 1995.

94. John Newmeyer, interview with author, San Francisco, 31 January 1995.

95. Sidney Brinkley, "AIDS Conference Focuses on Grassroots Issues," *Washington Blade* (29 March 1996), 17.

96. Andrew Holleran, "The Wrinkle Room," *New York Times Magazine* (1 September 1996), 60.

97. Ned Rorem, letter to the editor, *New York Times Magazine* (22 September 1996).

98. Arnie Kantrowitz, telephone interview with author, 22 November 1996.

99. Marshall Forstein, M.D., interview with author, Washington, D.C., 13 September 1995.

100. Torie Osborn, interview with author, Washington, D.C., 15 February 1995.

101. Lisa Keen, "Mississippi Governor Signs Marriage Measure," *Washington Blade* (14 February 1997), 1.

102. B. R. Simon Rosser, telephone interview with author, 14 August 1995.

103. Gabriel Rotello, *Sexual Ecology* (New York: Dutton, 1997), 244.

104. John Leonard, "Welcome to Gay City," presentation at the National Lesbian and Gay Health Conference, Seattle, 17 July 1996.

105. John Leonard, telephone interview with author, 2 January 1997.

106. Mark Mardon, "SFAF's Gay Life: A New Route to Prevention," *Bay Area Reporter* (30 April 1998), 1.

107. Peter Baker, "Clinton Equates Gay Rights, Civil Rights," *Washington Post* (9 November 1997), A18; Official White House transcript of the president's keynote address.

108. Peter Freiberg, "Commission: Federal AIDS Effort Stalled," *Washington Blade* (12 December 1997), 1.

109. Lou Chibbaro, Jr., "AIDS Funding Gets a Boost," *Washington Blade* (6 February 1998), 1.

110. John F. Harris and Amy Goldstein, "Puncturing an AIDS Initiative," *Washington Post* (23 April 1998), A1.

111. Sheryl Gay Stolberg, "President Decides Against Needle Programs," *New York Times* (21 April 1998), 1.

112. Unsigned editorial, "Cowardice on Clean Needles," *New York Times* (22 April 1998), A30.

113. John F. Harris, "Clinton Appeals to Science for an AIDS Vaccine," *Washington Post* (19 May 1997), A7.

114. Tim Weiner, "Military Discharges of Homosexuals Soar," *New York Times* (7 April 1998), A24.

115. Paul Duggan, "Texas Sodomy Arrest Opens Legal Battle for Gay Activists," *Washington Post* (29 November 1998), A3.

116. Peter Frieberg, "Study Verifies Teen Suicide Data," *Washington Blade* (8 May 1998), 1.

117. Marc Peyser, "Battling Backlash," *Newsweek* (17 August 1998), 50–52.

118. Hanna Rosin, Thomas B. Edsall, "Religious Right Targets Homosexuality," *Washington Post* (15 July 1998), 1.

119. First quote is from M. Jane Taylor, "An Ever-Shifting Landscape," *Washington Blade* (13 February 1998), 1; second quote is from Peter Freiberg, "Gay Hate Crimes Rise 8 Percent," *Washington Blade* (4 December 1998), 14.

120. J. Jennings Moss, "Capitol Gains," *Out* (April 1998), 112.

121. Lou Chibbaro, Jr., "Plans for March Unveiled," *Washington Blade* (6 February 1998), 1.

122. David W. Dunlap, "Gay Images, Once Kept Out, Are Out Big Time," *New York Times* (21 January 1996), 29.

123. Daniel Harris, *The Rise and Fall of Gay Culture* (New York: Hyperion, 1997), 270.

124. Charlie LeDuff, "At Parade, Proud Mix of the Blue and the Gay," *New York Times* (30 June 1996), 27.

125. David Richards, "Anita Bryant, Reconstituted," *Washington Post* (12 May 1996), F1. A generation after Bryant's "Save Our Children" campaign succeeded in removing sexual orientation from the Dade County (Florida) human rights law, the Miami-Dade County Commission voted seven to six to reinstate it on December 1, 1998. Eleven states, twenty-seven counties, and 136 cities now had laws protecting gay people against discrimination (see the unsigned [lead] editorial, "A Close Vote on Gay Rights," *New York Times*, 3 December 1998, A30).

126. Brian O'Connell, "*Native* Stops Publishing After 16 Years," *Washington Blade* (17 January 1997), 14.

127. Sheryl Gay Stolberg, "Gay Culture Weighs Sense and Sexuality," *New York Times* (23 November 1997), 4-1.

128. Larry Kramer, "Gay Culture, Redefined," *New York Times* (12 December 1997), A39.

129. Edmund White, *States of Desire: Travels in Gay America* (New York: E. P. Dutton, 1980), 260.

130. Robert N. Bellah, et al., *Habits of the Heart: Individualism and Commitment in American Life* (Berkeley: University of California Press, 1985), 153.

131. Cleve Jones, interview with author, San Francisco, 2 February 1995.

132. Rodger McFarlane, interview with author, New York City, 4 March 1995.

133. Paul Akio Kawata, interview with author, Washington, D.C., 24 March 1995.

134. Apuzzo interview.

135. Reggie Williams, telephone interview with author, 25 August 1995.

136. Fenton Johnson, interview with author, San Francisco, 31 January 1995.

137. Benjamin Schatz, interview with author, San Francisco, 2 February 1995.

138. Kantrowitz interview.

139. Arnie Kantrowitz, "Friends Gone with the Wind." In John Preston, ed., *Personal Dispatches: Writers Confront AIDS* (New York: St. Martin's Press, 1988), 24–25.

140. Johnson interview.

141. Bruce Patterson, interview with author, New York City, 2 March 1995.

142. John Preston (Michael Lowenthal, ed.), *Winter's Light: Reflections of a Yankee Queer* (Hanover, N.H.: University Press of New England, 1995), 115–24.

143. Patterson interview.

144. Andrew Holleran, *Dancer from the Dance* (New York: William Morrow, 1978), 42.

145. Steven Schwartzberg, telephone interview with author, 22 June 1995.

146. Rofes interview.

147. Quoted in Larry Kramer, *Reports from the holocaust* (New York: St. Martin's Press, 1989), 277.

148. Kantrowitz interview.

Index